# Neuropsychotherapy and Community Integration

## Brain Illness, Emotions, and Behavior

# *CRITICAL ISSUES IN NEUROPSYCHOLOGY*

*Series Editors*

Antonio E. Puente
*University of North Carolina at Wilmington*

Cecil R. Reynolds
*Texas A&M University*
*and Bastrop Mental Health Associates*

---

*Current Volumes in this Series*

CONTEMPORARY APPROACHES TO NEUROPSYCHOLOGICAL ASSESSMENT
Edited by Gerald Goldstein and Theresa M. Incagnoli

DETECTION OF MALINGERING DURING HEAD INJURY LITIGATION
Edited by Cecil R. Reynolds

FAMILY SUPPORT PROGRAMS AND REHABILITATION:
A Cognitive–Behavioral Approach to Traumatic Brain Injury
Louise Margaret Smith and Hamish P. D. Godfrey

HANDBOOK OF CLINICAL CHILD NEUROPSYCHOLOGY, Second Edition
Edited by Cecil R. Reynolds and Elaine Fletcher-Janzen

HANDBOOK OF NEUROPSYCHOLOGY AND AGING
Edited by Paul David Nussbaum

INTERNATIONAL HANDBOOK OF NEUROPSYCHOLOGICAL REHABILITATION
Edited by Anne-Lise Christensen and Barbara Uzzell

NEUROPSYCHOLOGICAL EXPLORATIONS OF MEMORY AND COGNITION:
Essays in Honor of Nelson Butters
Edited by Laird S. Cermak

NEUROPSYCHOTHERAPY AND COMMUNITY INTEGRATION:
Brain Illness, Emotions, and Behavior
Tedd Judd

THE PRACTICE OF FORENSIC NEUROPSYCHOLOGY:
Meeting Challenges in the Courtroom
Edited by Robert J. McCaffrey, Arthur D. Williams, Jerid M. Fisher, and Linda C. Laing

---

A Continuation Order Plan is available for this series. A continuation order will bring delivery of each new volume immediately upon publication. Volumes are billed only upon actual shipment. For further information please contact the publisher.

# Neuropsychotherapy and Community Integration

## Brain Illness, Emotions, and Behavior

Tedd Judd

*Neuropsychological and Psychoeducational Services*
*Bellingham, Washington*

Kluwer Academic / Plenum Publishers
New York, Boston, Dordrecht, London, Moscow

# Preface

The first time I walked onto a neurology ward during my graduate training I was shocked (much as family members of people with brain illnesses probably are). I had learned a great deal in class about aphasia, amnesia, agnosia, apraxia, and other cognitive disorders, but I had not been prepared for the behavioral disorders I was to encounter, for the severe physical disabilities, for the indignities of the patient role. Bit by bit I overcame this shock. I learned to look people in the eye who seemed to have more tubes than the New York subway system, people whose faces had been scraped off the pavement and who were drooling, incontinent, and severely dysarthric. I learned to see beyond what frightened and repulsed me to the human beings within.

I wish I could say that I saw in each person a deep human soul yearning to breathe free and to love, an essence, an intrinsic goodness, a wholeness; I did not. Rather, it seems like each and every unique element of human behavior, one's abilities, and one's desires can be destroyed by some brain lesion, while leaving a uniquely human person behind. Not only are there losses, but behaviors emerge at times that are not seen in people with intact brains but which still reveal a human attempting to cope. I do feel that I saw and still see in each such person something intrinsically human, but not the same thing in each. Some yearn, some merely respond. Some emote, some cogitate indifferently. Some try, some do not. I found that to be human is not one thing, but a collection of things that can be distorted and partially destroyed in endless variations and combinations by the dreaded diseases and injuries that can afflict our brains.

In my work, then, there is an element of faith—that I will find in each person (however fractionated) a valuable being, worthy of respect, and deserving a place in society. There is also an element of science—I need to find out who that person is, what is that value, and, together with that person, what is that place in society. Without the science I cannot find the person, the value, or the place in society—instead I will see my image of the person that I project; a false empathy. Without the faith, I risk losing my own humanity, not in a neurological sense but in a moral one. It is my hope that I have been able to infuse this book with both that faith and that science.

When I began training in clinical neuropsychology, the practice mostly involved diagnosis and disposition. I soon was disillusioned by a field in which the common practice was to put the hopeful person through hours of difficult and frustrating tests, only to give feedback which was, essentially, "Yes, you have brain damage, alright, and of a particularly interesting kind. Good luck!" Lacking significant guidelines, I began my own feeble attempts to provide something more substantial and useful. Over the years I found that my clinical intuitions matched those of other neuropsychologists and findings emerging in the literature, and that I had a systematic way of presenting these ideas that made them accessible to the non-neuropsychologist. At that point, the idea for this book was born.

Another formative experience in the development of this book was teaching neuropsychology in Central America. Since 1986 I have intermittently taught clinical neuropsychology most frequently in Nicaragua and in Costa Rica, where neuropsychology was all but unknown. The need to make my field accessible and practical in situations of great need and few resources honed my priorities and my delivery. This led to the development particularly of much of the material in Part 3. These experiences continue to open my eyes to the needless tragedies that result from senseless warfare and violence, malnutrition, preventable diseases, and economic injustice, and the devastating effects these outrages produce on brains and on lives. The real motivation and drive behind this book, then, is to take a few steps toward making the esoteric knowledge of neuropsychology practical and useful for the many people in the world who have thus suffered from our human failings.

Many worthy and relevant topics had to be excluded in choosing material for this book. Application of these materials and approaches to children is worthy of its own book and is not discussed here, although the alert clinician will find many adaptable ideas (see Blosser & DePompei, 1989; Horton, 1994; Lehr, 1990; Rosen & Gerring, 1986; Savage & Wolcott, 1994; Spanbock, 1992; Waaland & Kreutzer, 1988; Ylvisaker, Feeney, & Mullins, 1995). Although many examples in this book come from cross-cultural experience, explicit cross-cultural applications are not discussed (see Cavallo & Saucedo, 1995; Dikengil, Jones, & Byrne, 1993; Galanti, 1991; Lynch & Hanson, 1992; Ramirez, 1991; D. W. Sue & Sue, 1990; Werner, 1990). Ways of coping with the use and abuse of alcohol and illicit drugs in people with brain illnesses is also a specialized area which had to be excluded (see Corrigan, 1995; Corrigan, Lamb-Hart, & Rust, 1995; Gualtieri, 1991; Langley, Lindsay, Lam, & Priddy, 1990; Miller, 1993).

In accordance with the desires of many groups advocating for the rights of people with disabilities and the guidelines set forth by the American Psychological Association (1994), people with brain illnesses will generally be referred to in that manner to put the person first (rather than aphasics, amnesics, head injury victims, survivors, brain-injured people, etc.). "Brain illness" here will be taken to include traumatic brain injury. The terms "client" or "patient" will be used when reference is to those social roles. I have alternated a generic "he" with a generic "she" chapter by chapter.

The ideas presented in this book were a long time in development. I benefited substantially from discussions with Mary Pepping, Barry Willer, Jordi Peña-Casanova, Federico Montero, Frida Madrigal, Fernando Acosta, Marcela Solano, Marlene Koss, Idealda Lazo, Adriana Cortés, George Prigatano, and Bob Sbordone. My students in Nicaragua, in Costa Rica, in Spain, and in the United States have repeatedly challenged me to clarify, generalize, qualify, and demonstrate my ideas. An anonymous woman who had had a traumatic brain injury coined the concept of emotional rehabilitation, which was passed on to me by Lloyd Cripe. The able staff at Good Samaritan Hospital in Puyallup, Washington provided a cognitive rehabilitation framework, much feedback and discussion, and many opportunities to try out ideas. Among those many fine people to whom I am particularly grateful are Katie Mateer, McKay Sohlberg, Brian Baird, Jerry DeVore, Cindy Stoffel, Fred Silver, Sarah Raskin, Kim Kerns, Dennis Williams, and Suzanne Geyer.

Elizabeth Sequeira "midwifed" the birth of the idea for this book at the first Latin American Neuropsychology Congress in Buenos Aires in 1989. Together we elaborated many of the fundamental concepts, such as the continuum of responsibility, and refined their communication through workshop presentations. Her tireless collaboration and support have been an inspiration, for which I am continually appreciative. *¡En solidaridad!* Jill Winegardner shared with me and later extended our teaching in Nicaragua. She coauthored earlier versions of portions of Part 3 as part of our *Manual de Neuropsicología Práctica* [Manual of Practical Neuropsychology], and allowed me to use them here. Her sensitive collaboration and high sense of purpose have helped to keep me focused, for which I am most grateful. *¡La lucha sigue!*

My son, Robin Judd Walker, provided able editing, commentary, and patience, and learned more about APA style than he ever wanted to know. He monitored my warning signs of cognitive fatigue and intervened with meals and with physical exercise to prevent the onset of irritability. *Muchas gracias, mijo.* School psychologist and counselor, my colleague, illustrator, coauthor, and life companion, Roberta DeBoard, listened patiently; challenged and corrected my thinking; tolerated late night writing sprees; read and edited the manuscript; never shrank (to my knowledge) from offering criticism, correction, or coffee when I needed it; and maintained faith in me and the project throughout it all. To her I offer my heartfelt thanks and a well-deserved vacation. *¿Sabes qué?* The errors and shortcomings that all of these generous helpers failed to ferret out remain fully my responsibility.

The thousands of people with brain illnesses and their families and friends with whom I have worked and shared triumphs, disappointments, and frustrations over the years have given me the experiences and inspiration that made this book possible. It has been a privilege to have their trust and to have a glimpse into their lives, so often at moments of great vulnerability.

*Tedd Judd*

# Contents

List of Tables .......... xvii

List of Figures .......... xxi

List of Cases .......... xxiii

Chapter 1
INTRODUCTION .......... 1

What Is Neuropsychotherapy? .......... 3
Who Is Neuropsychotherapy For? .......... 6
What Problems Does Neuropsychotherapy Treat? .......... 6
Why Is Neuropsychotherapy Needed? .......... 8
Who Is the Neuropsychotherapist? .......... 8
When Is Neuropsychotherapy Needed? .......... 9
How Is Neuropsychotherapy Done? .......... 14

**Part I. THEORY** .......... 15

Chapter 2
NEUROLOGY AND NEUROPSYCHOLOGY .......... 17

Type of Illness .......... 17
Time Course of Illness: The Continuum of Responsibility .......... 17
Factors of Personality and Emotions following Brain Illness .......... 26

Chapter 3
EDUCATION AND PSYCHOTHERAPY .......... 31

Education .......... 31
Family Involvement .......... 33

Approaches to Psychotherapy ........ 33
Neuropsychotherapy–Psychotherapy Balance ........ 36
Conclusions ........ 37

Chapter 4
COGNITIVE REHABILITATION ........ 39

The General Stimulation Approach ........ 39
The Functional Approach ........ 40
The Process-Specific Approach ........ 40
The Natural Recovery Approach ........ 44
The Problem-Oriented Approach to Neuropsychotherapy ........ 47
Where Cognitive Rehabilitation and Neuropsychotherapy Meet ........ 48

**Part II. PRACTICE** ........ 49

Chapter 5
ASSESSMENT ........ 51

Assessment as a Cognitive Problem-Solving Process ........ 51
Conducting the Neuropsychological/Neurobehavioral Assessment ........ 63
Formulating Conclusions ........ 77
Intervention Planning ........ 81
Feedback ........ 81
Adjusting the Conclusions ........ 82
Summary ........ 83

Chapter 6
FUNDAMENTAL ISSUES ........ 85

Causality and Blame ........ 85
The New Person ........ 85
Communication Style ........ 87
Naming and Normalizing the Problem ........ 90
Controlling Behavior by Controlling the Environment ........ 91
Problem Analysis ........ 91
Search for Solutions ........ 93
Educating Family, Friends, Employers, Teachers, and Others ........ 96
Ethical Issues ........ 104

Chapter 7
GENERAL TECHNIQUES OF NEUROPSYCHOTHERAPY
AND RELATED INTERVENTIONS ........ 107

The Therapy Journal ........ 107
Cue Cards ........ 113

Empathy ..... 118
Self-Awareness ..... 122
Telling Others ..... 134

Chapter 8
INTERVENTION STRATEGIES FOR PROBLEM FEELINGS AND BEHAVIORS: FROM CAREGIVER MANAGEMENT TO SELF-REGULATION ..... 137

Introduction ..... 137
Interventions ..... 138
Record-Keeping and Procedures ..... 146
Conclusions ..... 152

**Part III. SPECIFIC PROBLEMS** ..... 153
Chapter 9
PSYCHOLOGICAL REACTIONS TO ILLNESS ..... 155

Grief Reactions ..... 155
Denial ..... 156
Depression ..... 158
Anxiety ..... 166
Perplexity ..... 168
Frustration ..... 170
Embarrassment ..... 172
Catastrophic Reaction ..... 173
Post-Traumatic Stress Disorder (PTSD) ..... 174
Personal Reformation ..... 178

Chapter 10
ORGANIC EMOTIONAL CHANGES ..... 181

Emotional Communication:
Impaired Emotional Expressiveness and Comprehension ..... 181
Reflex Crying and Laughing ..... 184
Automatic Cursing ..... 187
Compensatory Exaggerated Emotional Expressions ..... 189
Emotional Reactivity: Impaired Reactivity ..... 189
Labile Emotions ..... 192
Irritability, Impulsive Anger, and Agitation ..... 194
Emotional Obsessiveness Sometimes Associated with Temporal Lobe Epilepsy (TLE) ..... 208
Changes in Types of Emotional Responses ..... 211

Chapter 11
EXECUTIVE FUNCTIONS ........ 213

Introduction ........ 213
Impaired Initiation (Abulia) ........ 216
Disinhibition ........ 221
Perseveration ........ 225
Concreteness ........ 230
Impaired Monitoring and Judgment and
Lack of Awareness of Deficits ........ 233
Impaired Planning and Organization ........ 237
Impaired Communication Pragmatics ........ 240

Chapter 12
COGNITIVE AND MEDICAL PROBLEMS ........ 245

Impaired Attention and Concentration ........ 245
Impaired Memory and Learning ........ 248
Language and Speech Disturbances ........ 252
Fatigue ........ 255
Hyperaesthesia ........ 257

**Part IV. THE SOCIAL DIMENSION** ........ 261

Chapter 13
THE FAMILY ........ 263

Effects of Brain Illnesses on the Family ........ 263
Evaluation ........ 284
Interventions ........ 287
Conclusions ........ 289

Chapter 14
THE COMMUNITY ........ 291

The Medical/Rehabilitation Community ........ 291
The Disability Community ........ 293
The Work Community ........ 295
School ........ 301
The Social Community ........ 302
Prisons ........ 309
The Homeless ........ 311

Chapter 15
CONCLUSIONS AND FUTURE DIRECTIONS ........................................ 313

Directions for Future Research ........................................ 314
Directions for Future Action ........................................ 317

Appendix A
CLASSIFICATION OF FACTORS AFFECTING
PERSONALITY FOLLOWING BRAIN ILLNESS ........................................ 321

Appendix B
CONTEMPORARY NEUROPSYCHOLOGICAL
PERSONALITY ASSESSMENT TOOLS ........................................ 327

General ........................................ 327
Specific ........................................ 329

Glossary ........................................ 333

References ........................................ 339

Index ........................................ 357

# List of Tables


1.1. Causes of Brain Dysfunction 7
2.1. Progression of Self-Control 20
2.2. Organic Disturbances of Emotional Functions 28
2.3. Disturbances of Activation 28
3.1. Possible Roles of Family Members in Neuropsychotherapy Processes 34
3.2. Cognitive Task Analysis of Client's Role in Reframing Negative Thoughts 34
4.1. Zone of Recovery 45
5.1. Assessment Hypotheses 55
5.1a. Types of Hypotheses in Neuropsychological Assessment of Emotions, Behavior, and Personality for Intervention Planning 55
5.1b. Common Symptom and Problem Hypotheses by Diagnosis 55
5.1c. Common Symptom and Problem Hypotheses by Lesion Localization 56
5.1d. Common Symptom and Problem Hypotheses by Severity 57
5.1e. Common Symptom and Problem Hypotheses by Onset 58
5.1f. Common Symptom and Problem Hypotheses, General 58
5.2. Common Sources of Information in a Neuropsychological Assessment 59
5.3. Costs and Risks of Psychosocial Evaluation 61
5.4. Classification of Cognitive Errors in Diagnostic Reasoning 65
5.5. Neuropsychological Review of Systems and Functions 68
5.6. Social and Emotional History 70
5.7. Evaluating the Adequacy of the Environment of Recovery 74
5.8. Risks of Psychosocial Intervention 82
5.9. Steps in Feedback Regarding Neuropsychological Evaluation 83
6.1. Sample Neuropsychotherapy Session Agenda 90

6.2. Sample Problem Behavior Tally Sheets 92
6.3. Sample Anxiety Journal Format 93
6.4. Techniques of Family Education 97
6.5. Mentoring Activities in Rehabilitation for Family Members and Others 99
6.6. Mentoring Selection Criteria 100
7.1. The Continuum of Responsibility and the Therapy Journal 108
7.2. Possible Therapy Journal Sections 108
7.3. Sample Strengths and Problems List 109
7.4. Sample Neuropsychotherapy Session Summary 111
7.5. Cue Card Uses and Examples 114
7.5a. Cue Card Uses 114
7.5b. Sample Cue Cards for Emotional Control 114
7.5c. Sample Cue Cards for Social Procedures 115
7.5d. Sample Cue Cards for Stressful Events 115
7.5e. Sample Behavior Flash Cards 116
7.5f. Sample Introductory Card for a Neuropsychological Problem 117
7.5g. Sample Cue Card for a Child with Fatigue and Irritability 117
7.5h. Sample Cue Cards for a Confused Person Who Wanders 118
7.6. Principle Techniques of Validation Therapy 121
7.7. Risks of Overestimation of Disability 123
7.8. Techniques for Working with Overestimation of Disability 124
7.9. Major Risks of Underestimation of Disabilities 126
7.10. Three Levels of Awareness of Deficits 126
7.11. Self-Awareness Training 132
7.12. Benefits to the Person with a Brain Illness in Telling Others about her Problems 134
7.13. Techniques for Telling Others about a Neuropsychological Problem 135
8.1. Problem Feelings and Behaviors with Sudden Onsets that can Result from Brain Illnesses 138
8.2. Strategies for External Management of Incidents of Problem Behaviors 141
8.3. Strategies for Self-Calming 143
8.4. Possible Preparations for Returning from Backing Off 144
8.5. Sample Incident Log 146
8.6. Example of a Completed Incident Log 147
8.7. Levels of Cuing 149
8.8. Progression of Self-Control in Interventions for Problem Behaviors 151
9.1. Symptoms of Depression and Confusable Neuropsychological Symptoms 159
9.2. Barriers and Solutions to Depression Testing in People with Brain Illnesses 163

9.3. Modifications in Cognitive Psychotherapy for Treating Depressed People with Brain Illnesses 165
9.4. Indications Favoring the Use of Antidepressant Medications in Depressed People with Brain Illnesses 165
9.5. Potentially Confusable Symptoms: Post-Traumatic Stress Disorder (PTSD) versus Traumatic Brain Injury (TBI) 175
10.1. Sources of Anger following Brain Illnesses 195
10.2. Characteristics of Organic Impulsive Anger 196
10.3. Possible Risk Factors Associated with Anger 199
10.4. Possible Warning Signs of Anger 200
10.5. Sample Anger Cue Cards 203
10.5a. Typical Anger Cue Card 203
10.5b. Anger Management Program Acronym 203
10.5c. Cue Card for a Man Picking up His Children from His Ex-Wife 204
10.5d. Cue Card for Telling Others about an Anger Problem 204
10.6. Sample Anger Journal Format 204
10.7. Personality Changes Thought to Be Associated with Temporal Lobe Epilepsy 209
11.1. Executive Dysfunctions 214
11.2. General Schema for Executive Dysfunction Intervention 216
11.3. Hierarchy of Initiation Cuing Systems 219
11.4. Possible Disinhibition Risk Factors, Warning Signs and Strategies 225
11.5. Possible Perseveration Risk Factors, Warning Signs, and Strategies 229
11.6. Possible Concreteness Risk Factors, Warning Signs, and Strategies 232
12.1. Possible Activities for People with Aphasia and Their Families 255
13.1. Family Grief Reactions to Acute Brain Illness 264
13.2. Possible Activities for the Person in the Second Stage of Alzheimer's Disease 269
13.3. Secondary (Psychosocial) Causes of Sexual Dysfunction after TBI 273
13.4. The PLISSIT Model of Levels of Intervention for Sexual Problems 274
13.5. Sexual Assessment Planning: Areas to Be Assessed 274
13.6. Sources of Overprotection and Clinical Strategies 283
13.7. Areas for Screening Families of People with Brain Illnesses 285
13.8. Evaluating the Family in Depth 286
14.1. Guidelines for Forming Brain Illness Support Groups 294
14.2. Principles of Brain Illness Vocational Rehabilitation 295
14.3. Challenges to Employment in People with Traumatic Brain Injuries 296
14.4. Vocational Rehabilitation Intervention Strategies 297
14.5. Continuum of Vocational Placement Options 297
14.6. Cognitive Compensations Adaptable to the Workplace 300
14.7. AABCCC Analysis of Disinhibited Sexual Behavior 305

# List of Figures


| | | |
|---|---|---|
| 1.1. | Interventions and Intervenors | 2 |
| 1.2. | Relationships among Psychotherapy, Rehabilitation, Cognitive Rehabilitation, and Neuropsychotherapy | 3 |
| 1.3. | Neuropsychotherapy versus Cognitive Rehabilitation | 4 |
| 1.4. | Continuum from Individual to Community Interventions | 5 |
| 1.5. | Factors of Personality following Brain Illness | 6 |
| 1.6. | Recipients and Intensities of Interventions | 12 |
| 2.1. | The Typical Time Course of Brain Illness with Sudden Onset and Gradual Recovery | 18 |
| 2.2. | The Typical Time Course of Progressive Brain Illness | 18 |
| 2.3. | The Typical Time Course of Brain Illness with Intermittent Presentation | 19 |
| 2.4. | The Continuum of Responsibility between Caregivers and Persons Recovering from Acute Brain Illness | 19 |
| 2.5. | The Continuum of Responsibility between Caregivers and Persons with Progressive Brain Illnesses | 22 |
| 2.6. | The Continuum of Responsibility between Caregivers and Persons with Intermittent Brain Dysfunction | 25 |
| 3.1. | The Balance between Neuropsychotherapy and Conventional Psychotherapy in Acute Brain Illness | 36 |
| 5.1. | Testing Thresholds | 60 |
| 5.2. | Assessment Thresholds for Intensive Rehabilitation 3 Weeks after a Mild TBI | 62 |
| 5.3. | Assessment Thresholds for Mental Status Screening in a Geriatric Population | 63 |
| 5.4. | Assessment Thresholds for Problem-Solving Counseling following Major Brain Illness | 64 |
| 5.5. | Assessment Thresholds for Group Education Regarding a TBI | 65 |

7.1. Awareness versus Disability, Sudden Onset, with Depression/Catastrophic Reaction 122
7.2. Awareness versus Disability, Progressive Onset, with Depression/Catastrophic Reaction 123
7.3. Awareness versus Disability, Sudden Onset, with Anosognosia/Denial 125
7.4. Awareness versus Disability, Progressive Onset, with Anosognosia/Denial 125
8.1. A Progress Chart 150
9.1. Example of a Visual Mood Scale Item 162
13.1. Typical Family Awareness of Disability, Sudden Onset 265
13.2. Family Awareness of Disability, Sudden Onset, Less Stable Family Member and/or Mixed Signs or Messages 266
13.3. Typical Family Awareness of Disability, Progressive Onset 267
13.4. Family Awareness of Disability, Progressive Onset, Less Stable Family Member and/or Mixed Signs or Messages 267

# List of Cases


| | | |
|---|---|---|
| Case 1.1. | Georgia: Who Says It's All Bad? | 10 |
| Case 1.2. | Fyodor: Dostoyevsky | 10 |
| Case 1.3. | B. B.: The Tough Case: How Much? | 12 |
| Case 3.1. | Raj: The School of Hard Knocks | 32 |
| Case 3.2. | Marcel: Whose Denial? Whose Reality? | 33 |
| Case 4.1. | Elizabeth: Zone of Recovery | 46 |
| Case 4.2. | Vigilio: Hypothesis Testing in Evaluation | 47 |
| Case 5.1. | Naricio: Clinical Reasoning | 52 |
| Case 5.2. | Abuela: "I Want to Go Home!" | 76 |
| Case 5.3. | Pepe: Crutches for Pepe | 77 |
| Case 5.4. | Salvador: Organizing the Information | 78 |
| Case 6.1. | J.D.: Repetition, Repetition. and Repetition | 86 |
| Case 6.2. | Sigmund: What Is Abstract? | 89 |
| Case 6.3. | Janaki's Mother: Socratic Dialogue | 101 |
| Case 7.1. | Gabby: Who, Me? | 117 |
| Case 7.2. | Douglass: Working with What You've Got | 119 |
| Case 7.3. | Peleo: Naming the Problem | 119 |
| Case 7.4. | Tillie: Validation Therapy | 121 |
| Case 7.5. | R.: The Selectivity of Anosognosia | 127 |
| Case 7.6. | Cerebra: To Know Is Not Enough | 127 |
| Case 7.7. | Juan: Negotiating Supported Failure | 128 |
| Case 7.8. | Ingrid: Who's in Charge Here? | 129 |
| Case 7.9. | J.D.: Mirror, Mirror, on the Wall | 129 |
| Case 7.10. | Elvis: And Now from Studio R | 130 |
| Case 7.11. | Thomas: Using Tests to Build Awareness | 131 |
| Case 7.12. | Raj: "You Just Don't Understand!" | 135 |
| Case 9.1. | Gigi: Prognosis? | 179 |

| | | |
|---|---|---|
| Case 10.1a. | A.L.S.: Report from the Land of ALS | 184 |
| Case 10.1b. | Support Group: Thank You, and Now for My Next Act | 184 |
| Case 10.2. | Ludwig: Where Is Inspiration Localized? | 190 |
| Case 11.1. | Groucho: Disinhibition or Sexual Harassment? | 215 |
| Case 11.2. | Dumi: Reveille | 220 |
| Case 11.3. | Portland: I Am NOT Concrete, I'm Flesh and Blood | 230 |
| Case 11.4. | Ludwig: Anosognosia, Denial, or Something Else? | 235 |
| Case 12.1. | Lu Tan: When Less Is More | 246 |
| Case 12.2. | Gramps: I Love You All, but One at a Time, Please! | 246 |
| Case 12.3. | P. T. A.: When to Tell? | 253 |
| Case 12.4. | Doris's Letter | 254 |
| Case 12.5. | Frank: Our Song | 255 |
| Case 13.1. | Oscar: Homophobia in Rehabilitation | 280 |
| Case 13.2. | Marilyn: Parenting | 281 |
| Case 13.3. | Emma: An Unusual Housemate | 282 |
| Case 13.4. | Tierno: Mommy Won't Let Me Come Out! | 284 |
| Case 14.1. | G. P.: Quick. Which Key Locks up the Cobra? | 301 |
| Case 14.2. | Mr. Bates: If It Feels Good . . . | 306 |
| Case 14.3. | SWF: Woman Seeking Man | 308 |
| Case 14.4. | Don: The Best Therapist in the World! | 309 |
| Case 14.5. | O.: The Story of O. | 310 |
| Case 14.6. | Nguyen: How Many Others? | 310 |
| Case 14.7. | Pega: Community Consultation | 311 |

# 1

# Introduction

Maria had a stroke that left her left side weak, although she was able to walk. She cried frequently but when her family asked why she was not able to say, so they took her to a psychiatrist. He asked her if she was sleeping well. Maria's weak side made it hard for her to move in bed, so she told him, "No". He asked her if she had lost weight or had lost her appetite. She had lost weight in the hospital, as the weakness in one side of her face made it hard to chew, and she was less active so she didn't eat much. She answered, "Yes". He asked her about her sex life and she said that she hadn't had sex since her stroke. She and her husband assumed that sex could cause another stroke. The psychiatrist told Maria that she was depressed, and he gave her an antidepressant. She didn't feel depressed, but figured that he knew more than she.

Maria slept better, but the crying didn't stop so her family took her to a psychotherapist, who noted that the crying had started when Maria was in the hospital. She asked Maria if she had ever been in a hospital before. Maria told her how she had cried at the births of her children in a hospital. She remembered that she had been taken to an emergency room as a child but she didn't remember much about it. After asking a lot more questions, the therapist told Maria that she thought she had been sexually abused as a child but had repressed the memory. She told Maria that she had a post-traumatic stress disorder that was reactivated by her hospitalization. Maria had noticed problems with her memory since the stroke and the therapist said that was more evidence that she had been abused. The therapist tried to get her to remember the abuse. They used guided imagery, read books, and tried hypnotism, which was all interesting, but Maria never remembered any abuse.

As she was still crying, her family took her to another therapist who asked her how she felt. She said she was discouraged that the psychiatrist and the psychotherapist hadn't helped her problem. The new therapist said that it was exactly those kinds of negative thoughts and learned helplessness that made her depressed. He helped her restructure her thought patterns toward optimism. This was easy and fun. After a few sessions he asked her if she still felt depressed. She answered, "Who, me? Depressed? I've never felt depressed!" He laughed and told her she was cured and sent her home. However, she still cried.

One day a neighbor came to visit. Maria didn't want to see her because she was embarrassed about her crying but Maria remembered that her neighbor's husband had a stroke and thought she might understand. She invited Maria and her husband to a stroke club meeting. Maria was embarrassed to go because of her crying, but her neighbor assured her that everyone would understand. When Maria got there she was introduced to a man who had had a stroke and they both burst into tears! Two other people were crying, too. No one made a big deal about it the way her family had. The man said, "I see you have the crying problem, too." They called it reflex crying and laughed about how it used to embarrass them. They recognized that she wasn't necessarily upset or sad when she cried. A few of them had experiences like hers with psychiatrists and with therapists. One person taught her a trick of looking at the ceiling and breathing deeply to control it. Another gave her a folder about it to show her family.

Soon her family accepted her crying as a quirky change from her stroke, no more serious than sneezing. They stopped worrying and kept talking when she cried. She learned to explain it to people and went out in public again. With the stroke club's encouragement, she asked her doctor and found it was fine to resume sex, which she promptly did, and it didn't bother her husband at all when she cried.

This fictitious story, a composite of clinical experiences, illustrates how neuropsychological phenomena can be misinterpreted as purely psychological. Well-meaning therapists may apply inappropriate treatments that waste resources or even cause harm. It illustrates a neuropsychotherapeutic intervention, not by a professional, but by a neighbor and by a stroke club.

The emotional and behavior problems of brain illness can be addressed by a range of interventions which can be effectively carried out by various professionals, paraprofessionals, and lay people (Figure 1.1). This book is directed not just

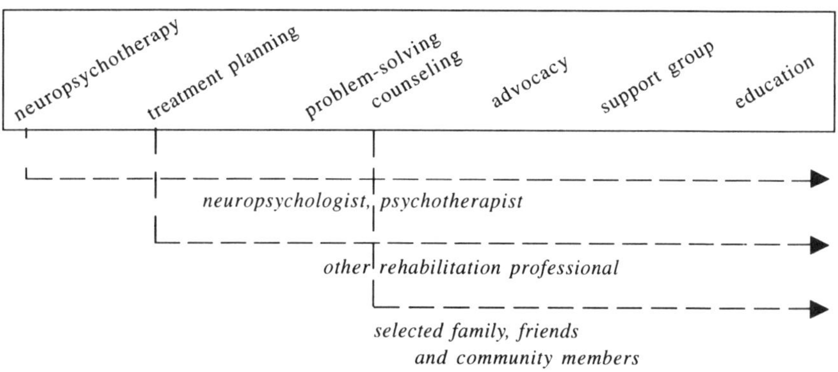


FIGURE 1.1. Interventions and intervenors. Formal neuropsychotherapy and rehabilitation planning requires the participation of professionals. Some problem-solving counseling is best done by professionals when specialized solutions to problems may be needed (e.g., rehabilitation services), but many laypeople can also perform competent problem-solving counseling when specialized solutions are not needed (e.g., transportation problems). Advocacy, support groups, and education can be provided by all.

at neuropsychologists and psychotherapists, but also at social workers, speech and language pathologists, nurses, support group facilitators, and whoever else is concerned with emotional and behavior problems resulting from brain illnesses.

## *WHAT IS NEUROPSYCHOTHERAPY?*

Neuropsychotherapy is the use of neuropsychological knowledge in the psychotherapy of persons with brain disorders. It can also include cognitive rehabilitation for impairments in executive functions (self-regulation) and in social intelligence (Figures 1.2, 1.3). However, brain illnesses often result in emotional, behavioral, and personality problems that require or respond best to interventions that go beyond neuropsychotherapy, such as environmental manipulations, behavioral programs, family therapy, group therapy, support groups, community and legal advocacy, and education for the person, her family, and the community.

Where formal, individual, (and billable) visits to a healthcare practitioner are the standard, efforts such as family interventions or community education may not be encouraged. This book emphasizes interventions nearer to the psychotherapy end of the spectrum (Figure 1.4), as they supply principles needed for other interventions. However, when more social interventions are preferred for reasons of efficacy, efficiency, or public health, these are also discussed.

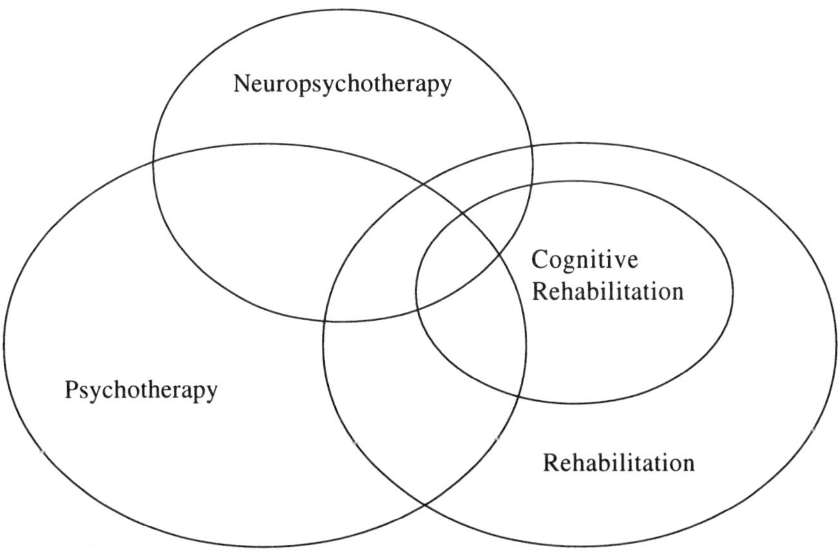


FIGURE 1.2. Relationships among psychotherapy, rehabilitation, cognitive rehabilitation, and neuropsychotherapy.

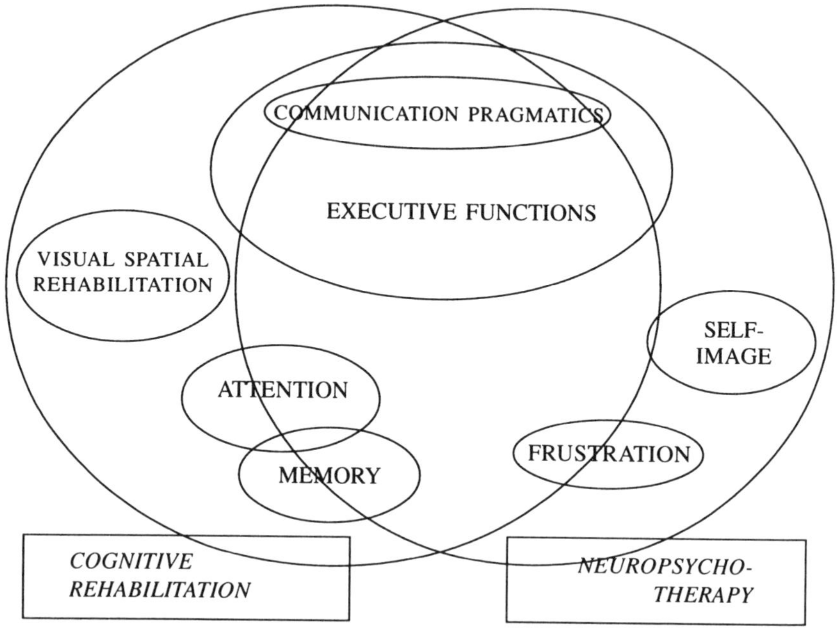


FIGURE 1.3. Neuropsychotherapy versus cognitive rehabilitation. Treatment of representative functions only is shown. For example, communication pragmatics, part of the executive functions, can be treated by both cognitive rehabilitation and neuropsychotherapy, with a few parts exclusive to each.

## *Neuropsychotherapy vs. Conventional Psychotherapy*

Brain illnesses often result in cognitive difficulties that may make conventional psychotherapy unproductive, frustrating, or even harmful. Neuropsychotherapy differs from traditional psychotherapy both in process and in content. The principal adaptation of process is the use of cognitive compensations, or techniques designed to circumvent cognitive difficulties. The principal adaptation of content involves a perspective of emotional rehabilitation, or the use of distinctive techniques to address changes in emotions and in behavior that are the direct result of brain disorders.

### *Cognitive Compensations*

Clients with organic amnesia are unlikely to remember much of what goes on in a psychotherapy session. They may need a therapy notebook. Those with impaired attention or organizational abilities may need extra structure in the session. Similarly, adaptations are needed to accommodate impaired communi-

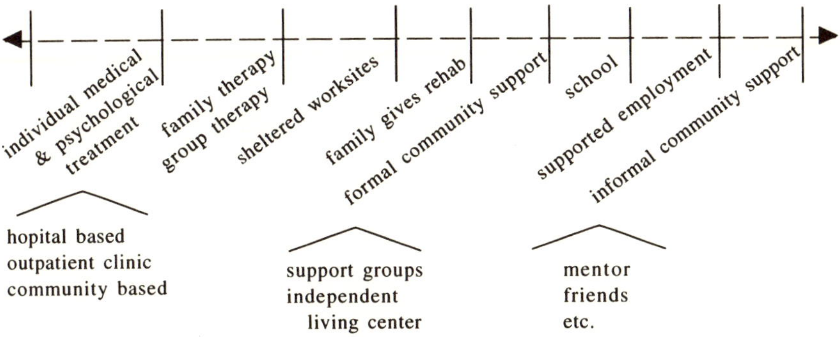


FIGURE 1.4. The continuum from individual to community interventions.

cation, initiation, and so forth. Without such cognitive compensations, the client who has little memory of previous sessions, or who wanders from topic to topic without encountering material of psychodynamic significance, or who cannot comprehend the therapist's grammatical constructions is unlikely to reap many of the benefits intended by the therapist, by the hopeful family, or by the third party payer (Becker & Vakil, 1993; Block, 1987; Hibbard, Grober, Gordon, Aletta, & Freeman, 1990; Lewis, 1991).

*Emotional Rehabilitation*

Three major factors contribute to the emotional state, behavior, and personality of a person with a brain illness (Figure 1.5, Lewis, 1991). The first factor is the pre-illness personality. The second factor is comprised of psychological reactions to the illness and its consequences, such as grief and post-traumatic stress disorders, which also occur with intact brains. Both of these factors can be understood via conventional psychological theories. Problems relating to them can be treated with conventional or with modified psychotherapy. The third factor, however, is not well explained by conventional psychological theories. It is the organic changes in cognition, in emotions, and in behavior that are the direct results of brain illness. For example, reflex crying (the case of Maria previously mentioned) may result from stroke. Similarly, organic impairments in emotional responsiveness or initiation (Blumer & Benson, 1975; Prigatano, 1992; Stuss & Benson, 1986; Stuss, Gow, & Hetherington, 1992) may be mistaken for depression.

Problems related to this factor require treatment based on a different understanding and on specialized techniques of emotional rehabilitation. As with physical and cognitive rehabilitation, emotional rehabilitation may use adaptation, compensation, or retraining. For example, someone with reflex crying may avoid

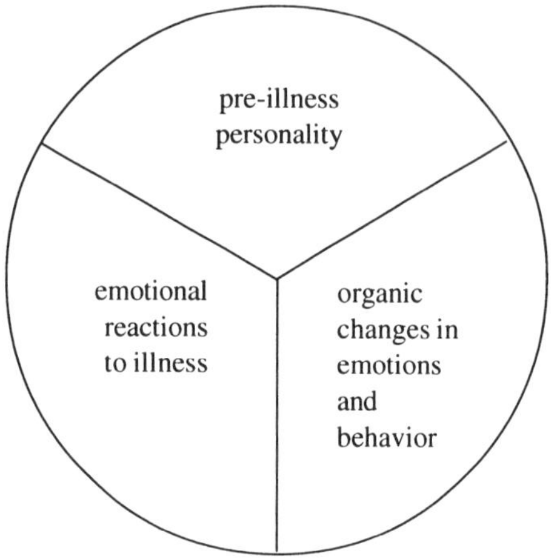


FIGURE 1.5. Factors of personality following brain illness.

situations that provoke tears (adaptation), provide explanations to those around her (compensation), or learn deep breathing to control crying (retraining). Emotional rehabilitation also involves correctly identifying the source of the problem. When an emotional or a behavioral problem is accurately recognized as organic, many fruitless and even harmful searches for other causes can be avoided, thereby defusing interpersonal conflicts and self-doubts. Although this does not relieve the person of responsibility for learning to cope with the problem, it does provide a firm foundation from which to begin that process.

## *WHO IS NEUROPSYCHOTHERAPY FOR?*

Neuropsychotherapy is for anyone with a brain disorder, regardless of its cause (Table 1.1), who has a problem in behavior, in emotions, or in personality that is an on-going concern. In addition, as biological psychiatry continues to discover brain and genetic bases of psychiatric disorders such as schizophrenia, manic-depression, and obsessive-compulsive disorder, these are being seen from a neuropsychological perspective. Neuropsychotherapy may be helpful for these populations.

## *WHAT PROBLEMS DOES NEUROPSYCHOTHERAPY TREAT?*

The core of neuropsychotherapy is treatment of organic changes in emotions and in behavior. What are those changes? Organic disturbances of emotion

**TABLE 1.1. Causes of Brain Dysfunction**

| |
|---|
| Traumatic injury |
| Vascular injury (occlusive strokes, hemorrhages, aneurysms, arteriovenous malformations, migraine) |
| Degenerative disorders (Alzheimer's disease, Parkinson's disease, Huntington's disease, multiple sclerosis, etc.) |
| Toxicities (alcohol, drugs, medications, industrial chemicals, heavy metals, pesticides, fetal alcohol syndrome, etc.) |
| Tumors of the brain |
| Infections (encephalitis, meningitis, malaria, AIDS, etc.) |
| Anoxia (from birth trauma, smoke inhalation, partial drowning, cardiac arrest, etc.) |
| Epilepsy |
| Hydrocephalus |
| Nutritional deficiencies (B vitamin deficiencies, Korsakoff's syndrome, pellagra, marasmus, kwashiorkor) |
| Metabolic disorders (hormonal disorders, kidney and liver diseases, hypoglycemia, etc.) |
| Autoimmune disorders affecting the brain |
| Electrical shock to the brain |
| Developmental disorders (mental retardation, myelomeningocele, cerebral palsy, Turner's syndrome, etc.) |
| Probable brain disorders: (learning disabilities, attention deficit disorder, etc.) |

can be both in the experience of and in the communication of emotion. These disturbances can be either a decrease or an increase in emotional reactions or communication. Among these changes are impulsive anger, catastrophic reactions, lability, indifference, reflex crying, and monotone voice.

Organic changes in executive functions or in self-control abilities often impact interpersonal and intrapsychic life. Most important are disturbances in self-awareness, such as a lack of awareness of one's organic deficits or the failure to recognize one's errors. Other executive dysfunctions are a lack of initiation; impulsivity; disturbances of judgment, planning, and prioritizing; rigid thinking; and a loss of empathy skills.

Finally, some losses unique to brain illness, such as major memory loss, produce unique emotional reactions. For example, when a person with brain illness forgets things she would not previously have forgotten or says one word when intending to say another, she may react with perplexity (Lezak, 1978), confusion, embarrassment, and distress caused by the unreliability and unpredictability of her own cognitive abilities.

All of these problems are potential foci of treatment in neuropsychotherapy and in related interventions. A clear understanding of the specific nature and causes of these problems is important for their effective treatment. This understanding needs to be united with intervention theory and strategies.

## *WHY IS NEUROPSYCHOTHERAPY NEEDED?*

Historically, it is often the physical manifestations of a brain disorder that are the first to be described in the scientific literature and to be clinically treated. Some decades later, the cognitive impairments are recognized. Finally, the emotional and behavioral changes are recognized. Yet, it is the emotional and behavioral changes that are the most significant barriers to effective functioning in family, in work, in school, and in other settings (Morton & Wehman, 1995). This has been the pattern with stroke, Parkinson's Disease, Huntington's Disease, brain trauma, multiple sclerosis, and many neurotoxicities.

The effects of brain illness on emotions and on personality has received increasing attention (Pepping & Roueche, 1991) but there have been relatively few guidelines for psychotherapeutic intervention (Carberry, 1991; Christensen & Rosenberg, 1991; Ellis, 1989; Feil, 1993; Hibbard et al., 1990; Langer, 1992; Lewis, 1991; Miller, 1993; O'Hara & Harrell, 1991; Prigatano, 1991; Small, 1980). For example, of the 4417 articles abstracted in *PsycSCAN: Neuropsychology* in 1994, only 14 were classified under Psychotherapy and Psychotherapeutic Counseling, and only 10 concerned psychotherapy for brain disorders. Neuropsychotherapy is needed, then, because brain disorders often produce significant and disabling behavioral and emotional changes that cannot be adequately treated with conventional psychotherapy and that, in general, do not yet receive recognition or intervention proportionate to their importance.

## *WHO IS THE NEUROPSYCHOTHERAPIST?*

The neuropsychotherapist needs preparation in psychotherapy and in rehabilitation, particularly cognitive rehabilitation, and a working knowledge of the cognitive and emotional changes resulting from brain disorders. Becoming a competent neuropsychotherapist takes dedication to the field and cannot be tacked on to preparation in one of the parent disciplines through a weekend workshop, for example. A neuropsychologist is in an ideal position to become an effective neuropsychotherapist. However, the neuropsychologist's extensive training in neuroanatomy, clinical neurology, psychological testing, and research methodology is not essential to effective neuropsychotherapy. A speech pathologist, occupational therapist, or other rehabilitation professional with experience in cognitive rehabilitation could become trained in psychotherapy and function as an effective neuropsychotherapist under the supervision of a neuropsychologist, a clinical psychologist, or a neuropsychiatrist. Similarly, a psychotherapist can study the cognitive, emotional, and behavioral changes resulting from brain illness and cognitive rehabilitation and become an effective neuropsychotherapist with appropriate consultation. Either type of crossover clinician will need to rely on a neuropsychologist for assessments.

Such preparation is an ideal, however. In the real world, neuropsychotherapy is often entirely missing from the treatment of the person with brain illness, or it is perfunctory due to the high volume workload and assessment orientation of the neuropsychologist's practice. Extensive psychotherapy is often referred out to psychotherapists who may or may not be prepared to work with brain illnesses. One purpose of this book, then, is to aid the psychotherapist who receives such referrals and the neuropsychologist who is advising that psychotherapist.

Many other professionals, paraprofessionals, and lay people can and should participate in interventions for emotional and behavioral problems resulting from brain illness. Rehabilitation team members can be trained to participate in behavior management programs and to integrate their work with the goals of neuropsychotherapy. Family members need training that is individualized to the problems they are facing. Support groups can identify their own needs and seek and share the training and information they find useful.

## *WHEN IS NEUROPSYCHOTHERAPY NEEDED?*

Neuropsychotherapy is needed when:

1. The person with a brain illness has significant behavioral or emotional problems resulting from that illness,
2. The problems cannot be managed or improved adequately or efficiently in and by the person's setting, and
3. Intervention is likely to reduce those problems.

The first of these conditions is typically determined through neuropsychological or through other mental health assessment, (see Chapter 5; Christensen, 1989; Judd & Fordyce, 1996; Lezak, 1995; Miller, 1993; Silver, Yudofsky, & Hales, 1994). The question as to whether or not problems are significant is a clinical judgment concerning whether or not they interfere with functioning. For example, one middle-aged man had not cried for 20 years prior to his stroke, which produced mild reflex crying. He thereafter cried at funerals, sad movies, and so forth. This was not an embarrassment for him; in fact, it provided relief. Therefore it was merely a change, not a problem needing treatment beyond brief education. Positive personality changes have also been reported with brain illness (Cases 1.1. Georgia; 1.2. Fyodor; Ranseen, 1990), most often aggressive people becoming more placid, or timid individuals becoming more assertive and outgoing.

The second condition for when neuropsychotherapy is needed—when the setting of the person is inadequate to cope with the problem—is currently also a clinical judgment (Chapter 5).

The third condition for when neuropsychotherapy is needed—when it is likely to be effective—suggests that practitioners should seek the best knowledge possible to assure that their services will be maximally beneficial. An inter-

*Who Says It's All Bad? Case 1.1. Georgia.* A painter with a mild anoxic brain injury had subtle changes in her visual perception. She reported that she saw scenes not according to the laws of perspective and how they would be depicted on canvas, but as if they were blotches of color on a sheet of glass. She then painted those blotches directly as she saw them, which gave her works a new, intriguing ambiguity. She also felt that she had lost some of her sensitivity to other people and switched from painting insightful portraits to impressionistic landscapes, which then sold better.

vention is equally ineffective when it is applied to someone who will recuperate at the same rate without it and when it is applied to someone who will not recuperate in spite of it. Conversely, an intervention may be effective even when the person gets worse if it slows functional deterioration from a degenerative disease. For example, medications may be considered effective treatments for cognitive and behavioral problems of Alzheimer's disease even though patients get worse on them if they get worse more slowly than on placebo. Similarly, emotional support for caregivers of persons with Alzheimer's disease may be considered effective when it postpones nursing home placement.

The concept of "ability to benefit" has implications not only for individual clinical decisions, but for research planning as well. If the development and testing of interventions is directed primarily toward certain groups (e.g., by culture, language, type of education, gender, or age), then other groups for whom the interventions are less effective will not be able to receive adequate services. For example, most research on cognitive rehabilitation has been directed toward young, English-speaking adults with at least a primary education. This puts clinicians in a dilemma. When faced with a client who falls significantly outside of those categories, they can refuse to offer services on the grounds that they have not been shown to be effective and thus will risk appearing biased, or they can offer services of questionable effectiveness.

*Dostoyevsky. Case 1.2. Fyodor.* Although still controversial, many authors maintain that a small minority of individuals with temporal lobe epilepsy develop specific interictal personality changes as a result of the seizure focus (Bear & Fedio, 1977; LaPlante, 1993). Among the reported manifestations are *hypergraphia*, or a tendency to write prolifically, and a religious or philosophical preoccupation (see Chapter 10). These tendencies are said to have contributed to the writings of the 19th century Russian author, Fyodor Dostoyevsky, and the contemporary U.S. writer, Thom Jones (Jones, 1993). The strong character of Dostoyevsky provides a useful mnemonic for remembering many features of this condition.

The ideal world of brain illness rehabilitation in which there is adequate knowledge about effectiveness of interventions is still a long way from being realized. Clinical decision-making requires extrapolation from available data and from clinical judgments based on informal and on formal empirical knowledge. The proper position regarding interventions that have not been adequately scientifically tested is not that they are ineffective but that their effectiveness is unknown (Malec, 1993). Much of the theory and the techniques that follow are in this category. Although extrapolation from available data and from clinical experience suggest that these interventions are effective, they await formal testing. The reader is cautioned to exercise particular care when deciding to apply such unproven techniques.

The question of when neuropsychotherapy is needed goes beyond offering or not offering treatment to also include how much and what kind of treatment to provide. The term *neuropsychotherapy* focuses attention on the special nature of the most intensive and specialized of those interventions, but these are only part of the menu of services and supports that can help an individual cope with such problems. The level of intensity and of intrusiveness of intervention should also be determined by what is necessary to get the job done.

Intervention can occur at the stages of acute hospitalization, rehabilitation, and community reintegration (Kay & Cavallo, 1994). It can occur at the level of the individual, the family, or the community. Intensity of intervention ranges from information and education through support, problem-solving restructuring, and advocacy to formal therapy (Figure 1.6). Kay and Cavallo maintained that "*All* families benefit from education and problem solving; *some* family members require longer-term formal treatment because of issues outside the event of TBI (traumatic brain injury) [emphasis in original]" (p 558). Although this applies to interventions with families, it is not fully appropriate as a rule for neuropsychotherapy. Some individuals with brain illnesses may not be able to benefit significantly from education or from problem-solving interventions because of the severity of their illnesses, amnesia, and so forth but may nevertheless benefit from other interventions.

The question of when neuropsychotherapy and related interventions are needed includes prioritizing treatment among many deserving people. In an ideal world, the capacity to prevent brain illness would be maximized and there would be far fewer such incidents to treat. That failing, an ideal world might include intensive, caring professional rehabilitation for every individual unfortunate enough to experience a brain illness. Such service, however, can be quite expensive. For example, recommended rehabilitation and care costs in the United States for a 41-year-old man with a severe TBI beginning 2 years after the injury were $209,000 for the first year and $90,000 per year thereafter, exclusive of 6 weeks of acute medical costs and 14 months of rehabilitation costs (Case 1.3, "The Tough Case," 1993). In part due to such costs, the real world falls far short of

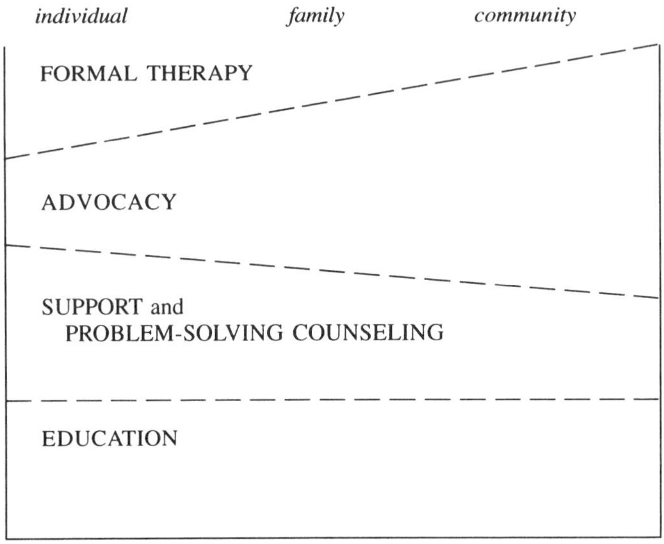


FIGURE 1.6. Recipients and intensities of interventions. Most people with brain injuries or illnesses, virtually all of their families, and selected members of the community (teachers, bosses, friends) need education about the condition. Most can benefit from supportive and problem-solving counseling, although this is generally less necessary the farther removed the recipient is from the person with the brain illness. Advocacy is frequently appropriate. Although advocacy is usually on behalf of the person with the brain injury or illness, sometimes on behalf of the family, and occasionally on behalf of a community organization or institution, it is usually directed toward some sector of the community and occasionally toward the family. Formal neuropsychotherapy, family therapy, individual psychotherapy for family members, or group therapy is sometimes required.

*The Tough Case: How Much??? Case 1.3. B. B.* ("The Tough Case," 1993). B. B. is a 41-year-old man evaluated 2 years after a severe TBI from a motor vehicle accident. He had 6 weeks of acute medical care, 9½ months of intensive, specialized inpatient rehabilitation, and 5 months of outpatient rehabilitation. At the time of the evaluation he was independent in activities of daily living, walked with a cane, and had right hemiplegia, right knee pain, diplopia, and dysarthria. His IQ was in the average range, and he had impairments in attention, in memory, and in executive functions, and had mood swings of depression and anger.

His neuropsychologist recommended a 1 year inpatient rehabilitation program for him and counseling for his family at a cost of $209,704. Costs for living at home thereafter were estimated at about $90,000 per year, versus about $94,000 per year for institutional care. These amounts were exclusive of the first two years of his medical and rehabilitation care costs.

these ideals. Only about 10% of individuals with TBIs in the United States receive adequate diagnosis and rehabilitation (Kreutzer, Gordon, & Wehman, 1989), as compared to about 1 to 2% of individuals in most other countries (Johnston & Tjandrakusuma, 1982; World Health Organization, 1981), especially those with poorly developed rehabilitation systems and even more inequitable distribution of those resources than in the United States. Further, in many medical systems, TBIs have a high profile and receive higher priority than strokes, dementias, toxicities, encephalitis, and so forth; care for these other conditions is probably even less adequate.

Therapists may find themselves advocating at a societal level for resources dedicated to treatment. These are choices of personal and of professional ethics. Should treatment be distributed according to the greatest need? According to ability to benefit? According to a mathematical "fairness" formula based on diagnosis (e.g., 10 hours of psychology services for a TBI, 5 hours for stroke)? According to how much the therapist enjoys working with the person or with his or her family? According to potential to return to gainful employment? According to ability to pay? According to race, gender, age, social class, or potential to contribute to society? According to the probability of reducing risks or costs to society? According to whether the person lived a responsible, cautious life prior to her accident or illness? According to whether someone advocates forcefully for the person? Most therapists have probably at least implicitly used most of these criteria at some time in making treatment decisions. If emphasis is to be on meeting needs, then practitioners will need to offer a menu of services with objective information on their risks and their potential benefits. Consumers, perhaps guided by care coordinators, will choose services most likely to meet their needs. As with any system that aims to distribute resources fairly, safeguards are needed to make sure that rehabilitation services adapt to the needs of all who require them, rather than preferentially serving clients of convenience.

Providing formal neuropsychotherapy by highly trained practitioners for all people worldwide who are struggling with neurologically induced emotional and behavioral problems would be very expensive, inefficient, and impractical. Sociologically and strategically, developing formal neuropsychotherapy services is a way to develop and to diffuse information about neurologically based emotional and behavioral problems and about ways to cope with them to other professionals, to paraprofessionals, to support groups, and, ultimately, to the general public. This goal is sufficiently idealistic that it is not likely to put neuropsychotherapists out of work any time soon. It is congruent with the World Health Organization's (1981) appeal that rehabilitation research and development be redirected toward ways of disseminating training and information to people with limited training and to the general public (Peat, 1991; Werner, 1990; Werner & Bower, 1982).

## *HOW IS NEUROPSYCHOTHERAPY DONE?*

This question is what is addressed in the remainder of the book. *Part I. Theory* covers theoretical backgrounds contributing to the development of this field. *Part II. Practice* includes neuropsychological assessment of emotional and behavioral changes, the formulation of treatment plans, and general principles of neuropsychotherapy, including techniques and cognitive compensations applicable to a wide range of neuropsychological problems. *Part III. Specific Problems* focuses on evaluation and treatment of specific emotional reactions, organic emotional changes, executive dysfunctions, and neuropsychotherapeutic considerations of the major categories of cognitive loss. *Part IV. The Social Dimension* deals with neurobehavioral problems in the context of the family and the community. The concluding chapter deals with directions for the future.

# I

# Theory

The theoretical foundations of neuropsychotherapy and of related interventions include knowledge of brain-behavior relationships, the nature of neurological illnesses and recovery, the theory of cognitive rehabilitation, and the theory of psychotherapy. The following chapters present the perspectives within each of these areas most pertinent to neuropsychotherapy and to related interventions. Readers generally familiar with these areas may still want to skim these chapters to become familiar with concepts used extensively in the rest of the book such as the continuum of responsibility, the conceptualization of problems of emotions and behavior following brain illness, a cognitive task analysis of psychotherapy, a natural recovery model of cognitive rehabilitation, and the zone of recovery.

# 2

# Neurology and Neuropsychology

## *TYPE OF ILLNESS*

A working knowledge of the type of illness the client is experiencing is critical to formal neuropsychotherapy and to many related interventions. It is quite important to know typical manifestations, the time course of the disease, medical treatments, how they are likely to be experienced, which symptoms indicate a recurrence or other problem needing further medical attention, what regimens need to be followed, and so on. This knowledge base can be found in neurology textbooks (cf. Brumback, 1993), in neurology texts for non-neurologists (cf. Cohen, 1993; Love, 1992; Wiederholt, 1988), in popular literature (cf. Mace & Rabins, 1991), and in neuropsychological texts regarding specific diseases (cf. Bennett, 1992; Hartman, 1995; Levin, Eisenberg, & Benton, 1989; Parks, Zec, & Wilson, 1993; Rao et al., 1991).

## *TIME COURSE OF ILLNESS: THE CONTINUUM OF RESPONSIBILITY*

Neurological illnesses can generally be divided according to their time course: sudden onset and gradual recovery, gradually progressive course, and intermittent presentation (Figures 2.1, 2.2, and 2.3, developmental disorders are not covered here). A few conditions, (e.g., multiple sclerosis, AIDS dementia, multi-infarct dementia) may be progressive or intermittent. Each time course has a common set of psychological consequences and therapeutic considerations.

The person who is unconscious or disoriented and confused is not responsible for his behavior, but his caregivers are. If and when he has fully recovered, he is fully responsible for his behavior. The process of recovery includes caregivers gradually turning over to the person responsibility for his own behavior along a

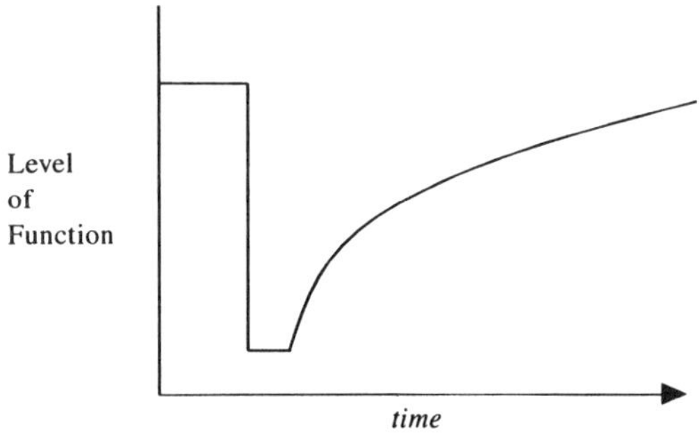


FIGURE 2.1. The typical time course of brain illness with sudden onset and gradual recovery. Examples include TBI, stroke, anoxia, acute infection, and acute toxicity.

continuum of responsibility (Figure 2.4, Sbordone, 1991). Neuropsychotherapy facilitates this process by educating participants about their roles.

Behavior problems in someone with severe organic impairment are dealt with via medication and by externally structuring his environment, with or without his understanding, cooperation, or even consent. By contrast, psychotherapy (Cicerone, 1991, 1992) is often used for problems of behavior and of emotions in mildly impaired people with brain illnesses. It is expected that such people will be able to control their own behavior by gaining insight and learning internal techniques such as systematic relaxation, self-talk, self-instruction, and so forth (Corsini & Wedding, 1995; Hibbard, Gordon, Egelko & Langer, 1987; Meichenbaum, 1993).

Although both behavior management and psychotherapy are valuable in neuropsychotherapy, both developed from work with relatively stable populations. The concept of the *continuum of responsibility* helps make the transition from one to the other understandable. For instance, behavior management may be applied in early stages of recovery from a severe TBI. As successful techniques are discovered, they are explained to the person as they are used, and written in the therapy journal (see chapters 4 and 7). As the person recovers, he is given specific roles in implementing the techniques. Cues from caregivers for

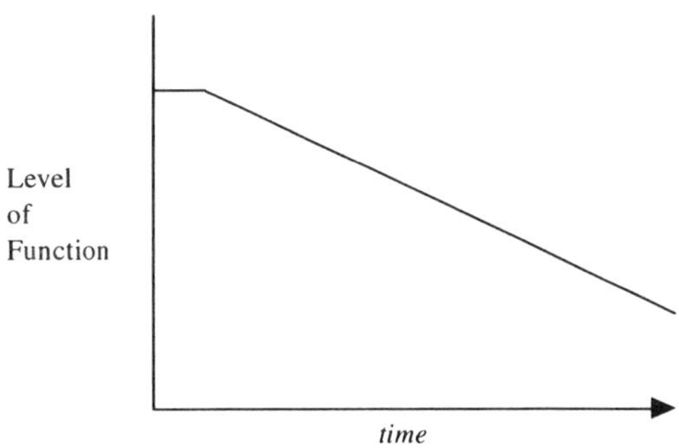


FIGURE 2.2. The typical time course of progressive brain illness. Examples include degenerative condtions such as Alzheimer's disease and Parkinson's disease, malignant brain tumors, and untreated infections.

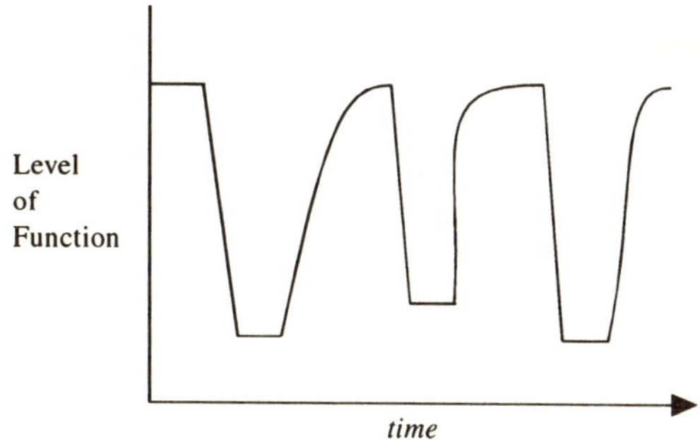


FIGURE 2.3. The typical time course of brain illness with intermittent presentation. Examples include epilepsy, some metabolic disorders, and some forms of multiple sclerosis.

using these techniques are gradually faded in favor of external compensations such as written instructions, avoiding certain situations, asking for help, and so forth. Finally, the therapist helps the person make the transition from external to internal techniques (Cicerone & Giacino, 1992; Meichenbaum, 1993). For transitions in the other direction in progressive illnesses, self-control techniques may be trained early to establish habits that can be directed by caregivers when the progress of the disease prevents independent use.

### *Sudden Brain Illness*

For the person recovering from an acute brain illness such as TBI, stroke, anoxia, toxicity, or infection, neuropsychotherapy passes through a series of stages along the continuum of responsibility (Table 2.1).

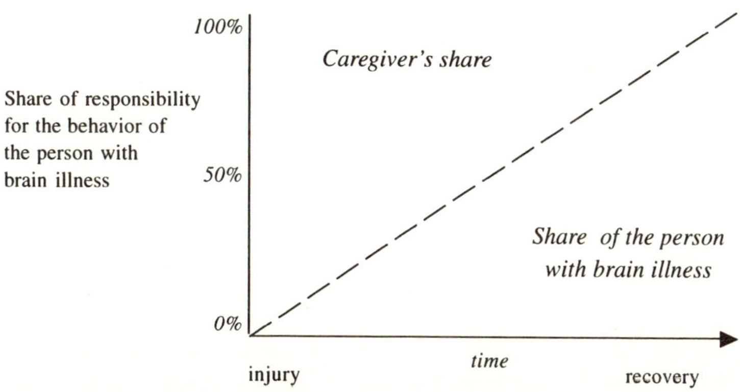


FIGURE 2.4. The continuum of responsibility between caregivers and persons recovering from acute brain illness. In this conceptual figure, the time dimension is an ordinal scale only, not an interval scale; that is, personal responsibility recovers progressively, but not necessarily linearly. For instance, someone might take a week to recover 90% of his or her responsibility for his or her behavior after a TBI, and six months to recover the remaining 10%.

**TABLE 2.1. Progression of Self-Control**

| Rancho level | Responsibilities | | |
|---|---|---|---|
| | Caregiver | Neuropsychotherapist | Person with brain illness |
| I. No response<br>II. Generalized response<br>III. Localized response | Provide for medical well-being, physical needs. Keep stimulation level appropriate. Manage finances in his or in her best interests. | Assess: find reliable communication, observe signs of potential and of problem behaviors. Educate and counsel the family and the staff. Establish trust through calm movements and tone of voice, reassuring touch, respect. | No responsibility. |
| IV. Agitated problems: Assaultiveness, escape, emotional lability | Responsibilities of Stages I–III, Keep surroundings safe (no weapons or dangerous objects, prevent escape). Give reassurance. Tell person frequently where he is and what has happened. Distract or redirect him when agitated. Monitor him continually. Use physical restraints as a last resort when necessary. | Responsibilities of Stages I–III. Behavioral analysis, empathy, and controlling behavior by controlling the environment. | Respond to immediate commands: "Let go of me, it hurts!" He cannot remember the request in the same situation later and cannot be asked now to do something later. |
| V. Confused, inappropriate, not agitated | Keep surroundings safe. Provide for medical well-being and physical needs. Give reassurance. Keep level of stimulation appropriate. Monitor frequently with someone always available. Tell the person frequently where he is and what has happened. Give appropriate directions about immediate situations. Manage finances. | Educate and counsel the person, the family, and the staff. Responsibilities of Stages I–III. Behavioral analysis, empathy, and controlling behavior by controlling the environment. Begin therapeutic alliance. | Follow immediate directions, but no carryover from one minute to the next is expected. He can recognize some behavioral problems and can agree to let caregivers structure the environment to cope with them through cues to rest, leave the situation, speak up, take a deep breath to calm down, and so forth. |
| VI. Confused, appropriate | Keep surroundings safe. Give person some choices as he participates in maintaining medical well-being and | Educate and counsel the person, the family, and the staff. Teach him to structure his own environment, recognize | Follow immediate directions with some carryover. Ask for help when needed. Learn to recognize problems. Respond |

| | | | |
|---|---|---|---|
| | physical needs. Give reassurance. Someone should always be available. Help the person to recognize and maintain an appropriate level of stimulation. Give appropriate directions and cues about immediate situations. Teach about the major problems and the strategies being used. Manage the person's finances with his consultation. | problems like fatigue, escalating anger, poor communication pragmatics, and so forth, respond to these problems when they arise, and compensate for cognitive impairments and personality changes. | appropriately to cues, use cue cards, and use some self-control techniques spontaneously. Participate in self-care and in financial decisions, but without controlling them. |
| VII. Automatic appropriate | Monitor medical well-being, physical needs and finances, overruling decisions when necessary. Someone should usually be available. Teach the person how to cope with difficulties. Cue self-control, fade cues as appropriate. | Educate and counsel the person, the family, the staff, and the community. Train and cue self-control strategies. Fade cues as appropriate. Work on generalizing strategies. Work on ways to tell others about his brain illness and about special understanding or accommodations he needs. | Maintain medical well-being, physical needs, and finances, asking for help when needed. Learn to use strategies and compensation techniques needed to cope with problems. Travel short distances alone in the community when caregivers know where and when. He may begin return to school/work. |
| VIII. Appropriate | Be available for consultation and support when needed. Finish fading cues. | Educate and counsel the person, the family, and the community. Finish fading cues. Fine tune self-control. Work on generalizing strategies. Work on telling others about his brain illness and about special understanding or accommodations he needs. Deal with subtle consequences of illness. | Maintain medical well-being, physical needs, and finances, asking for help when needed. Use strategies and compensation techniques needed to cope with problems. Be able to explain problems to others. Travel independently in the community. Return to school/work. |
| Recovered | No special responsibilities. | Be available for questions, for reflection, for personal reformation, and for coping with resulting life changes. | Maintain his own physical and emotional needs and finances. Travel and work independently. |

*Note*. This table is based on the Rancho los Amigos Cognitive Scale (Hagen, 1982) for people with TBIs. Levels of recovert (or decline) from other brain illnesses may differ.

### *Progressive Brain Illness*

The person with a progressive brain condition such as Alzheimer's, Parkinson's, and Huntington's diseases; malignant brain tumor; and so forth moves in the opposite direction through time along the continuum of responsibility (Figure 2.5). At first he is fully responsible for himself and his behavior; he gradually becomes less responsible as caregivers take over. Neuropsychotherapy techniques are less developed for these populations. The following principles are important:

#### *Grief Work*

Neuropsychotherapy can help the person with a degenerative condition to recognize and to accept that condition to the extent that he is able and willing. This can improve the remaining quality of life by helping the person with a degenerative condition to get closure on some life projects and relationships.

Grief work should be encouraged but not forced. The degenerative process may make the person less aware of his losses and decrease his ability to respond emotionally, leaving him less need to or ability to grieve. Alternately, the illness may make him emotionally labile, making grieving a frightening and unpredictable process as emotions careen out of control.

Grief work with caregivers and with other family members is also critical. They may need to deal with "unfinished business" while the person is still capable. Because losses are gradual, grief is often a gradual and progressive process.

#### *Establishing Preferences in Care*

Sometime within the first few months after the diagnosis of a degenerative neurological condition, it is often desirable to determine what kinds of care the

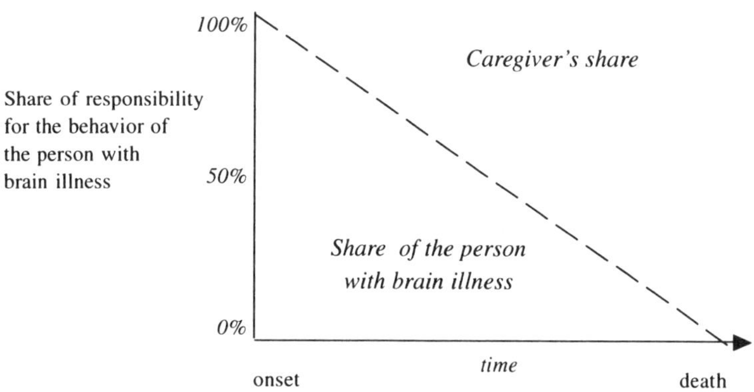


FIGURE 2.5. The continuum of responsibility between caregivers and persons with progressive brain illnesses. As with Figure 2.4, the time dimension is an ordinal scale.

person would like in the future. These decisions may include a living will, a conventional will, choosing where to live, and choosing caregivers. Although he may later change his mind and say so, knowing his preferences can comfort caregivers and family members who will be faced with decisions later for someone who may be unable to comprehend choices or to make or to express a decision. Expressing those desires can also reduce some of his anxiety about the future.

*Establishing Trust and Criteria for Future Withdrawal of Responsibilities and Privileges*

The person with a degenerative brain disease faces the gradual loss of many responsibilities and privileges such as a job, driving, managing finances, managing a household, parenting, and so forth. A professional who establishes a trusting and lasting relationship with him can ease the transition of those losses and family burdens. Discussions that begin with, "How will we know when it is time for you to (retire, have your wife manage the checkbook, stop hunting, stop taking walks alone, etc.)?" should have the answers written down for future reference.

*Establishing Techniques and Habits for Later Use*

Establishing a daily schedule early in the course of a degenerative disease can provide familiarity and security later. It is also the time to teach those involved how to use a predialed telephone, a microwave oven, a phone answering machine, a lifeline medic alert system, a message board, a memory book, and so forth.

*Stabilizing the Environment*

Impairments in new learning make changes in routine very difficult for the person with an advanced degenerative condition. Moving, household repairs, additions, adaptations, getting rid of unneeded possessions, and rearranging and reorganizing things are better done sooner rather than later.

*Establishing a Long-Term Relationship*

The neuropsychotherapeutic relationship with the person with a degenerative condition is ideally long term. There may be fairly intense treatment around the time of diagnosis that then tapers off. Transitions may bring him back to deal with new stresses. The relationship may be maintained through annual visits for limited testing to follow the progress of the disease and to address new practical issues. The trust built with a therapist early in the course of the disease may prove useful later when it may no longer be possible to establish such trust in a new relationship with a different therapist.

### *Care for the Caregiver*

The primary caregiver for the person with a degenerative disease, often an elderly spouse, is frequently under an enormous burden of 24-hour care without relief (Vitaliano, Maiuro, Ochs, & Russo, 1989). The physical and emotional strain is often overwhelming. Risks for illness, social isolation, anxiety, and depression are high. This issue should be addressed early and often. Adequate and consistent respite care and relief for the caregiver should be arranged to prevent caregiver burnout before rather than after disaster strikes. Support via support groups or via other arrangements is also important.

### *Respond to the Person's Emotional Reality*

People with degenerative dementias such as Alzheimer's disease frequently irretrievably lose their grasp on objective reality in the later stages of their dementia. Attempts to orient such individuals to objective reality are rarely successful and frequently result in conflict and distress. A more successful approach is to respond to their emotional reality, even when this means failing to correct or even affirming their incorrect beliefs and delusions (Feil, 1993; Jones, 1996). For example, when the elderly demented person asks emotionally, "When is my mother coming to take me home?" the caregiver can answer the emotional need with, "I'll take care of you," rather than trying to orient the person to reality with, "Your mother died many years ago. You live here in the Happy Days Nursing Home now."

## *Intermittent Brain Dysfunction*

Intermittent brain dysfunction can result from epilepsy, multiple sclerosis, migraine, some metabolic disorders such as diabetes, hypoglycemia, and severe premenstrual syndrome, some toxicities (including alcohol, drugs, and medication side effects), transient ischemic attacks, and so forth. It is more difficult to generalize about the continuum of responsibility with intermittent disorders (Figure 2.6) because much depends on the specific nature of the illness.

### *Responsibility for Avoiding Dysfunction*

The neuropsychotherapist may take the role of a health psychologist (Bishop, 1994; Brannon & Feist, 1992; Carroll, 1992), health educator, or substance abuse counselor, helping an individual establish systems and learn to take the steps necessary to prevent episodes of intermittent brain dysfunction. This may involve setting up a medication schedule or counseling to help him and/or his family to accept the reality of the illness or the chronic condition. It may involve teaching one to recognize the warning signs of an impending episode through an activity journal and to avoid high-risk situations or triggers and to abort impending episodes.

### *Responsibility for Dealing with Dysfunction*

A neuropsychotherapist may help someone with intermittent brain dysfunction to understand his condition and to take prudent precautions to minimize damage from the dysfunction. This may range from helping someone with uncontrollable epilepsy to give up driving, to encouraging the use of medic alert bracelets, or to educating people about responsible use of alcohol.

### *Accepting Lack of Responsibility*

Some people with some forms of intermittent brain dysfunction or their families may feel that the person can have greater control over the occurrence of episodes or of his behavior during episodes than is actually the case. There may be feelings of guilt or blame regarding things said during a hypoglycemic delirium or when recovering from anesthesia, or of shame regarding seizures witnessed by others. The therapist can help people to clarify such feelings of responsibility, guilt, and blame and find ways to deal with others regarding them.

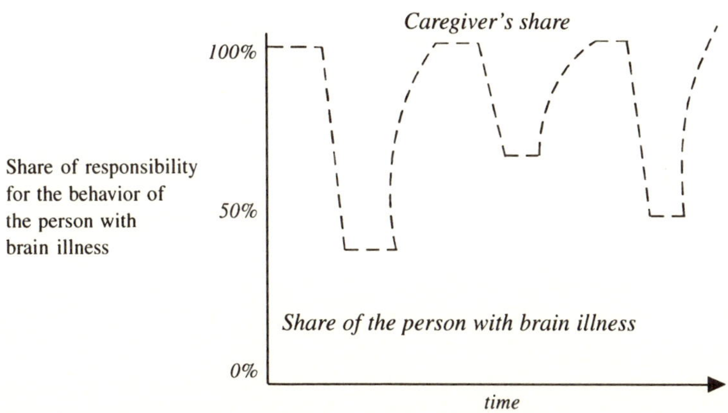


FIGURE 2.6. The continuum of responsibility between caregivers and persons with intermittent brain dysfunction. As with Figure 2.4, the time dimension is an ordinal scale. Because intermittent brain dysfunction is variable depending on the type of episode, this figure illustrates only a few representative types.

*Avoiding Scapegoating*

On the other hand, some people may inappropriately seek to avoid responsibility for their behavior by blaming intermittent brain dysfunction. "I couldn't help it, I was drunk," is one crude example. The use of hypoglycemia and premenstrual syndrome as defenses in murder trials is controversial. The therapist may need to confront inappropriate attempts to avoid responsibility on such a basis. Detailed knowledge of the specific disorder and of the circumstances is critical to such confrontations.

*Conversion Disorders, Factitious Disorders, and Malingering*

A minority of people with intermittent brain dysfunction also display episodes of pseudodysfunction resembling their actual episodes. Pseudoseizures, pseudodelirium, pseudoheadache, and so forth may be consciously faked to take on a sick role (factitious disorder) or other secondary gain (malingering), or may arise unconsciously (conversion disorder). Except for obvious malingering, these are issues for the skilled psychotherapist.

*Telling Others*

The person who experiences intermittent brain dysfunction may struggle with decisions about what to tell others. Important tools in this process are accurate information about the disorder and episodes, systematic reviews of episodes and risks, feedback from witnesses, and the experiences of others with the disorder.

## *FACTORS OF PERSONALITY AND EMOTIONS FOLLOWING BRAIN ILLNESS*

Catalogs or lists of personality changes resulting from brain illness (e.g., Pepping & Roueche, 1991; Prigatano, 1992; Sohlberg & Mateer, 1989; Williams & Long, 1987; Ylvisaker & Gobble, 1987) can give the impression that these changes are haphazard and chaotic. Although a unified and accepted theory of personality changes following brain illness is not yet available (Borod, 1992), nevertheless, some changes can be related to each other in a conceptualization that has more coherence and clinical utility than simple lists. The organizational scheme used in this book is described here generally, whereas the entire organization is presented in Appendix A. The specific problems are described in more detail in Chapters 9 through 12 or at the end of Appendix A.

There are three components of the personality of the person with a brain illness (Figure 1.3): the psychological factors of pre-illness personality and reactions to illness and the neuropsychological factor of direct, organic changes.

## *Psychological Factors*

Psychological factors influencing the personality, emotions, and behavior of the person with a brain illness can be understood from the psychology of people with intact brains.

### *Pre-Brain Illness Personality*

Because anyone can have a brain illness, the neuropsychotherapist must be familiar with the full range of human personalities. A common effect of brain illness is that the affected individuals become conservative in their coping strategies, resorting to primitive, tried-and-true defenses. Family members may report that the person has always been that way, even when his behavior is unusual for him. The person who copes regressively is, indeed, just like he always was, only more so. He becomes a caricature of himself.

The neuropsychotherapist is interested not only in pre-illness psychopathology, but also in normal variations in personality relevant to post-illness personality and rehabilitation. These may include coping style; family dynamics; religious faith; beliefs regarding brain illness, healing, disability, and causes of illness; and sources of self-esteem.

### *Psychological Reactions to Injury or to Illness*

Most brain illnesses are emotionally significant events that trigger reactions. Typical psychological reactions are well known from similar human experiences without brain injury (R. F. Antonak, Livneh, & Antonak, 1993), but in people with brain illnesses they are colored by changes in the ability to process emotions and information. Family members also typically have significant psychological reactions to the illness and to surrounding events.

## *Neurological and Neuropsychological Factors*

Neuropsychological or organic factors are those changes that result directly from brain lesions that change the functioning of the brain. These transformations in personality, in emotions, and in behavior are distinctive with brain illness and are often unlike phenomena in people with intact brains.

### *Emotional Changes*

Changes in emotions can be thought of as decreases or increases in various types of emotional communication (expression and comprehension of emotions) and of emotional reactivity (experienced emotions, Table 2.2). They are the focus of emotional rehabilitation.

**TABLE 2.2. Organic Disturbances of Emotional Functions**

| Function | Decreased | Increased |
|---|---|---|
| Communication | Monotone voice | Reflex crying |
| | Inexpressive face | Reflex laughing |
| | Impaired comprehension | Automatic cursing |
| Reactions | Diminished reactions | Impulsive anger |
| | Indifference | Catastrophic reactions |
| | | Lability |

*Changes in Emotional Communication.* Brain illness can produce dissociations between internal emotional experiences and outward manifestations of those experiences. The person may lose the ability to express emotions through tone of voice, words, or body language, or exaggerated emotional expressions may be produced.

*Changes in Emotional Reactivity.* Brain illness can produce modulations in the magnitude of emotional responses. These changes can affect all forms of emotional response equally, or can affect some more or less than others.

### *Executive Function Impairments*

The executive functions are the processes of self-regulation and of organization. Neuroanatomically, conceptually, and experientially, the executive functions stand at the interface of cognition and personality and are therefore categorized separately. Executive dysfunctions include disorders of activation (Table 2.3) and impaired awareness of deficits (anosognosia), of reasoning, of planning, of judgment, and of communication pragmatics.

### *Cognitively Mediated Changes of Personality*

The cognitive impairments resulting from brain illness are copiously documented in neuropsychology textbooks (Ardila & Rosselli, 1992; Hecaen & Albert, 1978; Heilman & Valenstein, 1985; Kolb & Wishaw, 1985; Luria, 1973; Walsh, 1978). Neuropsychotherapists need a thorough grounding in these impairments

**TABLE 2.3. Disturbances of Activation**

| Function | Decreased | Increased |
|---|---|---|
| Initiation | Abulia | Impulsivity, disinhibition |
| Termination | Perseveration | Impersistence |

based both in academic knowledge and in clinical experience. Some cognitive impairments create false impressions of changes in motivation or in personality. Some cognitive deficits can also be thought of as true changes in personality.

### *Medical Problems*

There are a number of medical problems that frequently accompany brain illnesses and injuries. The major principles for treating these disorders, however, are more properly part of behavioral medicine, and will not be dealt with in detail.

### *Interactions*

With so many different factors influencing personality following brain illness, the possibilities for combinations and interactions of features are enormous. It cannot be presumed that the various components of personality in an individual with a brain illness can be observed and measured independently, nor that their effects will simply be additive. Nor is it fully known just how such factors interact. Complex interactions are commonplace, as in the case of Maria at the beginning of Chapter 1. Evaluating such interactions accurately is a daunting challenge to experienced clinicians and to test developers.

# 3

# Education and Psychotherapy

## *EDUCATION*

Most clients' and families' previous experience with brain illness is not specifically relevant to the situation that brings them to therapy. Consequently, neuropsychotherapy almost always involves explicit and extensive teaching about the brain illness. Effective education is appropriate, accessible, and acceptable.

### *Appropriate*

Appropriate education is pertinent and relevant; it addresses the needs of the recipient. Although it is usually best for the learners to state their needs or questions first, the therapist often needs to teach information that the learners do not know they need to know. This can often be worked into answers to other questions. Approaching education with a rigid agenda risks the attention, learning, and trust of the learners. More than 5 minutes spent on neuroanatomy or on the normative base of testing suggests that either the therapist is off target or the real issues are being avoided.

### *Accessible*

Effective education is accessible to the learner: it should be offered in language she can understand, related to her experience, paced appropriately for her to understand, and active or interactive. Everyday words are preferable to technical terms (see the glossary). Easily understood metaphors, though not always strictly accurate, may approximate reality closely enough to be useful.

*Acceptable*

In many jurisdictions, the client has a legal right to know the results of her assessment (except when it would harm her). Nevertheless, news about brain damage in oneself or in one's loved one is usually emotionally difficult to receive and must be communicated sensitively. This lays the foundation of trust for future therapy. Evaluation and feedback are often therapeutic in themselves (Christensen, 1989).

Education is not a single event in therapy or in rehabilitation but is an ongoing process. This is because of the following:

1. Adjusting to and accepting the information requires time. Some information requires grieving, some requires real-life confirmation, and some requires adjusting cognitive frameworks or assumptions to be ready for other information (Case 3.1. Raj).
2. Some of the information is not known at the time of assessment, particularly in acute rehabilitation where the amount of recovery is not predictable with certainty (Case 3.2. Marcel).
3. Recovery (or degeneration) takes place over time. Education should be mostly geared toward the current and proximate stages.
4. There is usually too much information to learn in one session.
5. Impairments in memory and generalization slow learning.

The pacing of education can be critical. The therapist must be sensitive to how information is being received to know how much to say and how to balance priorities.

Sometimes education is the only intervention possible or necessary. Many people affected by brain illnesses are otherwise mentally healthy and resilient

*The School of Hard Knocks. Case 3.1. Raj.* Raj was a 32 year old finishing college engineering student when he experienced a mild TBI from a motor vehicle accident. He failed his final exams and took a leave of absence. He then opened a restaurant with considerable help from his wife. This enterprise failed, straining the marriage, with each partner blaming the other. Eighteen months after his accident, he was referred by a neurologist for neuropsychological assessment that revealed moderate impairments in attention, in memory, and in executive functions, as well as revealing impulsive anger. At the feedback session, Raj was very reluctant to accept this news, preferring to continue to blame his wife. He left the session before receiving recommendations, barely containing his anger. Before he left he was told that he would be welcome back at any time. The feedback session continued with his wife. The neuropsychological report was mailed to him, along with pamphlets on TBI, on cognitive changes, and on impulsive anger. Two months later he returned and began neuropsychotherapy and rehabilitation.

> *Whose Denial? Whose Reality? Case 3.2. Marcel.* Marcel was a 75-year-old man whose case was discussed at the inpatient rehabilitation team conference 1 week after a stroke had left him globally aphasic and severely apraxic. The team noted that his wife was "in denial," thinking that her husband understood most of what was said to him, and planning on his return to home and to driving, gardening, managing finances, and so forth. The team concluded that she would need "lots of education" to overcome her denial and to prepare for a difficult discharge. Within a week Marcel's condition had cleared into a mild aphasia and apraxia. The aggressive education that might have strained relationships with the rehabilitation team became unnecessary, as reality approximated his wife's view of the situation.

and have stable social support. Given adequate information they can work out their own adjustments. Others with financial or with other barriers must make do with limited professional services.

## *FAMILY INVOLVEMENT*

When the person with a brain illness is not fully responsible for her behavior, a family member usually takes up the slack. Even when the person regains personal responsibility, cognitive and emotional changes may unbalance family dynamics and family members need guidance; few people have models for coping with these changes. Neuropsychotherapists typically work with the focus person and with family members separately and together. Family members have several roles in therapy (Table 3.1).

Until and unless contrary evidence emerges, the therapist should assume that the family is healthy and functional but is coping with a tragedy. Emotional distress in a family is to be expected following the brain illness of a member; it does not necessarily reflect a dysfunctional family or a longstanding psychopathology. This is a different frame of reference than is typical for psychotherapists who are accustomed to searching for hidden psychopathology, often with good reason.

## *APPROACHES TO PSYCHOTHERAPY*

Appropriate psychotherapy techniques are chosen based on target problems, on therapists' abilities and preferences, and on clients' preferences and cognitive limitations. Neuropsychotherapy is compatible with many psychotherapies, but some approaches are not fruitful with certain conditions due to

**TABLE 3.1. Possible Roles of Family Members in Neuropsychotherapy Processes**

1. Informants about the behavior of the person with a brain illness in other settings.
2. Informants about the nature of the person's environment.
3. Informants about her personality prior to the illness.
4. Collaborators in treatment and/or as special members of rehabilitation team.
5. Recipients of education about the brain illness and its consequences, prognosis, and treatment.
6. Recipients of supportive counseling.
7. Participants in family or couples therapy.
8. Participants in support groups or in therapy groups for family members or in mixed groups with families and people with brain illness.

cognitive limitations. Client-centered therapy and free association are likely to go slowly for someone with impaired initiation and may run astray with someone who is disinhibited and disorganized. Concrete thinking may make psychoanalytic interpretations inaccessible. Visual imagery techniques are a poor choice when that capacity is impaired. Language-based approaches may be frustrating and confusing for aphasics.

A cognitive task analysis of expectations for the client can help determine if a technique is appropriate. Impaired abilities can sometimes be circumvented by compensations. For example, in Table 3.2, someone without adequate executive function and memory to carry out Parts 1 and 3 independently may still benefit from a limited and guided application of the reframing technique, provided she has some other motivation to use it. For instance, if she has a small repertoire of obsessive negative thoughts, with written notes and drilling she may memorize a few concrete reframings. However, the person with insufficient self-monitoring to learn to recognize her negative thoughts is unlikely to benefit from this technique.

### *Behavior Modification*

Classical behavior modification approaches, derived from the principles of classical and of operant conditioning, have considerable value in long-term be-

**TABLE 3.2. Cognitive Task Analysis of Client's Role in Reframing Negative Thoughts (Cognitive–Behavioral Therapy for Depression)**

1. Recognize that she is depressed (or that she has a problem)
2. Recognize her negative thoughts.
3. Understand the connection between her negative thoughts and depression.
4. Learn a schema for reframing negative thoughts.
5. Generalize the schema to a variety of negative thoughts.
6. Remember to apply the schema when she notices negative thoughts.
7. Write down this process and/or remember that she has applied it to evaluate it in future sessions.

havior management within controlled settings (Burke & Wesolowski, 1988; Eames, Haffey, & Cope, 1990; Howard, 1988; Jacobs, 1993), particularly for people with little ability to be responsible for their own behavior.

There are a number of challenges, risks, and limitations to implementing classical behavior modification programs with individuals with brain illnesses:

1. These approaches are conceptualized as externally imposed on a person, and in practice they often stay that way. This perspective requires vigilance to make sure that the program results in better self-control and more independence for the person with the brain illness.
2. In practice, such approaches tend to exclude other approaches that may also be of critical value.
3. There is often difficulty with generalization from the training situation to everyday life.
4. Behavior modification programs often require large investments of time, training, and resources in structuring a controlled environment that may outweigh the benefits.
5. Behavior modification programs often require a stability of institution and of a culture that allows for their implementation. Not all treatment settings, families, schools, and cultures are conducive to such programs.
6. Classical behavior modification programs are typically framed in a language many find alienating or confusing.
7. Classical behavior modification programs are based on research on learning in individuals with intact brains. Such results are not uniformly generalizable to damaged brains. For example, conditioning protocols are not useful in people in a confusional state (Eames, Haffey, & Cope, 1990).

### *Cognitive Behavior Modification*

Cognitive behavior modification contrasts with classical behavior modification in that its primary focus is on training people to regulate their own behavior, and it recognizes cognitive processes and emotional states as intervening variables (Meichenbaum, 1993). Cognitive behavior modification is less subject to the challenges, risks, and limitations listed previously for classical behavior modification, except for the last item.

The problem-oriented approach to neuropsychotherapy presented here is similar to behavioral and cognitive-behavioral therapy. Common goals are managing, compensating for, accepting, or overcoming specific problem feelings or behaviors.

### *Psychoanalytic Neuropsychotherapy*

Psychoanalytic neuropsychotherapy (Block, 1987; Ellis, 1989; Klonoff & Lage, 1991; Leaf, 1991; Lewis & Rosenberg, 1990; Miller, 1993; Prigatano,

1991; Small, 1980) is most appropriate for those with less severe illnesses, and for those who, prior to their illnesses, would have been receptive to psychoanalysis. A danger of psychoanalytic approaches is that, in seeking dynamic explanations of behaviors and feelings, organic determinants of the magnitude of those behaviors and feelings may be neglected. For example, Klonoff and Lage gave an astute analysis of narcissistic rage in two young men with traumatic brain injuries. However, they do not discuss the likely contributions of organic disinhibition to the magnitude of the rage, and their account suggests that several years of psychoanalytic psychotherapy neither gave these young men insight nor curbed the behavior.

Psychoanalytic approaches are complementary to problem-oriented neuropsychotherapy, although possibly less applicable to the full range of persons with brain illnesses.

## *NEUROPSYCHOTHERAPY–PSYCHOTHERAPY BALANCE*

The balance between neuropsychotherapy and psychotherapy is a function of the severity of the brain impairments and the prominence of brain illness

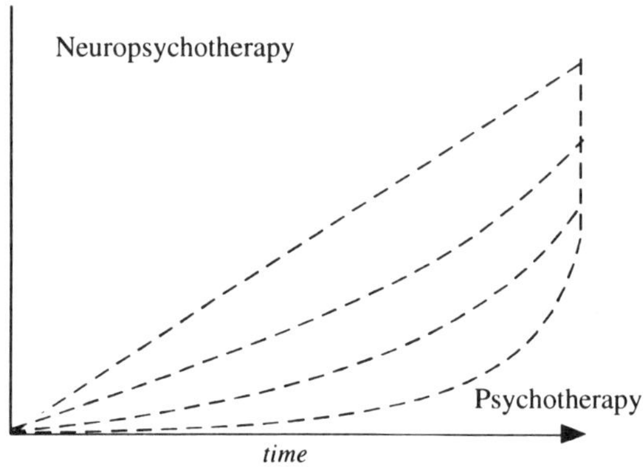


FIGURE 3.1. The balance between neuropsychotherapy and conventional psychotherapy in acute brain illness. In an individual with significant pre-illness psychological problems and/or adjustment difficulties from the brain illness, the balance between techniques and approaches that are specifically neuropsychotherapeutic and those that come from conventional psychotherapy is likely to follow the curve of the continuum of responsibility (straight line). At the outset, the focus will be on neuropsychological problems; with recovery, personality issues will become more prominent. For the person without significant pre-illness psychological problems or adjustment difficulties from the brain illness, the balance between techniques and approaches that are specifically neuropsychotherapeutic and those that come from conventional psychotherapy is likely to follow the rightmost line; that is, neuropsychotherapy will predominate throughout the course of recovery.

issues, psychological reactions, and pre-illness issues (Figure 3.1). This balance usually changes over time. For example, therapy early in recovery from a severe brain injury is almost purely neuropsychotherapy both in content or goals (behavioral/emotional rehabilitation) and in technique (cognitive compensations). As the person recovers and organic problems come under control, psychological reactions to illness, to discapacity, or to both may emerge and traditional psychotherapy may become more prominent. Someone with a mild brain injury may need few cognitive compensations in therapy, but may require considerable focus on emotional rehabilitation. Someone with a brainstem injury with major motor losses but with preserved cognitive abilities may need neither cognitive compensations nor emotional rehabilitation, but may benefit from conventional psychotherapy for coping with major losses. Someone with pure amnesia may need extensive notes to benefit from conventional psychotherapy for pre-illness problems. In someone with no psychopathology prior to her illness, there will be more focus on neuropsychotherapy techniques because coping with the brain illness will be virtually the only issue at hand. For the person who has had significant previous psychopathology, conventional psychotherapy may be needed sooner and may require more emphasis.

In an alternative analysis, Ben-Yishay and Lakin (1989) noted that many people with brain illnesses have lost the abstract attitude and some cognitive capacities necessary to maintain ego functions and to participate in psychotherapy. Those with sufficiently preserved ego functions are considered candidates for conventional, insight-oriented psychotherapy seeking to change behavior and lifestyle by changing attitudes. In neuropsychotherapy, the person is trained in changes in behaviors that later become internalized into changes in attitude, partly through witnessing the success of the behavior changes, and partly through exhortations of the therapist and of the therapy group.

## *CONCLUSIONS*

Many theoretical approaches to psychotherapy are compatible with neuropsychotherapy. What must come first, however, is a clear understanding of the nature of the person's problems and changes. In particular, organic changes in behavior and in feelings must be understood to be addressed appropriately. Cognitive impairments limit the ability to participate in therapy and the ability to change. Only when these factors are well understood can appropriate approaches be chosen for the individual.

# 4

# Cognitive Rehabilitation

Whereas disorders of emotion, of self-image, and of mood often affect the ability to think clearly, impaired thinking abilities may affect social skills, self-image, mood, and the reactions of others. The treatments of these changes or impairments through cognitive rehabilitation and through neuropsychotherapy also share many techniques and theory.

Four general theoretical approaches to cognitive rehabilitation are discussed, along with their relationships to neuropsychotherapy: the general stimulation approach, the functional approach, the process-specific approach (Sohlberg & Mateer, 1989), and the natural recovery approach (Judd, 1996).

## *THE GENERAL STIMULATION APPROACH*

This approach is often born from an enthusiasm for treating cognitive problems, along with limited treatment materials, ideas, theoretical analysis, and possibly assessment capacities. The feckless beginning cognitive therapist, believing that cognitive stimulation is good for a wide variety of cognitive problems, may attempt to tackle these problems using a small collection of general treatment tasks. Research on this approach is limited, but it is likely that such an approach has at least a significant placebo effect. For example, in the normal elderly, even a limited general stimulation approach is surprisingly effective in improving cognitive skills, especially for those in intellectually understimulating environments (Jutagir, 1992). However, when dealing with brain illness, this approach lacks the individual specificity and structure that leading practitioners of cognitive rehabilitation believe is necessary to optimize cognitive recovery.

The parallel of this approach in neuropsychotherapy would be the principle that some social stimulation is better than none. This is likely usually true, but it is rarely an adequate approach for resolving complex emotional and behavioral problems of significant brain illnesses.

## *THE FUNCTIONAL APPROACH*

Often a cognitive perspective is added to an already existing, functionally oriented physical rehabilitation program. This often results in a cognitive program oriented around functional goals, such as grooming, transportation, cooking, money management, and employment. Such programs may use a cognitive analysis of functional activities to generate strategies for overcoming cognitive difficulties that prevent those activities. For example, a person with a brain illness may have difficulty cooking. Neuropsychological testing and task analysis may determine that his main cognitive problem is attentional, and that he is distracted when trying to cook. He is then trained to minimize distractions in his kitchen and is given explicit written directions to follow to help him stay focused.

This approach has much to recommend it. It is congruent with the structure of many existing physical rehabilitation programs. It is individually adapted and focused on concrete goals of obvious value to the person, the family, and the payor. Its limitation is that skills retrained or compensated for in one context often do not easily generalize to other contexts (Lloyd & Cuvo, 1994; Raskin & Gordon, 1992; Sohlberg & Mateer, 1989; Webb, 1991). For instance, the person trained to cook in this manner may have difficulty generalizing these skills to another kitchen or menu or to other contexts needing attention abilities.

The functional approach is relevant to neuropsychotherapy in its individual adaptation and in its focus on concrete goals. However, neuropsychotherapy includes intrapsychic goals such as self-acceptance and is not exclusively focused on improving function.

## *THE PROCESS-SPECIFIC APPROACH*

The process-specific approach to cognitive rehabilitation (Sohlberg & Mateer, 1989) is founded in cognitive theory, which identifies specific cognitive processes disturbed by brain illnesses. These main processes are attention, memory, language, visual-spatial skills, motor programming, reasoning, and executive functions. Each area is sometimes further fractionated by specific brain lesions (cf. Lezak, 1995; Sohlberg & Mateer; Squire, 1987), and treatment can be highly focused on specific deficits (Riddoch & Humphreys, 1994). Because these processes are fundamental to a variety of activities, they are then treated in an individualized and prioritized manner. Clinical cognitive gains are applied to functional areas through generalization training. This approach depends on an accurate, theory-based assessment of cognitive processes to determine the configuration of deficits. Each cognitive impairment is approached through therapeutic strategies of compensation, adaptation, and/or restoration.

### *Compensation*

*Compensation* involves finding a way around a problem or a solution coming from outside the person to do cognitive jobs he cannot do. *Attention compensations* include reducing noise and clutter and avoiding crowds. *Memory compensations* include daily planners, "things to do" lists, and memory logs, where the paper remembers what the person cannot; alarms; and electronic personal organizers. *Organization compensations* include written agendas and instructions, labeled filing systems, and routines.

When applying compensation techniques, the therapist takes responsibility for the success of the system (Sohlberg & Mateer, 1989; Wilson, 1997). This means that the therapist chooses a system appropriate to the needs, abilities, and disabilities of the person; trains him (and family members when appropriate) in its proper use; and checks for generalization and maintenance of use.

Neuropsychotherapy uses these compensation techniques in emotional and in interpersonal realms, for example, with a therapy journal and cue cards (see Chapter 7).

### *Adaptation*

*Adaptation* involves using preserved cognitive abilities to carry out activities usually done using cognitive processes that are now disturbed. *Circumlocutions* are the adaptation of using preserved descriptive abilities to substitute for impaired word-finding abilities (e.g., saying "that long yellow fruit" when unable to think of "banana"). *Verbal self-cuing* is used to adapt to self-regulation deficits. For example, someone with difficulty sequencing movements might say, "left, right, cane, left, right, cane" with each movement while learning to walk with a cane.

Adaptation is used in neuropsychotherapy, with executive functions, interpersonal skills, and cognitive-behavioral psychotherapy techniques (Meichenbaum, 1993). Previously automatic processes often need to be relearned through explicit, conscious instruction and through self-instruction. For example, listening skills are retrained through instruction in active listening techniques. Looking at the ceiling is used to control reflex crying. Deep breathing and affirmative self-talk are used to cope with frustration.

### *Restoration*

*Restoration* is the direct regaining of disturbed abilities through practice and relearning. Cognitive rehabilitation uses logical, theory-based sequences of retraining procedures. These allow partial or full recovery of disrupted abilities when natural recovery processes and the existing environment have not or will not facilitate that recovery. For example, attention is retrained through a series of graded exercises for focused, sustained, selective, alternating, and divided attention (Sohlberg & Mateer, 1989). The appropriate level for working is identified through pretesting. The person begins with tasks that are mildly to moderately impaired, working at that level repetitively over several sessions until there is substantial improvement before moving on to the next tasks.

Much of neuropsychotherapy aims to restore pre-illness abilities, including self-regulation of behavior, social communication, and emotional reactivity and communication. Training for restoration can pass through stages of compensation and of adaptation. For instance, an individual with acquired difficulty speaking in public might initially read from a script prepared by the therapist (compensation). He might later learn to prepare the script (adaptation). Script use might gradually be faded to an outline, to a rehearsal spoken aloud, to an internal rehearsal, and finally to spontaneous speech, or restored ability.

The following general principles also apply to the process-specific approach: repetition, hierarchy of tasks, using preserved procedural learning, training generalization, using generalization probes, and knowledge of results.

### *Repetition*

Restoration of function is not the teaching of information, it is the retraining of cognitive skills. Repetition across time is necessary to establish and to maintain the skills as habits.

Repetition is also important in learning new skills and information in neuropsychotherapy. It must become a habit of communication style for the neuropsychotherapist (see Chapter 6).

### *Hierarchy of Tasks*

Training uses tasks of graded difficulty of target performances (for instance, speed and number of errors) and of task complexity. This hierarchy may be empirical (based on what the person finds most difficult), or it may come from cognitive theory. Hierarchization of tasks in neuropsychotherapy applies to both cognitive and to emotional difficulty of activities.

### *Using Preserved Procedural Learning*

In anterograde amnesia (impaired explicit learning of new information), procedural learning is often well preserved (Squire, 1987). *Procedural learning* is learning how to do something or how to carry out a procedure or a sequence of activities. This includes motor skills, such as learning mirror writing (Milner,

1962; Starr & Phillips, 1970), solving puzzles, carrying out mathematical procedures (Wood, Ebert, & Kinsbourne, 1982), mirror reading (Cohen & Squire, 1980), and learning how to sing or play particular pieces of music (Judd, 1988; Starr & Phillips). In some individuals, this learning is implicit. They have no conscious memory of the training, yet they retain improved task performance. This phenomenon is exploited in cognitive rehabilitation of memory impairments. Procedural learning is used to train routines and approaches to functional problems so the compensation (e.g., memory book use) becomes a habit (Baddeley, 1992; Sohlberg & Mateer, 1989).

In neuropsychotherapy, procedural learning is used particularly in training routines for coping with increased emotional reactivity and in training communication skills.

### *Training Generalization*

People with brain illnesses often have difficulty generalizing skills or solutions from one circumstance to another. For this reason, retraining skills involves a variety of activities involving those skills both in the clinic and in real life (Burke, Danick, Bemis, & Durgin, 1994; Lennox & Brune, 1993; Sohlberg & Mateer, 1989; Wilson, 1992).

Training generalization is critical in neuropsychotherapy. Communication skills learned in the clinic need to be tried out and refined in real-life. Retraining emotional control often needs to occur in real life situations when the problems do not come up often and cannot easily be simulated in the clinic.

### *Use of Generalization Probes*

The neuropsychological tests used to evaluate a function are different from the tasks used to train that function to be certain that the function has improved, as opposed to an ability on a single testlike task. For example, attention abilities might be trained using a visual vigilance computer program, and might be probed for generalization using a mental calculations test. Functional generalization probes are also used to see whether results from the clinic carry over to real life. This might be done through teachers' or family's ratings or through performance measures such as time spent on homework or work productivity.

Generalization probes in neuropsychotherapy include the following: case conferences, clinic notes, or rating scales indicating that skills learned in neuropsychotherapy have generalized to elsewhere in a rehabilitation program; self-ratings of mood states or of the number of episodic problems reported in a diary; interviews with family, friends, teachers, employers, and so forth; and functional achievements, such as productivity on frustrating tasks or making it through stressful social situations.

### *Knowledge of Results*

In restoration training, the therapist needs to know if work should continue, stop, or change, and the person needs to track his progress. This is done through progress records at three levels: the training tasks themselves, neuropsychological generalization probes, and functional generalization probes.

In neuropsychotherapy, keeping formal records of results at three levels is not always possible or necessary. Neuropsychotherapy emphasizes generalization of skills to functional settings, and work and record-keeping often begins at that level (Jacobs, 1993). For example, therapy may focus on angry outbursts that occur at home but not in the therapist's office.

Neuropsychotherapy record-keeping includes tracking subjective mood states. The person identifies one or more problematic moods and rates their intensity, often on a scale of 1 to 5. Ratings are not directly observable or confirmable by the therapist and are subject to many biases. Still, discussions of self-perceived mood allow the person to express feelings that he may believe are not being appreciated and force more careful self-observation and self-monitoring. This process reduces problem feelings in therapy clients with intact brains, and likely has the same effect for many people with brain illnesses (Meichenbaum, 1993).

## *THE NATURAL RECOVERY APPROACH*

The natural recovery approach to cognitive rehabilitation, like the functional and process-specific approaches, focuses on functional outcomes as the final goal. Like the process-specific approach, it emphasizes a cognitive and a neuropsychological analysis and identification of problems. Unlike that approach, it emphasizes working on those problems in natural contexts as early and as much as possible. In addition to principles described previously, the natural recovery approach uses the concepts of the zone of recovery and task analysis.

### *The Zone of Recovery*

In his social-interaction approach to child cognitive development, Vygotsky (1978) argued that children develop cognitive abilities not only by brain growth and maturation, and not only by learning to solve problems in their environment, but also by learning from other people. He studied interactions in which children learned and from this experience developed the concept of the zone of proximal development (ZPD). This zone is the level of difficulty of an activity just a little harder than the child can manage independently; the kind of task he can accomplish with a little help. It is in this zone, Vygotsky maintained, that the most learning takes place. The ZPD has been adapted to neurorehabilitation (Cicerone & Tupper, 1990) and is presented here as *the zone of recovery.*

If an activity is too easy, the person recovering from a brain illness may become bored by it and may even become resentful of being given a child's task (Table 4.1). The activity may not contribute much to recovery. If an activity is too hard he may become frustrated, angry, and discouraged. An activity facilitates recovery if the person is challenged and can do it with some help (physical help, directions, cues, or other cognitive strategies; Case 4.1. Elizabeth).

Encountering the zone of recovery is, in some respects, an art. Some people are very good at it, such as many parents and teachers; others are not. The rehabilitation professional can help people develop this skill by teaching them how to break down a task into components, how to find which components to attempt, and how, when, and how much to help. The rehabilitation professional can also help introduce specific cognitive techniques adapted to the person, the task, and the circumstances.

The zone of recovery is a moving target. The helper needs to reduce the level of help, of cues, and of supervision and increase the difficulty of the activity to keep pace with recovery. For example, someone progressively recovering social skills and tolerance might follow this sequence: receive one visitor at home; receive several visitors; visit one family member in their familiar home; go to small family gatherings; shop in a small, uncrowded store; go to a movie; go to a small public gathering; go to a small party; go to a shopping mall; go to a large public gathering. Such a sequence might also be extended by reducing the amount of supervision given.

In neuropsychotherapy the zone of recovery fits with the continuum of responsibility (see Chapter 2). In some contexts the concept strongly resembles the hierarchy of fear-provoking stimuli used in phobia desensitization, in which the person faces progressively challenging, fear-provoking situations while maintaining calm. A similar model can be used for relearning frustration tolerance, embarrassment control, assertiveness, and so forth. For example, someone embarrassed about word-finding difficulties might construct a hierarchy of potential embarrassment, from conversing casually with family through giving directions to a stranger, to public speaking. With guidance and support he might then attempt these challenges progressively, using word-finding techniques, self-state-

**TABLE 4.1. Zone of Recovery**

| | | |
|---|---|---|
| Boredom<br>Overprotection | Challenge<br>Can do it with some help | Frustration, Anger<br>Discouragement |
| Too easy | Just right | Too hard |

*Zone of Recovery. Case 4.1. Elizabeth (fictitious).* Elizabeth was a good cook before her TBI, but when she got home from the hospital and tried to cook dinner nothing came out right. She spilled and burned things, started making things she did not have ingredients for and could not substitute, and forgot to add spices or added them twice. Her husband said she had to keep trying, it was the only way. The next time she tried she got frustrated and threw a dish towel at the TV he was watching. Cooking dinner was not appropriate for her at that time; it was in her Frustration Zone.

Her husband switched tactics. He prohibited her from cooking, but made her wash all of the dishes, a big, boring job that she did well. This time a sponge hit the TV. This was not an appropriate task; it was in her Boredom Zone.

Finally, her son cooked dinner with her. He asked her what she wanted to make, then guided her in checking that they had the ingredients and in shopping for those that were missing. They planned what she would have to start first and when. He got her to use the recipe that she thought she had memorized and to mark each step as she did it. He reminded her to use a timer. When it went off and she couldn't remember what it was for, he had her look at the stove and figure it out. When dinner time got close and not everything was ready he pitched in to make a salad and got his father to set the table. After dinner she washed the dishes, he rinsed while they talked, and nothing hit the TV. This way of doing dinner was in her Zone of Recovery.

ments, explanations to others, cue cards, or other techniques that help him control his embarrassment.

### *Activity Analysis*

Using natural activities to facilitate recovery does not mean abandoning what is known about cognitive abilities and their rehabilitation. Instead, it means recognizing those abilities in natural contexts through activity analysis. (The more common term is *task analysis*, but this suggests goal-directedness and onerousness for activities that may have neither yet can facilitate recovery, such as playing with a young child.)

When someone's usual activities are no longer practical due to brain illness, the cognitive specialist observes and analyzes the activities in light of the person's known cognitive limitations. The person is encouraged to continue those parts of the activity still possible. The specialist tries to determine what obstructs the difficult parts and seeks appropriate compensations, adaptations, or restorations (Case 4.2. Vigilio).

Activity analysis also applies to neuropsychotherapy for helping the person to understand and overcome emotional and behavioral barriers. This analysis of

*Hypothesis Testing in Evaluation. Case 4.2. Vigilio.* Vigilio was a 35-year-old, right-handed Costa Rican police officer with 11 years of education who was disabled from a gunshot wound to the head 4 years earlier that was affecting the right temporal and left frontal lobes. He complained that he was no longer able to read recreationally.

Recreational reading can be disturbed by aphasia, by alexia, or by impairments in attention, in memory, or in visual-spatial skills, among others. Appropriate treatment depends on which one is responsible. It was hypothesized (based on the location of the lesion and the lack of evident aphasia in his speech) that visual-spatial impairments were responsible. When examined, it was found that he had a severe left neglect and constructional difficulties. When asked to read the newspaper aloud, he neglected words on the left and was poorly oriented to the page. With guidance, he was able to use a marker for the left side of the page and a line guide to allow him to read accurately. His family was trained to guide and to train him.

real-life events is very familiar to psychotherapists. For example, a psychotherapist might help a woman figure out her difficulty in asserting herself with her co-workers and how to overcome it. This analysis may be more art than science, especially for the neuropsychotherapist, who must consider cognitive losses, behavioral and emotional changes, emotional reactions, pre-illness personality, and context in analyzing why an activity is not succeeding.

Cognitive rehabilitation specialists recognize that the cognitive processes of people with brain illnesses are disturbed or distorted, not simply lost or damaged, and that they carry out cognitive activities by whatever means possible. They are differently abled, not disabled. This may produce inefficiency, failure, or idiosyncratic behaviors rarely seen in people with intact brains, such as perseveration, confabulation, paraphasias, unilateral neglect, and reading by letter tracing. Sometimes these attempts can be fruitfully harnessed and channelled; sometimes they interfere with efficient cognition and must be interrupted or eliminated.

This principle is also important for neuropsychotherapy. Brain illness produces not just a lack of behaviors, emotions, and abilities but new behaviors, emotions, and adaptations. It may be desirable to eliminate some of these, channel others, and merely recognize, acknowledge, and accept others.

## *THE PROBLEM-ORIENTED APPROACH TO NEUROPSYCHOTHERAPY*

The approach to neuropsychotherapy presented here draws on all approaches to cognitive rehabilitation. It is a problem-oriented approach based on identifying and treating specific psychological (emotional, behavioral, and cognitive) problems resulting from brain illness. Although these problems can be as many and as varied as the human condition, 30 or so main problem types (see Chapter 2) form the core of this approach. Problem-oriented neuropsychotherapy extends process-specific cognitive rehabilitation to include not only cognitive but also emotional and behavioral processes and their overlap in the executive functions. However, these problems are dealt with in their context as in the natural recovery approach.

Although the problem-oriented approach is useful for planning treatment, the neuropsychotherapist must see the whole person as more than a sum of their parts. The life problems someone with a brain illness confronts are more than a collection of individual cognitive impairments and behavioral and emotional changes. The psychological problems resulting from brain illness do not occur in isolation; they interact with who that person was prior to the illness and with personal and social expectations for his behavior. Impaired arithmetic abilities might devastate an accountant but would have little consequence to a laborer whose spouse handles the finances. Mild sexual disinhibition and impulsive anger might have little effect on an artist but could provoke a crisis of conscience and career in a clergyman. Problems also interact. For example, someone with impaired attention and impulsive anger might have catastrophic reactions to minor frustrations, whereas each of those problems alone might not produce that result. The person with anosognosia might not get depressed over severe deficits that would depress the individual with full awareness.

## *WHERE COGNITIVE REHABILITATION AND NEUROPSYCHOTHERAPY MEET*

Ideally, the junction between cognitive rehabilitation and neuropsychotherapy is seamless. In an integrated rehabilitation program with good communication and cross-training, occupational therapists, speech pathologists, and other therapists help deal with frustrations, anxieties, and anger. Psychotherapists reinforce cognitive training procedures and cue memory book use. Some therapists offer both services simultaneously.

However, training limitations and interdisciplinary rivalry sometimes prevent a seamless approach, and cognitive rehabilitation and neuropsychotherapy are not always in integrated programs. In such situations it is better to refer a problem than to practice beyond one's competence and to prioritize limited treatment resources based on functional problems, on a long-range perspective, on cost versus benefit, and on the likelihood of favorable outcomes.

# II

# Practice

# 5

# Assessment

The role of neuropsychological assessment in neuropsychotherapy and in related interventions ranges from fundamental to almost irrelevant, depending on the problem and on the intervention. It is very important to know the etiology and the prognosis of the condition and the causes and the manifestations of resulting problems for detailed, problem-solving counseling and neuropsychotherapy. By contrast, it may be enough to know the diagnostic category or the type of problem to recommend education and support groups. Some problems are so obvious that little assessment is needed. The clinician recommends how thorough an assessment is needed for the presenting problem and for the intended intervention and weighs costs of assessment and the risks of error in helping the client to make prudent use of professional resources.

Neuropsychological assessment of cognitive functions (Ardila & Ostrosky-Solis, 1991; Hanson & Tucker, 1992; Lezak, 1995; Puente & McCaffrey, 1992) and neurodiagnostic assessment (DeJong, 1979; Van Allen & Rodnitzky, 1981; Wiederholt, 1988) have been discussed at length many times and need no review here. This chapter focuses on the neuropsychological assessment of personality, emotions, behavioral problems, and executive functions for the purpose of intervention planning. Often these areas are well described in neuropsychological assessments, but sometimes further assessment is needed by the neuropsychotherapist. The assumption of this chapter is that an adequate evaluation of cognitive strengths and weaknesses is available and a neurological diagnosis has been given, although the more specific nature and possibly the diagnoses of emotional and behavioral problems may need further, more functional assessment.

## *ASSESSMENT AS A COGNITIVE PROBLEM-SOLVING PROCESS*

The diagnostician's cognitive processes include receiving preliminary information, generating hypotheses, refining hypotheses through information gathering, arriving at and confirming working diagnoses, intervening, and making further diagnostic refinements (Kassirer & Kopelman, 1991, Case 5.1. Naricio).

### *Hypothesis Generation and Refinement*

In neuropsychotherapy, preliminary information typically includes the client's age, gender, diagnosis, and presenting complaints. Hypotheses concern many types of information (Table 5.1). These hypotheses direct information gathering. Which hypotheses to pursue and whether to use a confirming or a disconfirming strategy depends on the relative probability and seriousness of each hypothesis; the ease, risk, and cost of gathering information; and the urgency, risk, and benefit of various interventions.

It is useful to jot down hypotheses before the assessment and modify the list as the assessment proceeds. The list becomes a useful planning tool for later parts of the assessment and evolves into a problem list for the conclusions.

As information is gathered, hypotheses are refined, rejected, or regarded as more or less probable than previously. New ones may be suggested. Hypothesis

*Clinical Reasoning. Case 5.1. Naricio.* The following is a schematic recounting of my unfolding thought processes in a clinical case presentation. The information is presented in the order in which I received it; my thought processes are in italics.

1. Naricio is a 15-year-old, Spanish-speaking, Costa Rican, left-handed ninth-grade student from a working-class family presented by his psychologist for a brief exam and intervention plan at a hospital outpatient clinic in Costa Rica. He had left frontal and parietal strokes 3 weeks previously from an attempt to embolize a nasopharyngeal hemangioma prior to surgery.
2. *He probably has aphasia and right hemiplegia. He is young and left-handed, and it is only 3 weeks since his stroke, so there is hope for substantial recovery from whatever we see today. With left-handedness, "all bets are off" on lateralization of language and other cognitive functions, so we need to examine typical right hemisphere functions as carefully as left hemisphere ones. Even so, aphasia is likely, because for left-handers, roughly one third have left hemisphere language, one third have right hemisphere language, and one third have bilateral language. Children with acquired aphasia typically have expressive aphasia regardless of lesion localization (within language areas). He is somewhat past childhood, but that is still the most likely aphasia.*
3. *Knowing this neurology department, he and his family likely received little information about his state and need education, reassurance, and advocacy to deal with the system. They are likely to be angry with the doctor. Undoubtedly they postponed surgery, so that is a potential future trauma. Now I want to focus on his mental and physical condition and on his family.*

*Case 5.1 (Continued)*

4. When his psychologist first saw him, 3 days after his stroke, he was not speaking but was able to follow one-step commands. He had a right hemiplegia. He seemed depressed and aware of and frustrated by his limitations. His mother was at his bedside. She was very concerned about his future and angry that they had not been told the risks of embolization. The psychologist learned that he had been a very good student, with no significant previous developmental, emotional, academic, or medical difficulties. He had many friends who were concerned about him, and a 6-year-old brother he was anxious to be with.
5. *This could be aphasia, or there could also be lack of initiation and/or voluntary mutism from emotional shock. Good awareness is a good prognostic sign. We will check depression. I wonder how much he understands of what happened to him. Checking aural comprehension is a high priority to know what else we can do with him. We should watch for family overprotection and model appropriate communication. I wonder how we might mobilize the help of those friends. We need to check on his family's anger and see if it will interfere or if it can be usefully channeled.*
6. In outpatient clinic 2 weeks after his stroke he spoke single words, followed two-step commands, and answered simple yes/no questions accurately. He was easily frustrated in attempting to communicate. He copied a sentence with well-formed letters, but he misspelled words. His copy of a complex drawing had mild organizational difficulties, but delayed recall for it was adequate. He had striking right neglect on a cancellation task.
7. *This is aphasia, although there may still be a minor lack of initiation and voluntary mutism. It seems to be clearing into expressive aphasia. We want to make sure his family knows how to communicate with him, maximizing his abilities and minimizing his frustration. We need to check reading to see if it can help him get around oral communication limits and how much rehabilitation it will need. Spelling errors in copying suggest that he does not comprehend well what he reads. His drawing disorganization and neglect suggest symptoms more typical of right hemisphere lesions, and of mixed lateralization, but it is still early. These may clear before he recovers enough physically for them to be significant functional problems. We should monitor them. Good visual-spatial memory is expected and is a good prognostic sign.*
8. *We will start the evaluation with him and his family together and check current problems and concerns, their understanding of what happened, and his functioning at home. Then we will test comprehension. If everyone is comfortable, we will continue our evaluation in front of the family, checking naming, reading comprehension, spontaneous writing, and neglect.*
9. He enters with his father half-carrying him. On inquiry, his family reports that he has begun physical therapy, but they have not been taught how to help him around. His parents and grandmother seem too intimidated by the medical setting to ask questions (a common socialization pattern for Costa Rica). They answer that he is independent in eating and toileting, and he reads the newspaper. They

*(continued)*

*Case 5.1 (Continued)*

see him as depressed and possibly suicidal. They claim to understand what happened and do not express anger about it; they are focused on his recovery.

10. As comprehension testing begins, his family watches carefully, pleased with each success, and concerned with each failure. Although his mother needs to be asked gently once not to help him with the tests, everyone is comfortable, so the evaluation continues in their presence. Comprehension and speech have improved substantially but are still very basic. He has major difficulties with phonetic reading, but reading concrete nouns is functional. Each new modality tested turns into a discussion with his family about how to communicate with him and what activities to encourage. The process of recovery is stressed, backed up with a handout. A possible return to school when vacation ends in 3 months is discussed, and Naricio brightens. He and his family deny that he has any vegetative symptoms of depression. He greatly appreciates expressions of empathy for his frustration and his anxiety. As home activities are discussed, it becomes clear that his family overprotects him, but they appreciate encouragement to let him do as much as possible for himself. The psychologist promises to advocate for him to see a language pathologist. She asks them to ask the physical therapist for training and to bring one of his friends to the next appointment to get involved in helping with his recovery.
11. *Overprotection is a problem, but there is plenty of help available that needs to be channeled properly. The health care system will not supply much rehabilitation. We need to advocate for him and to get his family to help him properly. Anger with the doctor appears to have passed, but that should be explored later to be sure. He is changing rapidly; any thorough assessment will be rapidly out-of-date. It is better to concentrate on helping him and his family understand what is likely to happen next. Reading simple stories to his 6-year-old brother may be a naturalistic way to work on reading, perhaps a few weeks from now. Getting his friends involved should help mobilize hope and motivation. His depression appears to be reactive and likely to respond to empathy, encouragement, good information, and progress. With his limited mobility, constant family attention, and his lack of predisposing history, suicide is not a high risk.*

ANALYSIS: Paragraphs 2 and 3 contain hypothesis generation for problems, prognosis, and interventions. Heuristics for age and lateralization are invoked. There is some prioritizing of the information gathering. By paragraph 5 there is some refinement of hypotheses and tentative planning of intervention so the evaluation itself can be therapeutic. In paragraphs 7 and 8 the hypotheses and plan for information gathering are further refined. In paragraphs 9 and 10, the assessment was pursued only as far as needed to establish working hypotheses for the priority interventions of the moment. In paragraph 11 working hypotheses are consolidated with plans for further information-gathering and interventions.

**TABLE 5.1. Assessment Hypotheses**

**TABLE 5.1a. Types of Hypotheses in Neuropsychological Assessment of Emotions, Behavior, and Personality for Intervention Planning**

What are the emotional, behavioral, and personality problems?
Under what circumstances are they present?
How severe are they?
What has caused them?
What real-life risks and functional problems do they present?
What is their prognosis?
What pre-illness experiences and personality characteristics are relevant to the situation?
What strengths, supports, and resources are available?
What types of interventions are likely to help?
What are appropriate intervention goals?

**TABLE 5.1b. Common Symptom and Problem Hypotheses by Diagnosis**

TRAUMA

*General*

- Impaired attention, especially attentional control
- Impaired memory, especially encoding and storage
- Impaired executive functions
- Focal signs from contusion or hemorrhage
- Headache
- Irritability, impulsive anger, agitation
- Sensitivity to alcohol
- Fatigue
- Perplexity/anxiety
- Anger with the source of the injury
- Guilt (person with the trauma and/or family members) about the cause of the trauma
- Substance abuse
- Posttraumatic Stress Disorder
- Contributing psychosocial stressors
- Impulsive or risk-taking personality style

*Accidental Cause*

- Suicide attempt
- Contributing medical condition (e.g., heart disease, diabetes, sleep or seizure disorder)

*Violent Cause*

- Aggressive personality features

STROKE

- Depression
- Reflex crying
- Medical nonadherence
- Psychosocial stressors
- Post-traumatic stress symptoms (concerning experience of stroke, helplessness, ambulance, intensive care, etc.)
- Guilt (person with stroke and/or family members) about not managing risk factors
- Focal symptoms

*(continued)*

**TABLE 5.1. *(Continued)***

ALZHEIMER'S DISEASE AND RELATED DEMENTIAS
- Memory impairment (encoding, storage, and retrieval)
- Generalized loss of cognitive abilities
- Lack of awareness of or hypersensitivity to cognitive impairments
- Caregiver stress and depression
- Family conflicts over diagnosis, severity, caregiving, safety, and independence

**TABLE 5.1c. Common Symptom and Problem Hypotheses by Lesion Localization**

FRONTAL
- *General*
  - Any of the executive function disorders
  - Any of the emotional changes
- *Dorsolateral*
  - Lack of initiation
  - Emotional indifference
  - Impaired emotional expression (especially right)
  - Frustration, catastrophic reaction (especially left)
  - Depression (especially left)
  - Perseveration
  - Impaired planning and sequencing
  - Concreteness
  - Lack of empathy
  - Lack of awareness of deficits (especially right)
  - Left neglect (with right lesion)
- *Posterior*
  - Dorsolateral symptoms
  - Motor impairments (contralateral weakness)
  - Expressive aphasia (especially left)
  - Impaired singing and musical expression
  - Apraxia (especially left)
- *Orbital*
  - Disinhibition
  - Lack of awareness of deficits
  - Concreteness
  - Lack of empathy
  - Insensitivity to social feedback
  - Disorganization
  - Confabulation (when amnesia is present)
  - Poor planning
  - Impulsive anger
  - Hypersensitivity to noxious stimuli
  - Anosmia (loss of sense of smell)

PARIETAL
- *General*
  - Contralateral sensory-perceptual impairments
  - Visual-spatial impairments
  - Impaired body schema

**TABLE 5.1. *(Continued)***

| |
|---|
| *Left* |
| Aphasia |
| Alexia |
| Agraphia |
| Apraxia |
| Left-right confusion |
| Arithmetic difficulties |
| *Right* |
| Left neglect |
| Impaired emotional comprehension, especially facial |
| TEMPORAL |
| *General* |
| Impaired auditory perception |
| Impaired emotional comprehension, especially prosody |
| Impaired memory, especially storage |
| Contralateral superior quadrantanopsia |
| *Left* |
| Fluent aphasia |
| *Right* |
| Impaired music perception |
| Left neglect |
| OCCIPITAL |
| Contralateral visual field defects |
| BASAL GANGLIA |
| Difficulty with initiation of thought and action |
| Slowness |
| Impaired emotional expression |
| Decreased emotional reactivity |
| Depression |
| Memory impairment |

**TABLE 5.1d. Common Symptom and Problem Hypotheses by Severity**

| |
|---|
| Mild |
| Attentional difficulties |
| Fatigue |
| Perplexity |
| Conflicts over not being believed |
| Conflicts over whether or not to tell others |
| Hypersensitivity and overreaction to impairment |
| Moderate |
| Struggles with family over safety, independence |
| Struggles over understanding of limitations |
| Guilt |
| Severe |
| Struggles over caregiving |
| Caregiver stress |
| Guilt |

*(continued)*

**TABLE 5.1.** ***(Continued)***

**TABLE 5.1e. Common Symptom and Problem Hypotheses by Onset**

| |
|---|
| Acute |
| Shock |
| Posttraumatic Stress Symptoms |
| Grief reaction |
| Progressive |
| Perplexity |
| Conflicts over not being believed |
| Conflicts over the diagnostic process |
| Family conflicts over diagnosis, severity, caregiving, safety, independence |
| Lack of focus for grieving |
| Intermittent |
| Perplexity |
| Anxiety about recurrence |
| Conflicts over not being believed |
| Conflicts over the diagnostic process |
| Family conflicts over diagnosis, severity, caregiving, safety, independence |
| Family conflicts over whether or not episodes can be controlled and how |

**TABLE 5.1f. Common Symptom and Problem Hypotheses, General**

| |
|---|
| Confronting mortality |
| Guilt or anger over the disease process |
| Search for life meaning of the disease process |
| Grief reaction to loss |
| Search for understanding |
| Struggle with change in abilities, responsibilities, roles |

generation and refinement come from the skilled application of extensive knowledge of functional neuroanatomy, clinical neurology, clinical psychology, neuropsychology, testing, learned associations of symptoms, and explicit and implicit heuristics (for example, the rule of thumb that if a person asks to be evaluated for Alzheimer's disease, suspect depression, whereas if a family member asks that a person be evaluated for Alzheimer's disease, suspect Alzheimer's disease). As in medicine (Kassirer & Kopelman, 1991), these skills seem best acquired through the practice of the cognitive processes of assessment and clinical reasoning, and through modeling and guidance of skilled practitioners.

### *Information Gathering*

Information gathering is directed by two complementary strategies, screening and probing. *Screening* covers information routinely gathered in all formal evaluations, either because it provides a baseline, or because the cost of checking is low, the condition is common, and/or the risks of the condition are high. There is substantial agreement on some screening information—demographics, previous medical conditions, alcohol and drug use, violence risk, and so forth—general agreement about some areas to be assessed—memory, attention, language, intellectual level, and so forth—and variable practice in other areas, such as test batteries.

A *probing* strategy is used when information gathering is directed by hypothesis refinement. For example, if one hypothesis is organic irritability, then the clinician may interview clients about irritability before and after the illness, watch closely for frustration during testing, and administer a personality test that is sensitive to irritability and related phenomena. Unfortunately, although cognitive processes of hypothesis refinement have been studied in general and in medical diagnosis (Kassirer & Kopelman, 1991), they are not well studied in neuropsychological assessment. Ways of refining common neuropsychological hypotheses regarding emotions and behavior are found in part 3.

No one test or assessment technique is adequate to assess the etiology of personality and emotional problems after brain illness. Several types of information are needed (Table 5.2; Ardila & Ostrosky-Solis, 1991; Lezak, 1995; Walsh, 1978).

At some point there is enough certainty to permit an intervention decision based on a working diagnosis. The degree of certainty needed for this decision depends on factors such as the urgency, the risk, the benefit, and the cost of intervention. Several principles apply to determining certainly about diagnostic hypotheses. These include adequacy, coherence, and parsimony.

### *The No Treatment/Test/Treatment Thresholds*

When the probability of a condition is low, no treatment is given. As the probability of the condition increases, there comes a point where it is worthwhile

**TABLE 5.2. Common Sources of Information in a Neuropsychological Assessment**

1. Medical history
2. Mental health history
3. Social history
4. Educational and vocational history
5. School, military, substance abuse, and legal histories
6. Interview with the person being assessed
7. Interview with an informant who knew person well before and after the llness
8. Reports from members of the rehabilitation team
9. Behavioral observations
10. Cognitive neuropsychological tests
11. Tests of personality and of emotional state
12. Evaluation of the person's environment, including home, school, and work visits and an assessment of family dynamics

to gather more information (Figure 5.1). That point is the *no treatment/assess threshold.* As the probability of the condition further increases, there comes a point where no more assessment is needed, and treatment can begin. This point is the *assess/treatment threshold.* These thresholds are movable, depending on the sensitivity and specificity of the assessment and on the risk/benefit ratios and the costs of assessment and treatment.

Neuropsychological assessment is frequently expensive and stressful. The decisions of whether, what, and how much to assess can influence the motivation of the person being assessed and their family and the availability of resources for intervention and for other uses. Although it is common to encounter admonitions that intervention should not proceed without a comprehensive, multidisciplinary evaluation, these exhortations often represent a conflict of interest for their advocates.

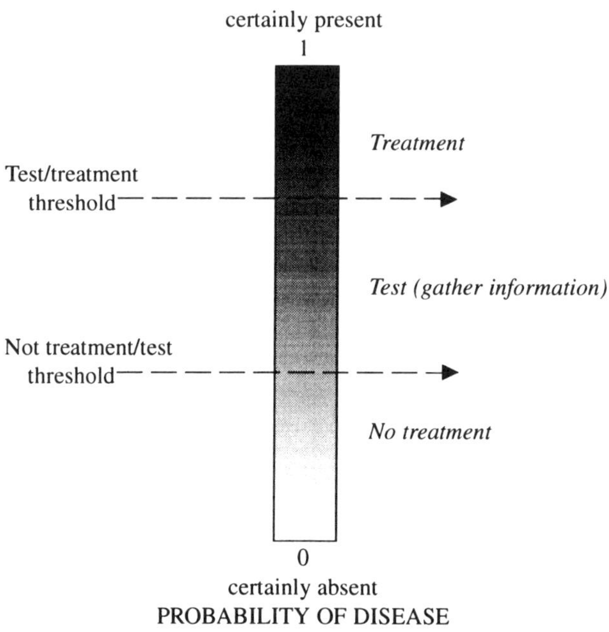


FIGURE 5.1. Testing thresholds (adapted from Kassirer and Kopelman, 1991). The probability of a specific disease (or neuropsychological problem) is represented on the vertical line from 0 (no probability) to 1 (certain). At the extremes, the course of action—no treatment or treatment—is clear. In the middle range of probability of disease a test (or other information gathering) is used to determine the presence or absence of the disease or of the problem and the course of actio. The boundaries are movable depending on test sensitivity and specificity, the risk/benefit ratio and the cost of tests and of treatments.

**TABLE 5.3. Costs and Risks of Psychosocial Evaluation**

| |
|---|
| Economic cost. |
| Psychological invasiveness may violate the client's sense of privacy or of autonomy. |
| Tests may be cognitively stressful and fatiguing and may precipitate frustration or a catastrophic reaction. |
| Tests can detract energy and resources from psychosocial interventions and from other aspects of rehabilitation. |
| Tests may reinforce the client's self-image as sick, weak, or crazy. |
| It may cause embarrassment. |
| It may cause alienation from psychosocial intervention and from rehabilitation due to alienation from psychosocial evaluation. |
| It may create an externalized locus of control and identity for the individual and/or the family. |
| It may be an emotionally difficult confrontation. |
| Results may generate despair or egotism. |

The clinical and financial cost/benefit analysis (Table 5.3) of assessment versus intervention can increase efficiency without increasing risks. The following questions can guide the assessor:

1. Are results of the next test, interview question, observation, or other means of inquiry likely to determine or to change my choice of intervention?
2. Is it better to spend our limited time and resources on more evaluation or on intervention?
3. Will the interventions I am planning be harmful or ineffectual if my hypotheses are wrong?
4. What are the risks and benefits of further evaluation?

To illustrate, the no intervention/assess threshold for intensive rehabilitation is high in the first few weeks after a mild TBI (Figure 5.2, Kay, 1995). Because most such people recover spontaneously, extensive evaluation is not called for, and early psychosocial interventions are best confined to education and reassurance. Rehabilitation is more appropriate for those who have not fully recovered after a few months. The no intervention/assess threshold is much lower, however, for mental status screening in a geriatric population (Figure 5.3). Mental status screening is inexpensive and benign, and the probability of a treatable problem is high in the elderly.

At the other end of this continuum, the assess/intervention threshold is moderate to high (Figure 5.4) for individualized education and problem-solving counseling—it could be quite harmful to tell someone that she has Alzheimer's disease when she does not, or that she can work or drive or care for young children when she should not, and the cost of such interventions is somewhat high. Likewise, psychoactive medications and formal therapy have moderate to high assess/intervention thresholds. General group education and printed materials about brain

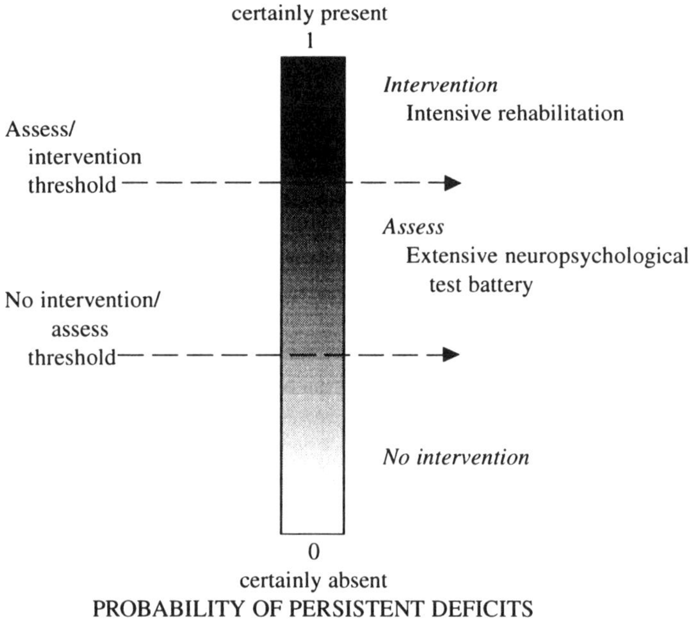


FIGURE 5.2. Assessment thresholds for intensive rehabilitation 3 weeks after a mild TBI. When the decision is whether or not to give an extensive neuropsychological test battery to determine the need for intensive rehabilitation 3 weeks after a mild TBI, the no intervention/assess threshold is high because the test is expensive and spontaneous recovery is common.

illnesses are benign and inexpensive interventions with a low assess/intervention threshold (Figure 5.5).

### *Diagnosis Verification*

A working diagnosis usually awaits further confirmation from treatment outcome. Treatment success tends to support the working diagnosis. Failed treatment may reflect a faulty diagnosis or inadequate treatment and needs to be carefully reconsidered.

### *Cognitive Errors*

Cognitive errors made by the diagnostician (Table 5.4, p. 65) can result from faulty knowledge bases or errors in reasoning processes.

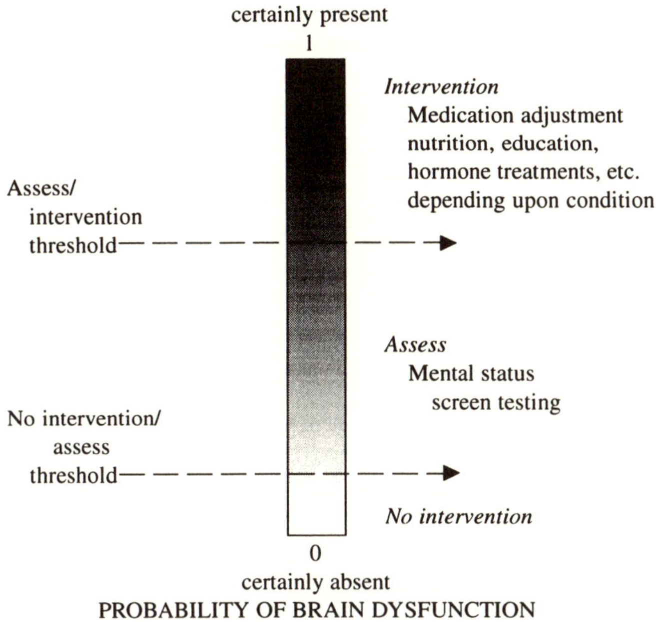


FIGURE 5.3. Assessment thresholds for mental status screening in a geriatric population. When the decision is whether or not to screen test for possible cognitive decline in a geriatric population, the no intervention/assess threshold is low because the test is inexpensive and low risk, and the probability of a condition needing intervention is relatively high.

## *CONDUCTING THE NEUROPSYCHOLOGICAL/ NEUROBEHAVIORAL ASSESSMENT*

Cognitive neuropsychological assessment is generally very test-oriented, but available data do not support such an approach for neuropsychological personality assessment. Neuropsychological tests of personality and of emotions are not well developed (Judd & Fordyce, 1996; Appendix B). This portion of the assessment must still rely heavily on interviews, behavioral observations, and other records.

### *Reviewing Medical Records*

The neuropsychotherapist reviews medical records with an eye for any indications of what the person's pre-illness personality was like. Difficulties with medical adherence and conflicts with care providers may indicate problems to be

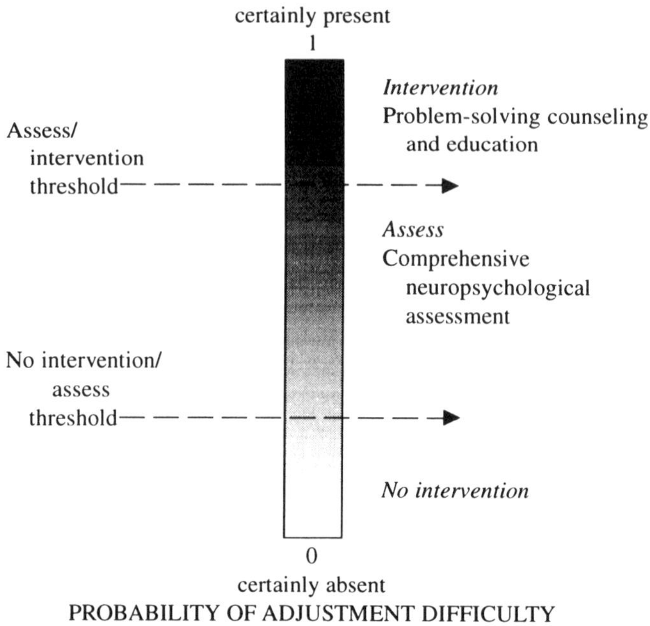


FIGURE 5.4. Assessment thresholds for problem-solving counseling following major brain illness. When the decision is what kind of counseling and education to give following a major brain illness, although testing is often expensive and may involve slight risk, the assess/intervention threshold remains moderately high because the risks of inaccurate information or of inappropriate advice are fairly high and the costs of counseling are moderately high.

addressed in therapy. A previous history of mental health treatment, substance abuse, or of family or sexual problems should be explored.

For diseases of potentially uncertain onset, such as the dementias, cerebral vascular disease, multiple sclerosis, infections, and metabolic disorders, indications of personality changes or of other problems prior to diagnosis may be hypothesized to have resulted from the unsuspected onset of the disorder. Exploring this hypothesis in interviews may allow both the person and the family to reinterpret previous actions.

The history of the illness itself should be explored for its time course, uncertainties preceding diagnosis, the time of diagnosis, stressful diagnostic and treatment procedures, and the loci of the lesions. All of these factors may illuminate the nature of the problems and the experiences of the person and of the family and may provide the basis for educating them about the disorder.

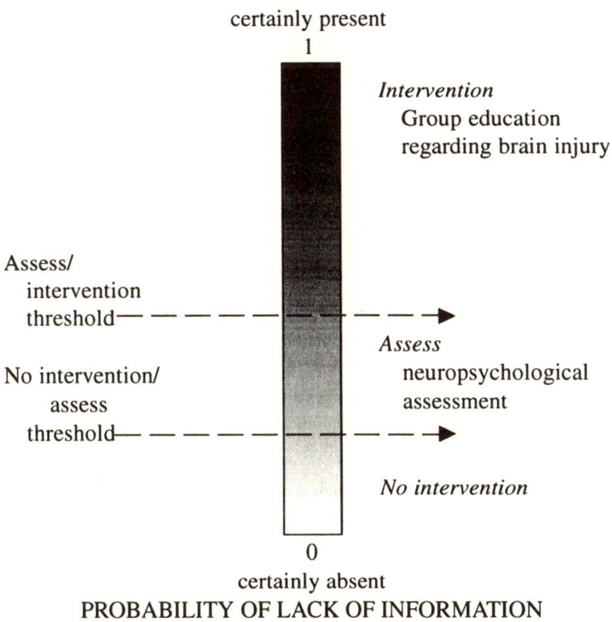


FIGURE 5.5. Assessment thresholds for group education regarding a TBI. When the decision is whether to give group education regarding a TBI the assess/intervention threshold is low because the risks and costs of education are low and the benefits are relatively substantial.

### *Interviews*

A variety of approaches to interviewing exist; this chapter describes an approach similar to that used in The Head Injury Family Interview (see Appendix B; Kay, Cavallo, Ezrachi, & Vavagiakis, 1995).

**TABLE 5.4. Classification of Cognitive Errors in Diagnostic Reasoning**

| |
|---|
| Faulty hypothesis generation |
| Faulty context formulation |
| Faulty information gathering and processing |
|   Faulty estimation of disease or symptom prevalence |
|   Faulty interpretation of a test result |
|   A faulty causal model |
|   Overreliance on a clinical axiom |
| Faulty verification |
|   Premature closure |
| "No-fault" errors |

*Note.* From *Learning Clinical Reasoning* (p. 38), by R. I. Kassirer and R. I. Kopelman, 1991, Baltimore: Williams & Wilkins. Copyright 1991 by Williams & Wilkins. Reprinted with permission.

*Preparing the Interviewees*

With few exceptions, it is critical to interview both the person with the brain illness and at least one other informant, usually a close family member. An informant is important because anosognosia, amnesia, and aphasia, each common in brain illness, can make the person an unreliable historian for critical information. Informants can also provide background on the person's personality before the illness, her social context, resources available, and problems the family faces.

Before beginning, the assessment process is described in full to the person being assessed and to the informant together. The expectation of conjoint and separate interviews should be stated orally and in the written informed-consent form. This routine lessens the likelihood of distrust by the person with the brain illness. If she is reluctant to allow an informant interview after this explanation, the therapist may choose to avoid confrontation and proceed with an individual or a conjoint interview and hope that enough rapport will be established to allow for an informant interview later. Occasionally, available information will indicate a need to confront the issue immediately, for instance, with someone with a known history of intentionally manipulating the medical system. Special care must be taken, however, to respect cultural differences in privacy and in family structure. For example, in some cultures it is considered inappropriate for a man to talk with another man's wife alone.

Conjoint and individual interviews allow the therapist to observe the nature of the interactions between the participants, but they also give each party privacy. Announcing at the outset that there will be individual interviews spares participants the anxiety of figuring out how to report something that is important but delicate in the presence of the other. If time does not allow, individual interviews are preferred over conjoint ones.

*From General to Specific*

Proceeding from general questions to specific ones minimizes any effect of "leading" the interviewee and gives greater validity to reported problems. Spontaneous complaints are more predictive of functional difficulties than are symptoms reported on checklists or similarly elicited responses (Gerber & Schraa, 1995).

It is useful to begin the conjoint interview by asking the person with the brain illness an open-ended question concerning the reason for the assessment, such as "What brings you here?" "Tell me what happened to you." "How can I help you?" or "Why are you in the hospital?" This type of a question can get at the person's understanding of her illness, her understanding of and feelings about her need for help, her ability to recognize and respond to the social situation, the priorities she identifies, her attributions of the problems, and her ability to organize her response. Starting by attending to the interviewee's rather than to the interviewer's agenda helps establish a rapport and helps the interviewee feel "listened to". This is the time for "telling the story" of the illness. The examiner may need to explain that he has, indeed, read the medical record, but wants to know exactly how the client sees these events. It is also a time to ask if the interviewees have questions they would like answered at the end of the evaluation.

*Problem List*

Questioning then moves to constructing a list of problems. "What other problems have you been having?" or a similar question is asked repeatedly until there are no problems left, though others may come to mind later in the interview. The list will overlap substantially with the hypothesis list. Each problem is explored for its severity, frequency, practical consequences, and how it is perceived by each interviewee. It helps to ask for examples to determine circumstances under which the problem arises, whether it was present before the illness, whether it is getting better or worse, and what is being done about it.

*Review of Systems and Functions*

Once the problem list has been explored, a review of systems and functions helps to make sure no areas are overlooked. The contents of this review (Table 5.5) vary according to the interviewer's preferences and the circumstances. For example, some areas may be skipped if they were covered earlier in the interview or by other clinicians or if the answers are very obvious. Each area in the review of systems is pursued to the degree necessary. Changes of functioning are emphasized to help the interviewer know what to attribute to the illness and how to set treatment goals. When problem areas are identified in the review of systems but not spontaneously this gives information about the extent of denial and/or the lack of awareness of deficits.

Some clinicians prefer a review of systems by questionnaire, following up on areas where difficulties are indicated in the interview. This approach has the advantages of thoroughness and consistency. The disadvantages are that it is less sensitive than spontaneous complaints, it may suggest symptoms for some, and base rate endorsement for common neuropsychological symptoms is high in individuals without brain lesions (Dikmen, McLean, & Temkin, 1986; Fox, Lees-Haley, Earnest, & Dolezal-Wood, 1995).

*Review of Emotional Status*

The review of emotional reactions and changes begins with general questions, such as "How are you feeling?" "How has your mood been?" and "Have there been any changes in your emotions?" Reported feelings or changes are

**TABLE 5.5. Neuropsychological Review of Systems and Functions**

- Systems
  - Attention
    - Concentration
    - Speed of processing
    - Distractibility
    - Multitasking
  - Memory
    - Immediate recall
    - Delayed recall
    - Retrograde amnesia
    - Duration of post-traumatic amnesia
    - Procedural memory
  - Executive functions
    - Awareness of problems
    - Impulsiveness/disinhibition
    - Initiation
    - Judgement
    - Problem-solving
    - Perseveration
    - Communication pragmatics
  - Language
    - Speaking
    - Word-finding
    - Understanding
    - Reading
    - Writing
    - Mathematics
  - Visual–spatial
    - Construction (mechanical/artistic-activities)
    - Way-finding
  - Emotions
    - Depression
    - Anxiety
    - Post-traumatic stress symptoms
    - Anger, irritability
    - Hallucinations, delusions, paranoia
    - Suicidal or homicidal thoughts or actions
    - Emotional communication (crying, comprehension)
    - Emotional reactivity
  - Sensory–perceptual
    - Vision
    - Hearing
    - Touch
    - Smell
    - Taste
    - Equilibrium

**TABLE 5.5.** ***(Continued)***

| |
|---|
| Motor |
| Strength |
| Coordination |
| Stamina |
| Tremor or other movement disorder |
| Medical |
| Fatigue |
| Pain |
| Seizures |
| Functions |
| Mobility |
| Dressing |
| Grooming |
| Eating and appetite |
| Sleep |
| Work |
| School |
| Money management |
| Driving |
| Getting around in the community |
| Cooking |
| Housekeeping |
| Shopping |
| Child care |
| Repairing things |
| Family relations |
| Sexuality and libido |
| Recreation |
| Socialization |
| Religious or spiritual involvement |

explored for their quality, intensity, frequency, time course, typicality, and examples of specific emotional episodes or displays.

More specific questions can then probe changes in crying, anger, laughter, and feelings of sadness, fear, happiness, frustration, and confusion. When there is an increase in displays of emotion such as crying or anger, it is important to ask to what extent the person actually feels upset when crying, and if she feels that her angry behavior is justified, appropriate, and in character. Changes in the intensity of feelings should be explored regarding to what extent they represent a change in circumstances versus a change in emotional responsiveness.

As in any mental status examination, it is important to note the presence of main symptoms of the major psychiatric disorders, such as delusions, hallucinations, paranoia, loose associations, suicidal or homicidal ideation, and so forth. Care must be taken to determine the nature and time-course of such symptoms, because each could be the result of a preexisting psychiatric condition, the recurrence of a psychiatric condition triggered by the brain illness, or a new symptom induced by the illness. For example, psychotic symptoms are common in delirium and in post-traumatic amnesia (Cummings, 1985) but generally pass rapidly as the sensorium clears. Psychotic symptoms are also common in Alzheimer's Disease and have characteristic and distinctive features (Gilley, 1993). Additionally, it is necessary to ask about emotional phenomena common to brain illness but rare with intact brains, such as changes in emotional communication.

### *Social and Emotional History*

Taking the social and emotional history of a person with a brain illness (Table 5.6) differs from taking the history of a person with an intact brain. It is important to distinguish what was characteristic prior to the illness from what is characteristic currently, including symptoms of progressive conditions that may have appeared prior to diagnosis. Also, when preparing for conventional psychotherapy there is often an assumption that the interviewer must find psychopathology. For neuropsychotherapy no such assumption can be made. All sorts of people have brain illnesses, many of them previously well-adjusted and with normal personalities. Although it is important to discover psychopathology when it exists, the therapist is not obligated to find pre-illness pathology to account for present problems.

The neuropsychotherapist is interested in much more than frank pre-illness psychopathology. Pre-illness personality style in the normal range can give invaluable information for intervention planning. For example, a history of sexual abuse (Raskin, 1997), as well as pre-injury personality features of overachievement,

**TABLE 5.6. Social and Emotional History**

| |
|---|
| Problems with pregnancy, birth, development |
| Cultural/ethnic/linguistic/acculturation background |
| Educational history, highest level, degree of success |
| Family constellation |
| Childhood traumas, abuse, neglect, parental divorce or death, moves |
| Legal difficulties |
| Work history |
| Significant adult trauma or major events (e.g., war experiences, assaults, major losses, immigration, etc.) |
| Mental health difficulties/treatment |
| Significant medical history |
| Alcohol and substance use/abuse |
| Personality style |
| Life goals |
| Recreations/hobbies |
| Social affiliations |
| Religious/spiritual background |

childhood emotional deprivation, dependency, subclinical "borderline" personality, grandiosity, and narcissism (Kay, 1992; Ruff, Camenzuli, & Mueller, 1996) have been identified as critical contributors to adjustment difficulties following a mild TBI.

### *Conjoint Interviews*

Beginning with a conjoint interview allows the clinician to apportion time efficiently for the individual interviews. By beginning with the person with the brain illness, her competence as an historian soon becomes evident. It is of value to note whether she defers to the informant readily, reluctantly, or not at all; whether the informant supplements answers appropriately or overprotectively; and whether conflict is evident between them. When there is much disagreement, most of the interviewing may need to be separate, covering most of the same information both times. If there is substantial agreement and comfort in the relationship, the separate interviews may be reduced to a perfunctory "Do you have anything to add to what was already said?" or "Is there anything you would like to add that perhaps you were not comfortable saying in (the other person's) presence?" In a few areas, such as sexuality, it is best to inquire separately regardless of comfort level in the conjoint interview.

Even when the person is severely impaired, a conjoint interview can be revealing. People emerging from a coma may show their strongest reactions and their best communication efforts in the presence of particular family members. The person who is hostile and resistive with rehabilitation staff may be tranquil and cooperative with family, or visa versa.

### *Interviewing Informants*

The informant interview follows the same pattern as the interview of the person with the brain illness, beginning with a chance to ask questions and to state concerns, going from general to specific, and including probing and a review of systems and of functions. The amount of redundancy needed between the separate interviews depends on how much agreement was seen between them during the conjoint interview, on the hypotheses considered, and on the no intervention/assess/intervention thresholds.

## *Cognitive Testing*

Formal cognitive neuropsychological testing (Lezak, 1995) helps to confirm or to disconfirm hypotheses generated previously, identify strengths, and identify what cognitive deficits need to be addressed in rehabilitation, adjusted to emotionally, and compensated for during neuropsychotherapy.

Neuropsychological testing is not always a benign procedure. Lengthy, stressful testing can be a devastating and impoverishing experience that may alienate the testee from further psychological intervention, but proper preparation can make it a significant therapeutic experience (Christensen, 1989).

### *Behavioral Observations*

Interview observations of quality of speech, organization of thoughts, pragmatics of communication, and emotional responsiveness are important, but the structure of the situation limits the sample of behavior. Qualitative features of behavior during testing can give further information about behavioral control; emotional adjustment; awareness of and responses to errors, failure, and frustration; impulsivity; initiation; effects of fatigue; and motivation. Observations in waiting rooms, in cafeterias, on wards, and in rehabilitation therapies may provide distinctive information. Home, school, and work visits and community excursions can contribute immensely to the ecological validity of an assessment in selected instances, especially when the setting is unfamiliar to the clinician or if informants are unavailable (Starch & Falltrick, 1990).

### *Personality Testing*

#### *Conventional Personality Tests*

Most conventional personality tests, such as the MMPI–II, the 16PF, the California Personality Inventory, the Rorschach, the Thematic Apperception Test, the Geriatric Depression Scale, and so forth, were not designed to be sensitive to the specific types of personality and emotional change that result from brain illness. Further, they generally do not distinguish between personality, emotions, and behavior before versus after illness. Many of these tests rely on self-report, and their validity in the face of an organic lack of awareness of deficits must be questioned (Gilley & Wilson, 1997; Youngjohn, Davis, & Wolf, 1997). For these reasons, these cannot be considered to be true neuropsychological tests.

In spite of their shortcomings, however, some of these tests, particularly the MMPI–II (Butcher, Dahlstrom, Graham, Tellegen, & Kaemmer, 1989), still play a role in many neuropsychological assessments, in part due to the relative lack of well-researched neuropsychological tests of personality. These tests have a legitimate use in neuropsychology, particularly with the client who has a mild or a questionable illness or the client whose illness was many years previous to assessment. Special cautions must be taken in their interpretation, however, due to cognitive and somatic items usually interpreted as reflecting personality features when responses to those items may actually represent consequences of brain illnesses (Alfano, Finlayson, Stearns, & Neilson, 1990; Bornstein & Kozora, 1990). For example, the SCL-90-R contains items that refer to having trouble remembering things, having difficulty making decisions, having trouble concentrating, having one's mind going blank, getting headaches, being easily annoyed or irritated, having to do things very slowly to ensure correctness, and feeling low in energy or slowed down (Woessner & Kaplan, 1995).

More useful are conventional measures of emotional state, such as the Beck (Beck, Ward, Mendelson, Mock, & Erbaugh, 1961), Hamilton (1960), and Zung (1965) Depression Scales, the Overt Aggression Scale, (Yudovsky, Silver, Jackson, Endicott, & Williams, 1986), and so forth. These measure the client's current state, which can then be compared to the inferred pre-illness personality and state. Nevertheless, cautions in their interpretation are still needed because of the effects of lack of awareness of deficits and the tendency of some neuropsychological symptoms to mimic psychopathological symptoms, as in the discussion of the woman with a right hemisphere syndrome at the beginning of Chapter 1.

### *Neuropsychological Personality Assessment Tools*

A number of neuropsychological personality assessment tests, inventories, rating scales, structured interviews, and other tools have been developed recently (annotated list in Appendix B; see Judd & Fordyce, 1996 for a review). Some are for a general neuropsychological population, whereas others are specific to particular conditions, such as depression, emotional communication, frontal lobe syndromes, or epilepsy. With the exception of the Washington Psychosocial Seizure Inventory (Dodrill, Batzel, Queisser, & Temkin, 1980) and the Neuropsychiatric Inventory (Cummings, 1997), none of these is as well-researched or accepted as the personality tests mentioned previously. However, they can have an important role in assessment for neuropsychotherapy and for related interventions when interpreted with clinical judgment.

## *Assessing the Environment*

The natural recovery approach to rehabilitation (see Chapter 4) implies a relatively new role for rehabilitation workers—evaluating the adequacy of the environment for facilitating recovery. Although rehabilitation workers have done this informally for many years, it receives little attention in rehabilitation texts, in research, and in training. Home evaluation is well-developed for related specific purposes such as wheelchair accessibility, but this is different from evaluating a home's potential for facilitating recovery (Starch & Falltrick, 1990). Paradigms for evaluating rehabilitation centers, convalescent centers, and transitional facilities (Peppard, 1991) usually come from an institutional perspective, such as certification, rather than matching a facility to a particular individual. They also do not necessarily allow for comparing the facility with alternatives such as the person's home.

Except in the case of imminent threat to life or to limb, the decision of where to pursue recovery is, in theory, the consumer's. The rehabilitation professional can contribute to this decision through a careful evaluation of the choices. In the absence of empirical data, how factors regarding the environment of recovery are weighed must be a subjective decision, but guidelines (Table 5.7) may help make sure that important factors are not overlooked. Evaluation of families and workplaces are discussed in Chapters 13 and 14.

**TABLE 5.7. Evaluating the Adequacy of the Environment of Recovery**[a]

THE PHYSICAL ENVIRONMENT

- Building setup
  - Wheelchair accessibility
  - Stairs
  - Access to outside
- Emergency preparation
  - Escape
  - Emergency equipment
  - Getting help
- Materials organization
  - Complexity of environment
  - Consistent location of materials
  - Labeling of materials
  - Accessibility of materials
  - Presence of distractors
- Memory and orientation
  - Calendars/appointment books/schedules
  - Clocks/alarms
  - Method for taking messages
  - Phone list/phone book/autodial phone
- Planning/follow through
  - Lists for money management, transportation, shopping, home maintenance, and so forth
  - Directions for specific tasks
- Recreation resources
  - Games
  - Sports
  - Hobbies
  - TV, video, music
  - Computer
  - Reading
  - Pets
- Productivity resources
  - Kitchen
  - Workshop
  - Craft area
  - Garden, animals
  - Desk/office
  - Computer

**TABLE 5.7.** ***(Continued)***

- Community access
  - Alone or accompanied, and availability of accompaniment
  - Means of transportation
  - Accessible community resources
  - Access via telephone, computer, mail, and so forth
- Risks
  - Alcohol/drugs
  - Weapons
  - Sharp tools
  - Power vehicles
  - Heavy machinery
  - Electricity
  - Toxic substances (insecticides, paints, glues, medicines)
  - Places (bodies of water, heights for falling, traffic)

THE SOCIAL ENVIRONMENT

- Who is present?
- What are their:
  - Attitudes toward disability and teaching?
  - Skills?
  - Relationships with the person?
  - Availability to be trained?
  - Availability to provide training/guidance to the person?
- Who comes to visit?
- Who is available in the community, and how?
- Expectations of the environment:
  - Family milieu and expectations (see chapter 13)
  - Physical, cognitive, emotional, and social job requirements (see chapter 14)
  - Physical, cognitive, emotional, and social expectations of school

THE PERSON'S FUNCTIONING WITHIN THE ENVIRONMENT

- Ability to attend to the environment
- Orientation within the environment and the community
- Independent living
  - Mobility in the environment
  - Self-care
  - Bathroom use
  - Safety
  - Meal preparation
  - Housekeeping
- Use of time within the environment
  - Use of schedule
  - Realistic scheduling
  - Pacing of rest breaks
  - Frustration tolerance
- Communication with others in the environment
- Awareness of expectations
- Ability to relate to others in the environment
- Use of and interest in each of the resources listed previously

[a] From "The Importance of a Home Evaluation for Brain Injured Clients: A Team Approach," by S. Starch and E. Falltrick, 1990, *Cognitive Rehabilitation*, *8*(6), 31–32. Copyright 1990 by Neuroscience Publisher. Adapted with permission.

It is important that the evaluator actually sees the person functioning in the environment to evaluate the person-environment fit (Case 5.2, Abuela). Homes, values, and lifestyles vary considerably. The major goal of rehabilitation is to restore the person to her previous level of functioning, not to convert her to the values and lifestyles of the rehabilitation team. Although some adaptations are inevitably necessary, they need to emerge from a collaboration between the rehabilitation team and the person and the family that will use them (Case 5.3, Pepe). The point of a home evaluation is not so much to adapt the home to rehabilitation but to adapt rehabilitation to the home.

Assessing the environment of recovery is not just for the purpose of choosing a placement. It is also done to adapt the environment to the person's needs and to prepare the person to cope with the expectations of that environment. Assessment is not just an event but is also a process. The details of the person-environment fit can only be known through trial and error. Environmental adjustments continue after the placement is made. "Life is a place-and-train venture" (Willer & Corrigan, 1994, p. 653).

### *Behavioral Record-Keeping*

At times it is useful to analyze a behavioral or an emotional pattern that is a focus of treatment by keeping a record or a register over time (Jacobs, 1993; see

*"I Want to go Home!" Case 5.2. Abuela.* Abuela was a 78-year-old woman with no education who was admitted to the National Rehabilitation Center in San José, Costa Rica for rehabilitation of a right hemisphere stroke and left hemiplegia. She lived with her extended family in a dirt floor shack several kilometers from Turrialba, a city 3 hours from San José by bus. The Turrialba hospital social worker reported that her family was very concerned for her, but none of them could afford the time or the money to visit her. Using a telephone to call her in the hospital was a rare and difficult experience for them. Abuela came from a segment of society that believed that people went to hospitals to die. Abuela rapidly became depressed, ate very little, and gave little effort in therapy, a clear change from her reported behavior in the Turrialba hospital.

The Costa Rican National Health Care System had no mechanism to facilitate her family's visit. The rehabilitation team decided to transfer her back to the Turrialba hospital where her family could visit her, and where she could at least receive physical therapy. The team made a home visit with her to educate the family about her care and to find what adaptations would be possible. In Turrialba her mood, appetite, and participation improved and she was discharged home. In this instance, although Abuela was in the "best" rehabilitation setting in the country, the person-environment fit was not conducive to recovery.

*Crutches for Pepe. Case 5.3. Pepe*[a]. David Werner, a trainer of health promoters, was visiting a rural Mexican mountain village when a father invited him home to see his 13-year-old son, Pepe, who had polio as a baby and had never walked. Werner asked if he had tried crutches. The father responded that they could not travel to the city to get some. Werner cut branches with a machete and made crude crutches. The father protested that they would not work, and when Pepe tried them they broke under his weight. The father took the machete and cut a more appropriate species of wood. Following Werner's example, he skillfully fashioned functional crutches. Within half a day Pepe was proudly walking for the first time in his life.

This episode illustrates a collaboration between a professional with specialized knowledge and a layperson with the knowledge and skills to adapt that knowledge to local conditions. The intervention would have been unsuccessful without this collaboration. With it, the father conserved his dignity.

A North American example relating to the same point comes from a motorcycle gang member in postacute TBI rehabilitation who refused/forgot to carry his large memory notebook with his name on it but then found and consistently used a smaller, leather-bound notebook chained to his belt. Here the collaboration was between the idea for a memory book that came from the rehabilitation center, and a format that was acceptable and workable that came from him.

[a]From *Disabled Village Children* (pp. A1–2), by D. Werner, 1990, Palo Alto, CA: Hesperian Foundation. Copyright 1990 by Hesperian Foundation, 1919 Addison St. #304, Berkeley, CA 94704. Adapted with permission.

Chapters 6, 7, & 8). Typically this takes place after the main part of the assessment and its conclusions and after the main problems have been identified.

## *FORMULATING CONCLUSIONS*

The science and art of neuropsychology converge intensely in integrating all of the collected information. Initial and subsequent hypotheses are reviewed and accepted, rejected, refined, or revised based on the information obtained. Hopefully, each idea present in the conclusions is confirmed from each major domain of information—the medical aspects of the disease process as manifested in this individual, the individual's self-report, the reports of informants, behavioral observations, and test results (Case 5.4. Salvador). When contradictions are encountered, these must be resolved, either by seeking further information or by entertaining new hypotheses.

Ideally, the conclusions identify all neuropsychological problem areas and pertinent strengths. For each problem area there is a description of its severity, its manifestations in this individual, its functional consequences, its relationship to problems observed by the injured person and by the informant, a prognosis, a plan, and functional goals.

*Organizing the Information. Case 5.4. Salvador.* Salvador was a 23-year-old, bilingual Salvadoran university student who was seen for neuropsychological assessment 2 months after a severe TBI and evacuation of a right frontal subdural hematoma. Given the lack of postacute neurorehabilitation in El Salvador, a home rehabilitation program using family and friends in a circle of support was recommended. The following table simplifies the major conclusions of the evaluation and how they were reached:

| *CONCLUSION* | *IMPAIRED INITIATION* | *ANOSOGNOSIA* | *IMPAIRED REASONING* |
|---|---|---|---|
| *Lesion* | Right dorsolateral frontal | Right frontal and diffuse | Right frontal |
| *Self-report* | He is unaware, but able to acknowledge the problem. | He recognizes only the memory problem, but acknowledges others. | He is unaware, but can recognize and acknowledge the problem. |
| *Mother's report* | He is very passive, watches TV most of the day, but will eventually go along with things if asked. | He sees nothing wrong but his memory, but recognizes some errors when they are pointed out. | He has trouble fixing food, sequencing brushing his teeth, understanding decisions. |
| *Behavioral observations* | He is very passive in conversation and in testing, but responds to questions and to structure. | He usually thinks he is doing well on tests unless errors are pointed out. He shows little self-correction. | He shows inefficient, impulsive task strategies and poor understanding of the rehabilitation process and of family decisions. |
| *Test results* | He shows impaired verbal and figural fluency. | He shows poor self-correction on Wisconsin Card Sort, Block Design, Rey Figure, and so forth. | His performance is very impaired on the Wisconsin Card Sort and reasoning subtests of Test Barcelona. |
| *Prognosis* | Fair, given his response to structure. | Fair, given his acknowledgment of errors that are pointed out. | Fair, given his ability to respond to correction. |

*Case 5.4. (Continued)*

| | | | |
|---|---|---|---|
| *Plans* | The daily schedule is structured and moderated by the family, with fading cues. | Feedback is built into all activities with members of the circle of support, into the problems and strengths list, and into the exercise of translating neuropsychological report to Spanish. | Daily structured discussion of news, soap operas, and novels; supervised math practice; review of college texts; household chores; computer work in the family business. |
| *Goals* | Return to household management, social life, college. | Collaborate with rehabilitation, learn to use compensations, avoid disabling depression. | Return to household management, social life, college. |
| *CONCLUSION* | *IMPAIRED MEMORY WITH CONFABULATION* | *REDUCED EMOTIONAL REACTIVITY AND EXPRESSIVENESS* | *MOTIVATED TO RECOVER* |
| *Lesion* | Diffuse and frontal | Right frontal | |
| *Self-report* | He reports taking exams, playing soccer, driving, and drinking alcohol without problems after injury. He says he has trouble remembering what he reads. | He has not noticed any change. He does not report enthusiasm for any current activities(but does not report other symptoms of depression). | He reports that his goal is to go back to college and resume his social life. |
| *Mother's report* | None of the post-injury activities he reported actually occurred. He does not remember events or instructions well. | His reactions are muted compared to pre-injury,and his voice is less expressive. | He collaborates with suggested activities and is interested in his college career. |

*(continued)*

*Case 5.4. (Continued)*

| | | | |
|---|---|---|---|
| *Behavioral observations* | He forgets earlier conversation rapidly and forgets earlier tests. | He shows a somewhat flattened tone of voice, few gestures, and modest enthusiasm. | He responds well to structure, refuses rest breaks, and is persistent in the face of failure. |
| *Test results* | His performance in mildly impaired on Rey Figure recall, moderately impaired on Wechsler Memory stories, Test Barcelona stories, word list learning, drawing memory, and he shows gross confabulation on recall. | He shows mildly impaired emotional expressiveness, which improves somewhat to imitation. | |
| *Prognosis* | Fair, given his awareness of impairment and willingness to use compensations and to accept feedback. | Good | It can be used to help maintain rehabilitation program if connections between activities and goals are kept explicit. |
| *Plans* | Use a memory book, get feedback on confabulation, and check his "sense of knowing" during structured discussions. | Progressive social reintegration, focus on previously enjoyed activities, and get feedback by video. | Keep tasks as related to goals as possible, and start early with textbook study and social reintegration. |
| *Goals* | Manage household, study. | Resume social life. | |

There also needs to be a dynamic formulation that identifies the ways that the various problems interrelate. When a collection of symptoms fits a syndrome, this should be noted. However, the dynamic formulation also needs to identify patterns of reaction. For example, "Mr. H.I.'s difficulties with complex attention are particularly seen under time pressure and social observation; for example, in store checkout lines. Cognitive failures frustrate and irritate him, which further impairs his thinking. Always a sensitive person, his embarrassment compounds the situation. He withdraws socially to avoid such situations, but this exacerbates his depression." Such formulations help to identify strategies and priorities for intervention.

Sometimes it is useful and/or necessary to give a psychiatric diagnosis in addition to a neurological one. The *Diagnostic and Statistical Manual*, (4th ed., DSM-IV), of the American Psychiatric Association (APA,1994) provides useful broad categories. It recognizes that symptoms must produce significant functional disruption to be considered a disorder. It also recognizes that personality changes can result from neurological injury. Nevertheless, the DSM-IV presents a limited number of categories, so a diagnosis alone is not adequate for specifying interventions. Further, the DSM-IV largely attempts to incorporate neuropsychological changes into an existing psychiatric typology. This is like the ornithologist who encounters a bat and tries to decide what type of bird it is. For these reasons, even a detailed, 5-axis DSM-IV diagnosis often is not an adequate description of a neuropsychological disorder.

## *INTERVENTION PLANNING*

The simplified model presented in Figure 5.2 suggests that the decision to intervene is based simply on the probable presence or absence of disease and on the risk/benefit ratio of intervention. However, the probability of benefit from a intervention is not simply a property of that intervention, but also of the person receiving the intervention, the social context of that intervention, and the severity of the condition. Interventions are proposed as hypotheses regarding what will help a person's problem. These hypotheses can be pretested by dynamic assessment techniques, which directly evaluate the person's ability to respond to instruction, to training, to rehearsal, and to cuing, and to maintain appropriate interactions (Rees & Storry, 1996). These hypotheses are more fully tested by the actual intervention. When the goals of the intervention are concrete improvements in functioning, the success of the intervention can be judged and the intervention can be adjusted as needed.

The intervention plan is typically oriented around the problem list. The choice of interventions is based on the availability and the acceptability of the intervention, its suitability to the problem, and so forth. Although the benefits of intervention are often elaborated, risks also need to be considered (Table 5.8).

## *FEEDBACK*

Assessment is an intervention in itself (Christensen, 1989). Giving proper feedback to the evaluee and/or to the family is usually a legal and an ethical obligation of the evaluator and a crucial part of the assessment. Feedback helps

**TABLE 5.8. Risks of Psychosocial Intervention**

| |
|---|
| General Risks |
| Economic cost |
| Detract energy from other aspects of rehabilitation |
| Develop dependency |
| Develop sick role |
| Self-image as sick, weak, or crazy |
| Rejection from significant others |
| Embarrassment |
| Alienation from rehabilitation due to alienation from psychosocial intervention |
| Alienation from intervention at a more appropriate time |
| Externalized locus of control and identity for individual and/or family |
| Emotionally difficult confrontation |
| False hope or sense of security if treatment is not effective |
| Psychological treatment for medical problems preventing adequate medical attention |
| Education |
| Can be misinterpreted or misapplied |
| Support Groups |
| Can reinforce stereotypes and helplessness |
| Can expose individuals to risks from aggression, seduction, impulsiveness, drugs, and so forth from other members of the group |

guide decision-making, assists rehabilitation and intervention planning, and provides education and support to the person and to the family (Gass & Brown, 1992). In neuropsychotherapy, feedback also begins the treatment of distorted self-awareness, facilitates grieving, and helps the person formulate a new self-image. Gass and Brown emphasized using accessible language for feedback (see Chapter 6) and summarizing recommendations in writing. Rather than a test-by-test review of scores, they suggested summarizing performance in each functional domain (Table 5.9) and then waiting for responses, so feedback becomes a dialogue, facilitates understanding, and allows the person to relate results to everyday life.

In neuropsychotherapy, feedback is not just an event, but is an ongoing process over many contacts and with many different methods (see Family Education in Chapter 6), especially for self-awareness distortions (see Chapter 7). An evaluator who will not be giving treatment should recommend how feedback should continue.

## *ADJUSTING THE CONCLUSIONS*

Most conclusions are working hypotheses. Situations change as people recover from their illnesses, or as their conditions progress or recur. New symptoms

**TABLE 5.9. Steps in Feedback Regarding Neuropsychological Evaluation[a]**

1. Review the purpose of testing
2. Define the tests
3. Explain test results and behavior
4. Describe strengths and weaknesses
5. Address diagnosis and prognosis
6. Make recommendations

[a] condensed from Gass and Brown, 1992.

and new information emerge. External life events, such as changes in family, employment, living arrangements, and so forth, also change the situation. Passing through stages of grief, understanding, and adjustment for both the person and the family often changes the situation considerably. Therefore, conclusions are not a timeless statement, but rather are a snapshot of one moment. If an intervention is not succeeding, it can be a signal to reconsider the conclusions.

## *SUMMARY*

Assessment of emotions and behavior after brain illness for the purpose of intervention planning is a dynamic, multidimensional, goal-directed process. Those goals are the identification not only of problems, but also of causes, of manifestations, of prognoses, of strengths, of resources, of strategies, and of goals. Understanding the evaluator's cognitive problem-solving processes, using cost–benefit analysis, and giving consideration to the no intervention/assess/intervention thresholds can make the assessment/intervention process more efficient and effective.

# 6

# Fundamental Issues

## *CAUSALITY AND BLAME*

In their search for a sense of control and meaning from the experience (Kushner, 1981), people with brain illnesses and their families may channel anger and blame in appropriate ways, such as prosecuting an assailant, suing a negligent party, or working with an organization such as Mothers Against Drunk Driving; they may lash out at any handy target; they may turn blame inward as guilt; or they may see the event as a punishment from God (Block, 1987). Health care workers need to recognize these tendencies as common and normal. Information about diseases and their causes and risk factors needs to be presented with sensitivity to timing, emphasis, delivery, and belief systems.

Health care workers also need to recognize these tendencies in themselves (Gans, 1983). When working with multiple tragic situations, health care workers may search for each person's flaw or mistake—what they did wrong (that I don't do) that caused this situation—to believe that "This won't happen to me."

## *THE NEW PERSON*

Brain illness is like few other experiences, because the people who experience it are often fundamentally changed in their personalities, emotions, and abilities. A primary psychological struggle is to redefine themselves (Direnfeld, 1991; Prigatano, 1991). They face a perplexing existential, spiritual question (Block, 1987; Bullis & Cherry, 1994; Linge, 1990): "Who am I?" Old answers no longer work. They must reconstruct meaning for their lives. Even when changes are positive (Ranseen, 1990), they must be understood and incorporated into a new self-image.

Three barriers to the reconstruction of self-image and of life meaning are particularly important. First, cognitive impairments make the task more difficult because interpreting, integrating, and remembering the information involved is more difficult. Second, anosognosia is a direct organic barrier to self-knowledge. Third, the self is a moving target as impairments diminish in recovery from acute illness or increase with degenerative conditions (see Chapter 2).

Reconstructing the new person requires time, experiences, and insights, small and large. Only a limited amount of the new information can be taught (Case 6.1. J. D.). The person also needs to interpret experiences, and to integrate them into a new self-image. The person can be helped through this process as follows:

1. Help the person identify and seek out people important to him who can contribute to the process.
2. Guide and structure experiences that permit self-discovery (while avoiding danger, discouragement, and overload).
3. Help the person to interpret the experiences through recognizing what happened and why, finding labels for it, and relating experiences to one another or to the experiences of others.
4. Help the person to mourn and grieve the losses discovered (Hibbard et al., 1990), to express and acknowledge safely any feelings that the losses may generate, and perhaps to channel those feelings into meaningful decisions or into action.
5. Help the person to integrate the interpretations. The integration may take the form of self-descriptions, a self-portrait, or a "personal narrative";

*Repetition, Repetition, and Repetition. Case 6.1. J. D.* J. D. was a 40-year-old disabled lawyer seen for neuropsychotherapy 3 years after a severe TBI. He had a full motor recovery and language and visual-spatial skills were almost fully recovered. He had only mild impairments in attention and in new learning, but had moderate impairments in organization, planning, judgement, and reasoning, and was moderately impulsive. He had made several unsuccessful attempts to return to work, and was progressively alienating his entire support system. He had received extensive rehabilitation and education concerning the TBI, including extensive psychotherapy.

In the first session he was given a simple, two-page handout describing executive function disorders. He was asked to read the entire handout when he took his medications every night for a week. Because of the extensive therapy and education he had received previously, I was a bit worried that this might be too basic for him. To my surprise, the following week he asked if he could have the same assignment again, because he said that each night as he read it he got something new out of it and saw a different way that it related to his own behavior. The assignment was eventually continued for an entire month.

that is, the story one tells oneself and others about one's life and experiences.

6. Direct the person toward others who have "been there," through individual contacts, therapy groups, support groups, Internet groups, literature, or art. Self-narratives following brain illnesses are found in the literature of support groups and their parent organizations, in *The Journal of Cognitive Rehabilitation, Mouth: The Voice of Disability Rights*, Brodal (1973), Fishman (1988), Kapur (1997), Linge (1980, 1990), Marshall and Ruff (1989), Meltzer (1983), and Williams and Kay (1991). Motion pictures, such as *Regarding Henry* and *Awakenings,* can also be useful.
7. Support and guide the person through the life choices that the new self-image suggests.

Reconstructing the self is lengthy and cannot reasonably take place primarily within formal therapy. In fact, formal therapy may not be necessary. Supportive individuals willing to listen attentively are often sufficient to facilitate this process. Formal therapy may be needed if the person is developing a maladaptive self-image or does not progress in this process.

## *COMMUNICATION STYLE*

Clinicians are responsible for modifying their communication style to cope with impaired language, communication pragmatics, attention, memory, and executive functions. Otherwise, treatment may be frustrating and unproductive: the person sees the therapist as someone who says confusing things and who does not understand them and the therapist sees him as resisting treatment. The most commonly used adaptations are to make communication slow, repetitive, concrete, accessible, and structured.

### *Slow*

Most people with brain illness have slowed thought processes. Neuropsychotherapy and related interventions must accordingly proceed slowly both in the pace of speech (Block, 1987) and of ideas and in the progress on problems. Attention, language, or reasoning impairments may necessitate short sentences and simple grammar. Some clinicians do this naturally; others need training. Skills can be evaluated by session taping or by observation by a skilled clinician. This skill can be developed by imagining that the listener has a bad phone connection and language needs to be careful and clear.

Timers or progression on the agenda can remind the clinician to slow down. To prevent overload and fatigue, it is better to focus on just a few issues per therapy session, conversation, or educational presentation. Otherwise, nothing may be remembered and the effort becomes wasted. Sessions should be short and frequent when possible (Block, 1987; Lewis, 1991).

*Repetitive*

People with amnesia may need to hear things many times before they remember, and may need to practice many times before they can do something. Repetition and practice need to be spaced across time within the session and from session to session (Case 6.1. J. D.).

Active learning is usually more effective than passive learning. Repetition of information should not be practiced just by the clinician, but also by the person with the brain dysfunction (Block, 1987). For example, the following statements make good routines during and at the end of therapeutic interactions:

- I want to be sure you (understood, remember) what I just said. Could you (repeat, explain) it back to me, please?
- That was an important (point, conclusion, insight) you just made. Could you repeat it so you don't forget?
- Would you summarize this session in your (therapy book, diary, laptop computer, tape recorder), please?

Such routines give invaluable feedback to the clinician; it is rapidly obvious when the message is not getting through. If the person has not understood, the message needs to be repeated, simplified, or reduced. When dealing with an aphasia where the person understands and remembers but cannot repeat, or repeats without understanding, the clinician can repeat and summarize, seeking confirmation from the person with aphasia.

The clinician needs to discourage and cut off guessing and confabulation and needs to provide enough cues, guidance, and hints to allow the person to summarize effectively and to exploit the benefits of errorless learning (Wilson, 1992). Taping the therapy session or the final summary is another way of repeating (Hibbard et al., 1990).

When skills are to be learned, such as explaining a disability to someone, recognizing and controlling emotional outbreaks, avoiding alcohol, or taking medications on time, practice and training are needed to generalize the skills to their contexts of use. By contrast, if information is to be learned, such as causes of an illness, factors that contribute to recovery, reasons not to drink alcohol, or names of medications, it can sometimes be taught relatively rapidly. If information is not learned easily or is not available when needed, then it may need to be trained like a skill, with practice to generalize to contexts of use. Alternately, the person can be trained to find the information when needed in a therapy book or by using another compensation.

Active repetition can also be adapted to group work. In group therapy and support groups, the summary can be a group exercise. Interactive group education can include audience repetition and illustration of the content and completing the thought. Handouts can include questions to check understanding.

### *Concrete*

Neuropsychotherapy and related interventions often need to concentrate on the here and now, on concrete behaviors, and on current and recent feelings. If the prognosis is uncertain, long-range planning may be difficult. Psychological issues from the remote past will be largely irrelevant to coping with changes resulting from brain illness. Theoretical formulations are often inaccessible due to impaired abstraction abilities, attention, memory, or language. Metaphors and myths may be more satisfying for the clinician than helpful to the client, although stories of the form, "I heard of a person with a brain injury who . . ." can be quite helpful. Nonverbal materials—diagrams, pictures, dolls, or creative arts therapies (Prigatano, 1991)—can help make communication more concrete, especially when there are significant language impairments.

"Concrete" is a relative term; "familiar" may be more accurate. People with concrete thought due to brain dysfunction may still be able to manipulate abstract ideas that they know well although they may have difficulty with new ideas or with applying old ideas to new areas (Case 6.2. Sigmund).

Although the clinician generally needs to maintain a concrete communication style, she does need to help expand the perspective of the person with a brain illness, particularly for the future. The person who feels overwhelmed and discouraged by his deficits needs to be educated repeatedly about the extended course of recovery and about available resources and support.

### *Accessible*

Technical language is a habit of efficiency and precision among clinicians, but it can confuse and alienate uninitiated clients. Educating families and survivors in this language should *not* be a high priority for neuropsychotherapy or for

> *What Is Abstract? Case 6.2. Sigmund.* An eminent psychoanalyst had a severe TBI. His motor and language abilities recovered, but he had severe amnesia, impulsivity, inappropriate behavior, and grossly impaired judgement concerning his own abilities. Nevertheless, he gave competent supervision to a psychiatry resident on a psychoanalysis case (within an uninterrupted session), and he manipulated the abstract concepts of psychoanalysis appropriately. In other words, he handled familiar abstract material at a high level, but was disastrous at managing unfamiliar situations.

rehabilitation. The Glossary gives useful "translations" of clinical jargon into everyday language. On the other hand, overcompensation in simplifying language can be patronizing and equally alienating, for example, when a clinician asks a man, "Do we need to use the little boy's room?"

The clinician needs to seek the proper register of language for each individual. Language register is a dimension of communication pragmatics covering level of vocabulary, regionalisms, figures of speech, level of formality (first names vs. titles of address such as Ms. or Dr.), use of slang versus newspaper-type language versus clinical language, sentence length and complexity, and base of reference (e.g., biblical quotes, sports metaphors, business metaphors). One way to find the proper register is to adopt the expressions used by the individual. For example, an adolescent boy who says his rehabilitation goal is "making it with chicks" may respond better to a clinician who can also use this expression than to one who transforms it to "resuming age-appropriate social relationships with peers." Inept attempts to use subcultural dialects can backfire, however.

### *Structured*

Techniques such as free association or client-centered therapy are likely to be unfruitful with people with impaired initiation, impulsivity, disorganization, and so forth. While being sensitive to the client's perspective and feelings, clinicians need to explain expectations clearly, explicitly, and frequently.

An explicit, written plan or routine for therapy sessions is often useful (e.g., Table 6.1), particularly for people who are overtalkative and for those with difficulty prioritizing. Responsibility for timing sessions by clock or by timer can be passed gradually from clinician to client to help restore time responsibility and prospective memory.

## *NAMING AND NORMALIZING THE PROBLEM*

Naming the problem in an accurate way that others can understand and accept is a powerful intervention that cannot be neglected or hurried. It is tremendously helpful for those involved to see how the problem relates to the brain

**TABLE 6.1. Sample Neuropsychotherapy Session Agenda**

| Time | Item |
|---|---|
| 5 min. | Review session agenda, including any special events since previous session that need attention. |
| 5 min. | Review notes from previous session and homework. |
| 5 min. | Review strengths and problems list. |
| 20 min. | Work on a new issue (or special event, if necessary). |
| 5 min. | Summarize session, including new homework. |

illness and how it has been manifested in others. This can remove much blame and guilt and clear the way for effective, cooperative intervention. This can be done through written materials, through stories of others with similar problems, or through support groups.

## *CONTROLLING BEHAVIOR BY CONTROLLING THE ENVIRONMENT*

Psychotherapeutic techniques that ask people with brain illnesses to analyze situations, remember techniques they have learned, and apply them spontaneously often emphasize their weaknesses in memory, initiation, reasoning, organization, and so forth, setting them up to fail. Often their behavior and feelings can be more successfully managed by controlling their environment, especially through concrete cognitive aids. Once successful techniques have been found for a particular person, he can be trained in their use, as he assumes greater responsibility for his behavior and feelings. Those techniques may then be internalized or replaced by self-regulation techniques.

This general principle applies to many techniques: regulating the level of stimulation; using orientation cues such as signs, calendars, watches, and so forth; using lists, signs, and recipes to sequence common activities; "childproofing" the house; asking others for help; restricting access to alcohol, drugs, inappropriate friends, car keys, and so forth; and external memory aids such as a memory book, a therapy journal, alarms, and similar devices.

## *PROBLEM ANALYSIS*

The literature on behavior management is quite extensive, and does not need to be summarized again here (Burke & Wesolowski, 1988; Eames et al., 1990; Howard, 1988; Jacobs, 1993). Instead, this section describes modifications and special considerations needed in applying behavior analysis to activities of people with brain illnesses. Many of these considerations can be applied equally well to analysis and management of experiences not easily described in behavioral terms, particularly emotional experiences such as embarrassment, perplexity, frustration, fatigue, anxiety, and other such experiences. Problem analysis and treatment is a collaborative experiment involving the active and willing participation of the neuropsychotherapist, the person with a brain illness, and sometimes others.

Analyzing problem behaviors and emotions is a critical step in learning to anticipate and to control them. In behavior therapy and in neuropsychotherapy this means observing the ABCs of behavior, or Antecedents, Behavior, and Consequences. However, with severe amnesia, consequences may be unimportant because amnesia may not allow learning from experience or by conditioning.

Similarly, orbital frontal lobe lesions can result in an inability to benefit from social experience or to respond to operant conditioning (A. R. Damasio, Tranel, & Damasio, 1990; Rolls, Hornad, Wade, & McGrath, 1994). In addition, not just antecedent events but also states, such as hunger, fatigue, pain, medication, and so forth, need to be considered. These may be more important with injured brains than with intact ones.

Some behaviorists, particularly those from specialized inpatient behavior management units (Eames et al., 1990; Jacobs, 1993) insist that precise baseline behavioral data must be collected, usually over 24 hours or more, and must be carefully analyzed before any intervention can begin. This is undoubtedly the case for an externally imposed, team-coordinated management plan for persistent and highly problematic behaviors. However, a more flexible approach is possible under other conditions. A problem behavior or emotion can often be analyzed informally through interviews and through direct observations. For example, it may take only a few questions to identify reflex crying, a few more to find what triggers it, and a few quick trials to find techniques that work to manage it. Structured interviews can be used when answers are less obvious. Discussion with family members or at a team meeting sometimes reveals patterns such as phobic reactions, perseveration, confabulation, or food hoarding with enough clarity to permit the efficient development of an intervention plan.

Other problems require the small experiment of systematic record-keeping over time. Hypotheses about what factors account for the behavior or the emotion are needed to know what to observe. For instance, if food sensitivities are thought to cause migraine headaches, then headache records need to include what specific foods were recently eaten. However, food can probably be safely ignored in records of sexual acting out, embarrassment in public, and so forth, whereas the social context of the episode should be included.

With the factors to record chosen, an incident report form or tally sheet is developed (Table 6.2). The easier and clearer the form, the greater the chances of a successful and accurate record. Who does the recording depends on who is available and competent, the nature of the problem, and the person's stage of recovery (see Table 7.1, p. 108). Problem behaviors are often better observed and recorded by others, whereas the person with a brain illness may be the better source on problem emotions (Table 6.3). For particularly persistent and problematic behaviors an even more structured approach is needed (Jacobs, 1993).

**TABLE 6.2. Sample Problem Behavior Tally Sheets**

| Date, Time | Anxiety Level 1–5 | Location | People Present | How Resolved? | Last Rest |
|---|---|---|---|---|---|
| Date, Time | Frustration Level 1–10 | Activity | Time spent on activity | Strategy used | |

**TABLE 6.3. Sample Anxiety Journal Format**[a]

| |
|---|
| Date and Time: |
| What Happened? |
| Anxiety Level (1–10): |
| What did I do? |
| What did I feel? |
| Did I back off? |
| What do I need to do now? |

[a] See chapter 8, Incident Log section (p. 146), for discussion.

Howard (1988) took a particularly pragmatic, eclectic, and useful approach to managing problem behaviors in people with brain injuries. He emphasized giving priority to emotional behavior, setting concrete goals, and building a caring environment around the person. He stressed that intervention plans should be structured, consistent, repetitive, practical, simple, generalizable, rewarding, and meaningful to the person. This perspective shows respect for the person and puts priority on social relationships for controlling behavior, which facilitates a later transition to self-control in the community.

## *SEARCH FOR SOLUTIONS*

Once the ABCs of a problem are identified, the search for solutions begins. These take many forms; this list is not exhaustive.

### *Fix the Biological Problems*

Treating biological problems that contribute to problem behaviors and emotions usually takes priority. This can include correcting drug reactions, correcting diet and medications, treating infections, controlling seizures, altering rest schedules, avoiding allergens, treating electrolyte or hormonal imbalances, treating pain, and so forth.

Psychoactive medications can also play an important role in managing problems of behavior and of emotions, but their use for injured brains is quite different from their use for intact brains (Gualtieri, 1991). Their use should also be integrated with non-medical interventions for the same problems.

### *Avoid Antecedents*

Sometimes it is easiest to avoid a problem by preventing the antecedent. This can mean keeping the person away from certain people, places, or situations. The decision to take this approach depends on how restrictive, practical or ethical the approach is. For example, if the person dislikes a certain staff member or a distant relative who rarely visits, and has a panic attack when that person is present, it may be easier to reassign staff or to ask the relative not to visit rather than to try to desensitize him to their presence. However, if he has such a reaction to all adults, then another approach is needed. Other avoidable antecedents are overstimulation, understimulation, fatigue, sudden changes, overly demanding tasks, and public failure. Once some success is achieved with this approach, it may be possible to train him or her to recognize and to avoid those conditions himself.

### *Modify Antecedents*

The person with a brain illness may have behavioral problems because he cannot anticipate. He may not read social cues well, learn from experience, or recognize that he lacks information and should ask a question. Even if he has been told recently of an upcoming event, he may not comprehend the message, integrate it into his prospective thinking, and/or remember it. Modifying antecedents, then, often consists of preparing for an activity properly through explanations, giving the person some choices or control over the activity, or developing a coping routine before starting (see Chapter 8). Frequently the person can be trained to take responsibility for such preparations.

### *Reinterpret Behavior*

Sometimes a behavior such as cursing is a problem for rehabilitation staff but is not a problem for the person or for his family or caregivers, or visa versa. Here the solution may be to encourage the staff (or the family) to be more tolerant. Sometimes a behavior such as reflex crying, mild irritability or a feeling like perplexity is a problem for the person and for his family until they understand and accept it as a relatively harmless effect of the brain illness. An explanation may be sufficient.

The person who is disoriented and agitated sometimes tries to escape from circumstances incomprehensible to him. When this is understood, it is often possible to avoid confrontation, provide frequent orienting information, and allow greater freedom, rather than increasing the restraints imposed, the sense of confinement, and the agitation.

Reinterpreting behavior does not exclude also trying to modify that behavior. It simply helps decrease anxiety and frustration among those trying to cope with the behavior and helps focus intervention priorities.

### *Modify Consequences*

Operant conditioning paradigms can sometimes be used to modify or to eliminate problem behaviors. Amnesia can make conditioning ineffective.

Memory testing gives some indication of whether or not conditioning is possible.

Possible approaches to modifying consequences include the following:

1. Extinction—removing a consequence that reinforces a problem behavior (not responding to inappropriate sexual remarks, removing someone from an enjoyable setting when the problem behavior occurs).
2. Differential reinforcement—reward a substitute behavior that occurs around the same time.
3. Overcorrection—the person must undo the damage done (fix something broken, apologize, return to do the work avoided).
4. Punishment—verbal reprimand, isolation, and so forth.
5. Response cost—the person must pay something for each occurrence of the unwanted behavior.

In rehabilitation, external behavioral controls should be thought of as steps on the way to self-control. Sometimes external control eliminates a problem behavior present during recovery and it does not recur. In other instances, the potential for the behavior persists. In such cases, self-control strategies can be taught to reinforce the control learned and to generalize it to other circumstances. With self-control in place, structured, external behavioral management controls can be gradually withdrawn.

### *Stages of Recovery*

Predicting specific outcomes of brain illnesses is still not very accurate on an individual basis. Therefore, any predictions made, especially shortly after an injury or a diagnosis, should be quite tentative. The clinician might state a range of possible outcomes, an honest approach that leaves room for the hope to maintain motivation while allowing the person to begin to contemplate and to prepare for a possible lifelong disability. For example,

> It has been only 3 months since your brain injury; you are still recovering. A few people with injuries like yours get almost a full recovery. We hope that that will happen with you. You could become able to walk and run normally and return to your old work. You might be able to recover most of your memory abilities so you could take courses again. You may learn to control your anger like you used to. That kind of recovery would probably take many months or years, and lots of work. But it is more likely that you will continue to have significant problems for a very long time with walking, with memory, and with controlling your temper. If you are able to return to work, it will probably be at a lower level. There is even a chance that you might not get a lot better than you are now.

Even though individual recovery cannot be predicted with precision, knowledge of stages of recovery can be used to anticipate potential problems. For example, someone with impaired self-awareness may pass through stages of anger or depression while recovering awareness and discovering limitations. Warning him and his family of this will leave them more alert to seeking out help before the problem gets too big. Follow-up appointments can be made around the time when problems might be anticipated; for example, when struggles may arise over being left alone, returning to work, driving, and drinking alcohol.

## *EDUCATING FAMILY, FRIENDS, EMPLOYERS, TEACHERS, AND OTHERS*

Educating the people in the social world of the person with the brain illness is a fundamental intervention for problems of emotions and of behavior. This is usually the family, but it may include friends, employers, teachers, schoolmates, other program participants, and others, depending on their need to know, ability to learn, the teaching resources available, and so forth. How much to teach and to whom is the decision of the person with the brain illness, when competent, whose right to confidentiality is paramount. The education process is similar for all of these groups.

### *Process*

Family education is a continuous process because of the variable rates at which family members understand the effects of the brain illness, their emotional adjustment, and the person's stages of recovery. New information should be prioritized and paced at a rate at which it can be absorbed. Often, in the early stages of an illness, it is best to teach the family only about what to expect in the next few weeks. Information delivered at the wrong time may not be heard or may alienate the family. The education needs to meet the family's perception of the problems and priorities. Although the clinician has basic information to cover, the initial focus should be on answering questions. In other words, the contents listed in the following sections may represent a long-term goal or agenda for the clinician, but the educational process should be shaped by the needs of the family.

### *Content*

Education should include the nature of the disease process, the strengths and problem areas of the person with a brain illness, strategies for dealing with the problems, the roles of the family and of medical professionals in treatment, the nature of rehabilitation and recovery, the prognosis and the course of the illness, the experiences of families, and community resources.

### *Techniques*

Learning is generally most effective when it is active, so teaching should be interactive. In most circumstances, teaching should be explicit (Table 6.4). If family members are to pay attention to modeling, if they are to be coached in specific skills, and if they are expected to read literature and to come to group meetings, then they need to be oriented to these roles and to their importance. Otherwise, they may resent "intruding" professionals who try to tell them how to deal with their own family members. Some few people may strongly resist any explicit attempts at education. For them it may be better to make information available through literature racks, posters, implicit modeling, and contact with other family members.

#### *Answering Questions*

Answering people's questions is a very good place to begin education. This process is most effective when it encourages follow-up questions and includes confirmation that the message has gotten through. Asking, "Do you understand?" is usually inadequate. "Does that answer your question?" is a little better. Repeating the question back to the person is still better. For example, "You asked when he will go back to school. Now what do you think about when he might go back to school?"

**TABLE 6.4. Techniques of Family Education**

| |
|---|
| Answering questions |
| Modeling |
| Coaching |
| Mentoring |
| Individually written materials |
| Printed materials |
| Visual aids |
| Socratic dialogue |
| Story telling |
| Metaphor |
| Support groups |
| Group discussion |
| Lectures |
| Videos |
| Teaching to teach others |
| Observing testing |
| Test results (drawings, writing samples, scores) |

*Modeling*

For many problems it is especially effective to demonstrate to the family or to model for them how to manage the problem, for example, communicating with someone with aphasia, dealing with reflex crying, calming down someone who is upset, cuing a time out, or directing relaxation. Modeling can be carried out in formal therapy sessions or in informal settings such as at bedside, in the dining area, in the waiting room, or at home. All interactions with the person with the brain illness that occur in front of the family and the staff are modeling, whether intended or not.

*Skill Training*

It is not always sufficient just to model skills; they may need to be explicitly taught. An effective way to teach specific helping skills is to model them and then have the family member analyze what took place and copy it. This might be done live or with videotape of management of specific behaviors. When techniques are broken down into explicit steps and strategies, the family member can remember and apply them more effectively. Skills can be practiced through role-play and can then be used with the person while the therapist coaches.

*Coaching*

Observing family members interacting with the person can present an opportunity for coaching. This consists of praising them for what they are doing right, gently correcting what is wrong, redirecting what is partly correct, suggesting or modeling alternatives, and so forth. There is no substitute for hands-on experience in learning skills; many such experiences should be part of any extended family education program.

*Mentoring*

Mentoring is a process in which a clinician, or sometimes a support group member, develops an extended relationship with a family member, teaching, training, and guiding that person in how to deal with the person with the brain illness. This process may include elements of all of the techniques listed in this section. Blosser and DePompei (1995) noted that a mentoring relationship in rehabilitation (Table 6.5) differs from traditional information-giving family education. They listed selection criteria for mentors and for protegés (Table 6.6). They noted risks of mentoring (jealousy, misunderstandings, overinvestment), and described the design of formal mentoring programs (administrative support, needs assessment, interest, plan, objectives, resources, recruitment training, evaluation). They suggested that mentoring be fostered in other relationships besides that of clinician to family member.

### *Individually Written Materials*

Notes, report summaries, letters, treatment plans, lists of things to do, names and addresses, and summaries of educational sessions may take extra effort to prepare but are usually greatly appreciated. They frequently improve the effectiveness of messages delivered orally. Such materials are often then shared with other family members and with friends, multiplying their impact.

### *Printed Materials*

Printed materials are often easy and inexpensive to obtain. They can be individualized by writing on them, underlining, and so forth to increase their usefulness and the chances that they will be read. They help people see that their experience is not unique. They should be distributed somewhat sparingly so they

**TABLE 6.5. Mentoring Activities in Rehabilitation for Family Members and Others[a]**

| Activity | Characteristics |
|---|---|
| Informal contact | This usually occurs during hospital visits. Give permission to ask questions. Give limited general information. |
| Interactive dialogue | Make the family comfortable in rehabilitation. Involve the family in treatment. Involve the family in giving information and observations. Get the family thinking about the future. Maintain the family's motivation and hope. |
| Role modeling | This can occur during therapies, team meetings, interactions with staff and with visitors, telephone calls, and in-service meetings. The family learns how to talk with professionals and how to describe the situation of the person with the brain illness. |
| Demonstration | The therapist demonstrates techniques, including communication, behavior management, praise, and so forth; the family member copies techniques; the therapist gives feedback. |
| Observation and feedback | This takes place after the family member participates in therapy activities, teaching another family member, telephone calls to agencies, team meetings, interacting with staff, informal contact with person with brain illness, and so forth. This ventilates the family's feelings, refines their skills, and builds their confidence. |
| Direct assistance | Help organize rehabilitation systems, materials, information, and home setup. |
| Long-term planning | This includes problem-solving assistance, referrals, community services, and financial aid, networking with support groups and with other families, help in reconnecting with friends, and help in organizing roles of different family members in continued rehabilitation. |

[a] Adapted from Blosser and DePompei, 1995.

**TABLE 6.6. Mentoring Selection Criteria**[a]

| Role | Criteria |
|---|---|
| Mentor | Experienced<br>Good interpersonal skills<br>Good instructional skills<br>Available |
| Protegé | Eager to learn<br>Able to learn<br>Emotionally stable<br>Available |
| Mentor–protegé match | Compatible personalities |

[a] Adapted from Blosser and DePompei, 1995.

actually get read and so that they are directed toward specific situations, rather than giving an overabundance of literature that may not be entirely relevant or that may even be misleading.

*Visual Aids*

Drawings, diagrams, recovery curves, and so forth often help make a point more concrete and memorable. For example, the continuum of responsibility in Figures 2.4-2.6 (pp. 19, 22, 25) can be used to discuss where the family member thinks the person is. Posters and other materials are often available from support groups, from their national organizations, and from health education publishers. Art might be solicited or purchased from art therapy program participants for the clinic walls.

*Socratic Dialogue*

Socratic dialogue, named after the Greek philosopher who used it, is a method of questioning that allows the person questioned to discover his own knowledge. It consists of asking leading questions that help to structure the person's thought processes. The technique can be used for cognitive reframing (Meichenbaum, 1993) of a situation. In this way it sometimes crosses the lines between assessment, education, and problem-solving counseling (Case 6.3. Janaki's mother).

*Story Telling*

Story telling has a deservedly rich and ancient tradition in education because it is involving and memorable. It is used in professional clinical education

*Socratic Dialogue. Case 6.3. Janaki's Mother (fictitious).*

*Janaki's mother*: I'm worried. Janaki doesn't seem to want to do anything. She just spends all of her time in front of the TV.

*Neuropsychotherapist*: Is this different from before her accident?

*M*: Oh, yes! Sure, she watched some, but she used to be very active. She played baseball, had pen pals, helped with the chickens and pigs, she was always off with her friends.

*N*: So why do you suppose she doesn't do those things now?

*M*: I don't know. I'm worried she may be depressed.

*N*: Does she say she's depressed, or sad, or down in the dumps?

*M*: No, she doesn't say much, but if you ask her she says everything is fine.

*N*: Does she act sad?

*M*: No, she usually doesn't show many feelings at all, but when there are people around she's cheerful and kind of silly.

*N*: Is she pessimistic?

*M*: No, she says she's looking forward to school starting, and she still talks about becoming a doctor.

*N*: People who are depressed often have trouble with their sleep and appetite. Has she had any problems in those areas?

*M*: Well, she sleeps about an hour more than she used to, but that folder said she would after a brain injury. She doesn't get herself snacks like she used to, but she eats everything I put in front of her. She has just about gained back the weight she lost in the hospital.

*N*: So do you think she's depressed?

*M*: It sure doesn't sound like it.

*N*: I agree. When I talked with her she didn't seem to me to be depressed. You said this is different from before the accident?

*M*: Yes, it does seem like the accident caused it. What is it?

*N*: Well, we talked before about . . .

*M*: We made that list. Here it is, let's see, "Problems Initiating." Could that be it?

*N*: Let's find out. If someone suggests something, will she do it?

*M*: Oh, yes. If her brother starts a game, she'll play. And when her friends visit she has a good time with them. Sometimes she helps me with the housecleaning when I ask, but then that's not much different from before.

*N*: And what did you say about her appetite?

*M*: She doesn't make snacks, but she'll eat what's prepared for her. I see what this means now. She'll do things, she just won't do them on her own.

*N*: That's right. So what can you do about this problem?

*M*: Well, I guess we can all make an effort to ask her to do things.

*N*: Exactly. Why don't we talk with her about what things she'd like to be doing and make a plan . . .

in the form of case examples. When used in family education, case examples need to be made pertinent to the situation. It is also important that they be engaging, that they introduce a conflict or problem with drama and feeling, and that they arrive at some resolution. Humor and a bit of acting or role-playing helps move education beyond a dry discussion of facts, and it gives family members permission to express their feelings. Story tellers must be careful to convey respect toward those whom they describe. Even when describing someone of the therapist's own experience, confidentiality in story telling must be maintained, for example, by the formulation "I once heard of someone with a brain illness who . . ."

### *Metaphor*

Metaphors can be extremely useful in getting someone to understand a phenomenon, but they can backfire if wrongly applied. It is important to make sure that the metaphor is drawn from a familiar source and to check that it is properly understood. For example, someone with impaired initiation is like a car with a dead battery that needs a push from friends to roll start it. However, for a child not familiar with cars, a better metaphor might be to say that Daddy is like a wind-up toy. He won't come down off of the shelf to play with you all by himself, but if you wind him up, he'll play. To check on understanding one might then ask, "So if Daddy is sitting in the living room and you want to play with him, what would you do?"

Simple medical metaphors can often be useful. For example, cognitive and emotional rehabilitation prosthetics and orthotics are metaphors for their physical counterparts, although it is often better to present them more concretely. For example,

> When your wife reminds you of what you need to do or sings for you to help you calm down, that's like having her push you around in a wheelchair. When you use your memory book or your cue card, that's like using a cane. It helps you to do it on your own.

### *Support Groups*

Families should be referred to support groups whenever possible. The people in these groups often have experiences that the clinician does not have. Their experience has more validity for those who discount the opinions and knowledge of professionals. These groups are usually fairly familiar with community resources.

### *Group Discussion*

Many rehabilitation centers organize group educational programs for families. These differ from support groups in their organization and their direction. It is often preferable that these be carried out by health educators with formal teaching training. Clinicians without such training may want to seek the advice of a professional educator or educational literature (Lazes, Kaplan, & Gordon, 1987; Werner & Bower, 1982) on how to prepare for such an audience. Given the many unknowns about such a group, it is wise to spend time at the beginning exploring their needs, questions, and level of knowledge through introductions, "break the ice" games, question sessions, written questions, and so forth. Sometimes the best presentation is no formal "presentation" at all, but consists of an extended question-and-answer session.

*Lectures*

Formal lectures often give a very good initial impression but are frequently very ineffective in the long run. Families may be impressed with the knowledge and the vocabulary of the lecturer, but they may retain little if they cannot relate it to their needs and use it to change their own behavior. If a formal lecture is the only format possible, then it should at least relate as much as possible to everyday life. As Werner and Bower (1982) noted, "To start with anatomy is the kiss of death" (pp.5-12).

*Videos*

Educational videos and carefully selected motion pictures are excellent tools for making information lively and memorable and for generating discussion. Videotaping of the person with the brain illness engaged in an activity, possibly with a family member helping, can be used to discuss specific problems, abilities, and training techniques.

*Teaching to Teach Others*

Immediate family members who receive the bulk of the education at the clinic often have to educate extended family members, friends, teachers, and others. Family education programs should facilitate that process. Written materials, story telling, and metaphor can be easily passed on to others. Explicit discussion of teaching others may also be needed. This can be directive ("Be sure to tell his friends and teacher that . . ."), or it can be part of problem-solving counseling ("What do you think his school needs to know?"). This component of family education can even go as far as role-playing or preparing notes together.

*Observing Testing*

In some circumstances it is helpful for the family to observe some of the testing or a reproduction of the testing. This can be useful especially when the presence of the family member calms the person and allows him to give a better performance, when the presence of the family member does not disrupt testing, and when standardized test administration is not a priority. Tests of left neglect, emotional communication, and aphasia are particularly useful for demonstration. Permission from the test-taker is required.

*Test Results*

The technicalities of test scores and the normative base of testing is of much more interest to neuropsychologists than to family members. Although this information should be shared, concentrating on such data keeps the discussion firmly in the control and area of expertise of the clinician and may tend to discourage questions, fuller understanding, and relating results to everyday life. Drawing and writing samples and specific item responses can illustrate points dramatically and concretely.

*Integrating Neuropsychotherapy with the Family and the Treatment Team*

The person with a brain illness, the treatment team, and the family should all work from the same list of strengths, problems, strategies, and goals. Much of the neuropsychotherapist's time is spent consulting with the treatment team and educating the family. Some of this should be done in the presence of the person so this coordination of care is understood.

Responsibility for care coordination can be shared between the neuropsychotherapist and the person with the brain illness according to the continuum of responsibility. At one end of this continuum, for example, inpatient rehabilitation, the therapist may coordinate the intervention plan with the rehabilitation team, training team members in behavior management techniques and in record-keeping as necessary. In the middle of the continuum, such as postacute outpatient rehabilitation, the therapist might coordinate overall plans and goals and seek feedback and data from team members, whereas the person with the brain illness would be responsible for explaining specifics of his anger management plan to team members and to family members and for asking for their cooperation in following it and for their help in keeping an anger log. At the other end of the continuum, for example, outpatient neuropsychotherapy for a mild brain trauma, the person with the brain injury might be fully responsible for explaining to the family and to friends what problems he is experiencing, what he is doing about them, and what support he would like from others.

## *ETHICAL ISSUES*

The continuum of responsibility for behavior implies a continuum of competence to make decisions and to carry them out. The person with a brain illness may be competent for one type of decision or activity and not for another. He may be competent to delegate authority, or to make or to participate in a decision provided the relevant information is appropriately structured and presented, but may not be competent to manage the situation independently. The clinician needs to remain clear about who is the client, and should generally function as an advocate for the person with the brain illness and for his autonomy and rights.

Impaired clients have the right to refuse treatment and to refuse communication with family members or with others about their condition and about other confidential information. These rights should always be respected. If the clinician believes that the person's competence to make such decisions is impaired and the disclosure of information is at issue, the clinician should err on the side of protecting confidentiality. At the same time, general information about brain illness is not protected information. Family members can be educated about the general effects of brain illness without necessarily having the permission of a family member who happens to have a brain illness.

In the United States, by law, clinicians must obtain the informed consent of their patients before giving treatment. The phrase "informed consent" acknowledges the social reality of the passive patient role, although the economic fiction is that the patient not only consents to but actually requests the treatment. This can pose a dilemma for the neuropsychotherapist, particularly when dealing with anosognosia. Why would someone consent to treatment for a problem he does not know he has? How can the clinician respect the wishes of the client when those wishes are confused, unrealistic, or delusional? In extreme cases it may be necessary to go through the cumbersome legal process of having someone declared incompetent, having a guardian appointed, and then invoking involuntary treatment, a process which in itself may render progress highly unlikely. However, it is often possible to circumvent such procedures through an attitude of respect, patience, and accurate empathy, as described in the next chapter.

# 7

# General Techniques of Neuropsychotherapy and Related Interventions

## *THE THERAPY JOURNAL*

A therapy journal (or a diary or a recovery book, etc.) is a cognitive compensation for extended neuropsychotherapy for people with memory or organization impairments (Ellis, 1989). It may be a section of a cognitive rehabilitation memory book (Sohlberg & Mateer, 1989). It is for the client (and possibly the family), not for the therapist, whose clinical notes are separate.

A journal written by others for the person with an acute brain illness when that person is still confused or amnesic may later help the person get a perspective on her recovery. This may be a forerunner to a therapy journal or a memory book. Keeping such a journal helps family members gain perspective, process experiences, and direct productive energy at a time when they may feel helpless. Such a journal is a suggestion only, not a burden assigned to an overstressed family or busywork to keep family out of the way of therapists. It is hard to know in advance which people will be curious about their early illness and early recovery once they emerge from confusion or from post-traumatic amnesia and will want to read such a journal, and which ones will be indifferent. Alternately, a family may use photography, video, audio recording, or drawing to make a record of this time.

### *The Continuum of Responsibility*

The continuum of responsibility applies to use of the therapy journal. The sequence of patterns of use (Table 7.1) requires individual variations depending

**TABLE 7.1. The Continuum of Responsibility and the Therapy Journal**

The following is a sequence of possible stages of therapy journal use between a therapist and a person with a brain illness over the course of recovery of cognitive abilities and of responsibility.

1. Therapist and others write in the journal and read it to the person.
2. Therapist and others write, including ideas that the person contributes. The person reads the journal with assistance.
3. The person writes in the journal; the therapist and others contribute ideas and help organize the journal and the ideas, sometimes dictating exact wording. The person reads the journal alone as an assignment.
4. The person writes in the journal with oversight from the therapist, and without supervision as assignment. The person reads the journal as an assignment and spontaneously. The journal becomes private between the therapist and the person, moves out of the memory book into a separate book.
5. The person takes full responsibility for the journal, writing down session summaries and homework assignments spontaneously and using feelings journal when needed. The person shares session summaries freely with the therapist, but chooses which parts of the feelings journal are relevant to treatment and need to be shared.
6. The person continues to keep a journal without maintaining session summaries, sharing only what is relevant to treatment.

on reading and writing ability, cooperation, and so forth. It is the therapist's task to choose appropriate levels of responsibility for therapy journal use.

## *Sections*

No single journal will have all of the possible sections discussed here (Table 7.2), and other sections are possible.

### *The Neuropsychological Report and Other Medical Records*

A neuropsychological report (or summary) and other medical records may help the person remember what has happened and improve self-awareness.

**TABLE 7.2. Possible Therapy Journal Sections**

| |
|---|
| The neuropsychological report |
| Other medical records |
| Strengths and problems list |
| Session plan |
| Session summary |
| Homework |
| Reading assignments |
| Behavioral management records |
| Feelings journal |

*Strengths and Problems List*

The therapy journal should include a list of strengths, problems, strategies, and goals. This list is derived from the neuropsychological assessment, the evaluation by the rehabilitation team, the person with a brain illness, and the family. The list is written and prioritized by the neuropsychotherapist and by the person with the brain illness (Table 7.3).

*Strengths.* The strengths part of the list is important for self-esteem, for hope, and to help all involved to stay aware of available resources. When faced with someone with impairments in all neuropsychological areas, the therapist may feel challenged to find convincing strengths to list. It helps to reach beyond neuropsychological domains to strengths such as a supportive family, adequate income, strong religious faith, a sense of humor, and so forth. Strengths come from the perspective of the person and from that of the family. Some characteristics are seen as strengths by the person but not by the therapist; for example, stubbornness or resignation. It is best to list more strengths than problems.

*Problems.* The problems part of the list is short at first (3-5 items), addressing only the most prominent problems or those that the person is able and willing to recognize and to work on. More items may be confusing or overwhelming. The

**TABLE 7.3. Sample Strengths and Problems List[a]**

| STRENGTHS | | |
|---|---|---|
| Language Skills | | |
| Physical strength | | |
| Coordination | | |
| Sensation and perception | | |
| Motivation | | |
| Family support | | |
| Faith in God | | |
| Support of church | | |
| Sense of humor | | |
| **PROBLEMS** | **STRATEGIES** | **GOALS** |
| Poor concentration and distractibility | Attention training, reduce distractions | Driving, work |
| Memory difficulties | Memory book, Attention training | Work |
| Irritability | Time outs, anger log, cue card | Get along |
| Trouble understanding other people | Active listening | Maintain marriage |
| Alcohol | Alcoholics Anonymous, no alcohol in house, support of family | Complete sobriety |

[a] This list would result from several neuropsychotherapy sessions.

list is expanded as trust and awareness develop. Problems are removed as they are resolved. The list generally includes neuropsychological and related deficits and reactions, such as memory problems, irritability, distraction, embarrassment, headache, and so on. It can include other problems such as medical, social, or economic difficulties if this helps the person with the illness to "own" the list.

*Strategies.* The strategies section contains an abbreviated outline of a treatment plan from the perspective of the person with the illness. It is written in the first person, and it mostly refers to the person's own role and responsibilities in rehabilitation.

*Goals.* The goals section uses the functional language of rehabilitation (see Table 5.5, p. 68), referring to life functions such as walking, driving, work, relationships, money management, and so forth. It can be better to postpone goals if the prognosis is uncertain or if the person has limited awareness of her deficits.

### *The Treatment Contract*

An individualized, written treatment contract provides useful structure to formal therapy and provides feedback for the person with impaired self-awareness (for examples see O'Hara & Harrell, 1991). The strengths and problems list can serve this role.

### *Session Plan*

A written session plan or agenda helps build comfort, trust, and progress, particularly for individuals with difficulties with time regulation, self-control, and organization (see Table 6.1, p. 90).

### *Session Summary*

When dealing with problems of memory or of organization, each session should begin with a review of the previous session(s) and with an overview of the current session plan. Each session should end with a review of that session (Lewis, 1991), summarized in the therapy journal (Table 7.4).

### *Homework*

The review should also contain any agreed-to therapeutic homework. Although it may be difficult to get someone with a brain illness to complete homework, it should not be assumed that memory lapses or failure to appear for appointments, to complete assignments, or to bring the memory book are due to resistance to therapy. The therapist is responsible for finding compensations that allow the person to remember to complete assignments. This may involve placing notes on the bathroom mirror, the refrigerator, or the pill bottle; getting a family

**TABLE 7.4. Sample Neuropsychotherapy Session Summary**

(The following is what would get said in summary time in the session.)

Today we talked about how I yelled at Sue about dinner when she didn't deserve it. I didn't remember to take a time out, but when Sue signaled me I remembered and took a walk. The time out worked! I read my cue card, relaxed, apologized, and talked about it. My anger signs were when I clenched my jaw, yelled, and stood up. This episode happened because of my irritability, my frustration, and my trouble understanding other people. I still need work in these areas.

We talked about what Sue has gone through in the 6 months since my injury. She worried I would die, and then had to take care of the kids and the house, visit me in the hospital, work, and deal with insurance and less money. She took care of me when I came home. I was angry a lot. I don't remember a lot of that.

Last week I didn't take a time out when I needed to. I only wrote in my feelings journal and reviewed my journal 3 nights instead of every night. I only took two practice time outs instead of every day. That was better than the week before. Reading my journal helped me remember to take practice time outs.

To help me remember I will put this note on my pill bottle that says "Read, Write, Set Alarm," so I remember to read my therapy journal and handouts, write in my feelings journal, and set my alarm to take a practice time out the next day every evening when I take my pills. I will set a time to talk with Sue. Before we talk I will reread the Active Listening handout.

I will review my therapy journal with her. Then I will ask her what the last 6 months have been like for her and practice active listening while she tells me. Afterwards I will write down what I can remember. This is to help me to understand her.

(This is how the summary would get written in the therapy journal.)

5/22/91 Yelled at Sue. Took TO, her signal. TO worked! Used card. Anger signs: clenched jaw, yelling, standing. Due to irritability, frustration, problem understanding others.

Sue's burden—I almost died, kids, house, hospital visits, work, insurance, less money, my anger, I don't remember that.

Homework:

Forgot to take TO. Read and wrote X3, Practiced TOs X2.

This week:

1. Note on pill bottle. Read and write every night!
2. Set alarm for Practice TOs.
3. Set talk time with Sue. Reread Active Listening. Review journal with Sue. Ask her what last 6 mo. have been like for her. Write down afterward.
4. Next appointment, Wed., 5/29, 10am.

member to give reminders; calling the person; setting a daily alarm; putting a therapy and homework schedule in the memory book schedule, and so forth. The therapist is responsible for choosing assignments that the person can accomplish (within her zone of recovery). Finding that level can also be an exercise in self-awareness, with the person predicting what will be possible.

### *Reading Assignments*

Reading assignments should be matched to the person's cognitive abilities. It is often best to start with short, simple assignments, that contain less than two pages, with emphasis on re-reading the same material daily for several weeks (see Case 6.1. J. D., p. 86) and reading the therapy summary for the previous session each day. The strengths and problems list should be reviewed daily for several weeks. It is important to check that reading assignments are comprehended, remembered, and applied before advancing to more difficult or lengthy material. If not, more active ways of processing the information are needed, such as writing summaries of the material, giving examples, or explaining it to someone else.

### *Behavioral Management Records*

Behavioral management program records can be kept in the therapy journal. This makes the program explicit, understandable, and participatory to the person, and it facilitates transition from caregiver control to self-control. Because the therapy journal is kept with the person, the records will be convenient to record-keepers, producing more timely and accurate records.

### *Feelings Journal*

A feelings journal is appropriate for people who enjoy writing or who have previously kept journals, and for people with changed emotional responsiveness. The person writes down recent feelings at the moment or at set times, such as bedtime. The writing can be free-form or it can follow a format (see Table 6.3). A feelings journal helps people understand changes in their feelings, shows the therapist which techniques are effective, and helps directly in managing feelings, for example, by writing during a time out to clarify thoughts and to choose future actions.

## *Cultural Considerations*

A therapy journal is an unfamiliar undertaking for most people. Much of the world's population is illiterate or has limited literacy. Many people who are able to read functionally do not habitually write extended, independent thoughts. A therapy journal can still be an important tool for them. Indeed, something written specifically for and about them by a professional may be more significant for them than for habitually literate people. For those with limited literacy, independent writing, although welcome, should not be an important therapeutic goal or tool. Much of the therapy journal can be just as effective if the therapist does the writing.

Wide cultural variation can also be expected in the acceptability of the previous sections. A session agenda may be too directive for some cultures, or it may not fit with their attitudes toward time. Homework and reading assignments, behavioral management records, and a feelings journal may be unrealistic in some cultures. Privacy and family involvement in the therapy journal and in the therapy process will vary across cultures.

### *Alternatives to the Therapy Journal*

A therapy journal can easily be on a computer. For people with literacy limits, a tape recorder can be used for session summaries, for homework, for the feelings journal, and for reading assignments.

## *CUE CARDS*

Cue cards are cognitive compensations for coping with difficult events. They summarize strategies and techniques that have been worked out, explained, and practiced in therapy. Cue cards are best written cooperatively by the therapist and by the person, and possibly by a family member. They are individualized to the person and to the problem and cannot be prewritten or mass-produced.

Cue cards can be written or typed on index cards or Post-It notes, or can be written on the palm of the hand. Each cue card for a specific function for an individual should have its own distinctive color to make it easy to grab the right one at the right time. They can be carried in or on the memory book or the therapy journal, in a pocket, or in a wallet or a purse. They can be taped to wheelchair arms, lap trays, steering wheels, doors, mirrors, refrigerators, pill bottles, school books, purses, and so forth to be seen when needed. It is a good practice to make several copies of a cue card to be put in all of the appropriate places, with a copy on file for replacements.

Electronic memo-recorders are alternatives to cue cards, especially for people with reading difficulties, or when the emotional tone or the voice of a certain individual is particularly effective. Such devices present a different configuration of privacy issues and potential embarrassment with public use.

For most uses, cue cards should be brief. Titles and lists should prevail over narrative and complete sentences. Concrete, active wording and imperative voice usually work best. Exceptions are when scripts are needed, or when explanations to others take the form of a card or a letter to be handed to the other person.

### *Uses (Table 7.5a)*

#### *Emotional Control*

Cue cards can contain action plans for coping with episodes of problem emotions such as anger outbursts, panic attacks, and perplexity. They can contain instructions, informative reminders, and self-affirming statements (Table 7.5b).

#### *Procedures and Routines*

Cue cards are a common cognitive rehabilitation tool to help people remember the steps of a procedure, such as a list of a bathroom routine on the mirror, a list of things to take to work each day by the front door, or social procedures. This may be an actual script, an outline, or general reminders (Table 7.5c).

**TABLE 7.5. Cue Card Uses and Examples**

**TABLE 7.5a. Cue Card Uses**

Emotional control
Procedures and routines
Stressful events
Reminders
Behavior flash cards
Explanations to others
Wandering
Incidental functions

**TABLE 7.5b. Sample Cue Cards for Emotional Control[a]**

ANXIETY CUE CARD
My Anxiety Signs
- Tapping fingers, foot
- Fast breathing, heart
- Sweating
- Tense muscles
- Fussing and fidgeting

Relaxing Break
- Alone, quiet, dark
- Close eyes
- Breathe slowly, deeply
- Relax muscles
- Let go of worried thoughts
- Picture beach

SUDDEN DEPRESSION CUE CARD

Signs of Depression:

1. Negative thoughts
2. Crying
3. Thoughts of drugs and suicide
4. Things on TV that remind me of my life and children and pregnancy

When I Feel Depressed or When Fred Tells Me I Need To:

1. Tell myself: "I'm getting better. I can learn to control this myself!"
2. Distract myself:
   A. Watch Fred and the others
   B. Draw
   C. Write
   D. Nintendo
   E. Clean
   F. Cook
3. Ask Fred for help

[a] These are individualized cue cards for specific problems and strategies.

**TABLE 7.5c. Sample Cue Cards for Social Procedures**

BUYING FOOD AT JACK'S
- Stand in line
- Order food & drinks, 1st person
- Pay, 1st person, take receipt
- Get drinks, 2nd person
- Find table
- Get condiments from rack
- Listen for my number
- Take receipt to go get food, give receipt
- No tip, leave plates, etc.

ACTIVE LISTENING
- Quiet, alone with other person
- No TV, radio, music
- Not doing anything else
- Face other person, eye contact
- Don't interrupt or react (bite tongue)
- Repeat other person's feelings

### *Stressful Events*

Cue cards can be used to help prepare for predictable stressful events such as interviews, phone calls, parties, or public speaking. These cards may combine steps of cognitive procedures and reminders of emotional coping tools (Table 7.5d).

**TABLE 7.5d. Sample Cue Cards for Stressful Events**

PUBLIC SPEAKING
- Use written outline
- Practice alone and with friend
- Have friend in audience
- Short relaxation before going on
- "I can do it! I know my stuff. They are friendly and want to hear me."
- Find friend in audience
- Speak to back of room
- Slowly and clearly
- Smile!

TALKING TO A PHONE ANSWERING MACHINE

Hello, this is Wanea White with a message for Maria Sanchez. The head injury support group meeting will be on Friday, May 24th at 7 pm at the Mt. Zion Baptist Church. Call me if you have any questions at 639-4275. I hope to see you there.

*Reminders*

Brief, individualized reminders of emotional coping strategies can be posted in places where they will be seen frequently; for example "Relax!" "I can do it!" "There must be another way to tackle the problem," "Listen," "Think before acting," and so forth. A note on a pill bottle or a toothbrush might remind the person at the appropriate time to read an assignment, write in a feelings journal, or review the day.

*Behavior Flash Cards*

Behavior flash cards serve any of the previous four functions, except that they are very brief (usually four words or less), they are written large to be read from a distance, and they are presented to the person by someone else to cue a specific behavior (Hopewell, Burke, Weslowski, & Zawlocki, 1990). They are part of an agreed-on plan for dealing with a specific problem; they symbolize rather than fully describe the behavior. They should be brief to minimally interrupt the flow of action, conversation, and so forth. (Table 7.5e). They may be color-coded for fast identification. Symbols, numbers, or drawings can be used instead of words, especially for people with reading problems. Gestures or objects can be used with an agreed-on meaning but their use should be practiced before depending on them (Case 7.1. Gabby), especially if the person has memory problems.

**TABLE 7.5e. Sample Behavior Flash Cards**[a]

| |
|---|
| Smile |
| Time Out! |
| Relax! |
| Stop talking |
| You're repeating yourself |
| Speak up! |
| Softer |
| Eye contact |
| Ask a question |
| Listen |
| What is she feeling? |
| Best choice? |
| Stay focussed |
| Stop and Think |
| What is my goal? |
| Think ahead |
| Another way to do it? |

[a] Each line represents a separate card.

*Who, Me? Case 7.1. Gabby.* A 30-year-old man had executive dysfunctions due to myelomeningocele, among them excessive talking. While at dinner with another couple, his wife gave Gabby a little kick under the table to let him know that he was talking too much. This was not a signal that was previously agreed to. Congruent with his limited social judgment, he did not get the hint. Instead, he embarrassed her by asking indignantly, "What did you kick me for?" Thereafter, they agreed on and used signals for such situations.

Behavior flash cards and signals are particularly useful for problem-solving and for social situations. They can be used to train restoration or for compensations. They work well in classrooms. Families can develop signal systems for chronic problems ranging from "You're drooling," to "Change the topic," to "Come here."

### *Explanations to Others*

Cue cards can allow people who have difficulty expressing themselves because of aphasia, tracheostomy, and so forth to explain critical aspects of their condition to others. These cards can range from a brief outline of topics to a script to a letter of explanation that can be handed to someone (Table 7.5f–g).

**TABLE 7.5f. Sample Introductory Card for Neuropsychological Problem[a]**

To my friends:

My stroke makes me cry and laugh at times when I am not feeling particularly upset or amused. Please don't be frightened by it, and remember that I'm still the same me underneath that. Sometimes when I cry I will look up, or when I laugh I will rub my mouth. That helps me control it. If I cry, please just keep the conversation going, I'm really alright. If I laugh, you can laugh a little, too, but don't keep going just because I am, that only makes it harder for me to stop. Thanks for your understanding.

Emilio

[a]This card was written with and for a man with severe dysarthria, reflex laughing, and reflex crying from a brainstem stroke.

**TABLE 7.5g. Sample Cue Card for a Child with Fatigue and Irritability**

Since her accident, Kim gets tired easily and doesn't always realize it. If she starts to get cranky, please suggest a quiet rest and find her a place without distractions. Thanks. (signed by parent, physician, or therapist, as most appropriate)

**TABLE 7.5h. Sample Cue Cards for a Confused Person Who Wanders**

| |
|---|
| Joe, Call Home.<br>Phone Number: 268–8743<br>Stay calm, don't walk away.<br>Ask for help.<br>Love, Sue |
| Joe, Ask someone to show you the main entrance and meet me there. |

### *Wandering*

For people who wander and/or get lost, for example, some people in the early stages of Alzheimer's disease, a simple cue card (Table 7.5h) or identity bracelet with name, phone number, and "Memory impaired" (Mace & Rabins, 1991) may help.

### *Incidental Functions*

In addition to explicit cognitive compensation functions, cue cards serve secondary functions. As physical objects, they symbolize both a problem and a solution, increasing the generalization of self-awareness to a variety of contexts. Cue cards posted at home educate household members about the problem and the strategy. Posting the card is a statement to the household, an admission of the problem, and a commitment to work on it.

People do not think clearly in times of emotional distress. It can be difficult to remember and to employ therapeutic techniques for managing distress. Cue cards can help overcome this problem.

## *Cultural Considerations*

Cue cards are extraordinarily effective in a variety of cultures, even if psychotherapy is not prominent in the culture, and even if literacy skills are limited (Cases 7.2. Douglass; 7.3, Peleo). Reference to concrete behaviors helps acceptability. Cue cards can sometimes be adapted to illiteracy with drawings.

## *EMPATHY*

Accurate empathy for persons with brain illness is helped by knowledge of neuropsychology, clinical skills, and experience with this population. Brain illness is a foreign and bewildering experience; accurate empathy can be a tremendous relief. Because it is also often confusing to families, the person with a brain

*Working with What You've Got. Case 7.2. Douglass.* A 50-year-old, 5th grade educated laborer was referred for assessment 3 months after a mild TBI. He complained of irritability and sensitivity to noise and to activity, particularly noise from the upstairs neighbor. He was afraid that his anger would get him in trouble.

Douglass was initially somewhat suspicious of the evaluation (most probably due to ethnic and to class differences with the examiner) and was circumspect in giving his history. Testing revealed moderate impairments in attention and in memory. In the feedback session he warmed up as he felt himself being understood (he later described this experience). He was given a very simple cue card (because of limited reading abilities) for anger, but he was not interested in a follow-up appointment.

He called 2 months later for an appointment, mostly seeking repeat reassurance that he was not crazy. He reported that he had rewritten the cue card larger, had put it on his kitchen table, and it had taken care of his problem.

This case illustrates the importance of accurate empathy. It also demonstrates the effectiveness of the physical symbol of a cue card, even with limited reading ability, and in an individual who did not appear to be a promising psychotherapy candidate.

illness may feel misunderstood or cut off from her usual support. Acute care medical personnel may sometimes treat her more like an object or a case than a person with feelings. Establishing credibility and trust through accurate empathy is often the first task of the neuropsychotherapist or of the other helper.

It is easy to arrive at pseudoempathy by saying to oneself, for example, "If I

*Naming the Problem. Case 7.3. Peleo.* A 31-year-old, 6th grade educated laborer was seen in Costa Rica for treatment 1 year after a severe TBI. He had moderately impaired memory, attention, and executive functions, and a moderate left hemiplegia. He walked with a cane and had not been able to return to his previous job, so he sold lottery tickets on the street.

His wife reported separately that he was quite aggressive and violent at home and in public, and that he often assaulted her and got into fights. This had been his pattern before his injury and it had not changed. She was almost ready to leave him because of his violence, although he was unaware of this.

He felt that his aggression was justified and understandable because he felt that he had no control over it. Nevertheless, he expressed a strong interest in stopping his violence and his aggression, in part because of the harm it did to others, and in part out of fear for his own physical vulnerability now that he was disabled.

Although he had considerable difficulty understanding the concepts, he was given a cue card for time outs to control his aggression. At the second session his wife reported separately that his aggression was greatly reduced due to his use of the cue card, and she was very pleased. He was also aware of and pleased by his progress.

couldn't read, control my bladder, walk, dress, or feed myself, I'd sure be depressed." Yet such projections are often inaccurate with anosognosia. Such a person may well truly be more concerned about a TV show than her deficits because she does not recognize or worry about her own condition. Attending to the person's true concern may help establish a working relationship (Bergquist & Jacket, 1993).

Another type of pseudoempathy is the superficial relating of the person's experience to one's own experiences. A common complaint at brain trauma and Alzheimer's support groups is of the well-meaning friend who remarks, "I forget appointments and lose things, too." These types of remarks discount and minimize the person's distress.

Often the clinical skill of "active listening" (Rogers, 1980) must be more "active" than "listening," especially with people with aphasia, physically constrained communication, or impaired initiation. This adapted technique involves surmising or anticipating the person's feelings and then seeking confirmation. For example, the therapist might say to someone with a tracheostomy who appears distressed, "People with brain injuries like yours often feel confused and frightened. Is that how you feel?" To a crying person with severe expressive aphasia, a clinician might say, "Many people who have had strokes like yours cry often. Does that happen to you?" [Head nod]. "Often they don't mean to cry." [Head nod]. "They may cry when they are not upset. Does that happen to you?" [Head nod]. These can be leading questions; the therapist needs to avoid being led astray by a desire to please or by a "yes" response set. If language comprehension is limited or questionable, questions need to be restated to confirm that they are understood, for example, "Do you mean to be crying?" "Do you cry when you don't mean to?"

With care, slow but meaningful therapy can take place with people who are only able to reply "yes" or "no", like a game of 20 Questions. Such extra effort is worth the trouble. There are few experiences more frightening and confusing, and in need of accurate empathy and communication, than being locked in one's body by a brain illness with little or no way of acting on one's own behalf.

Another powerful way to show empathy is to refer to others with similar experiences. This lets the person know that the experience is due to the brain illness, that she is not alone in the experience, and that the therapist is experienced and understanding.

For those with language difficulties, nonverbal communication becomes more important. Appropriate touch, getting physically close, and eliminating distractions often help with more severely impaired individuals. With a person with left neglect or with eye movement difficulties it helps to move into her line of sight to establish eye contact.

Another neuropsychological variation of accurate empathy is in validation therapy (Table 7.6) for Alzheimer's disease and for other dementias (Feil, 1993). In this therapy active listening is refined into an almost pure focus on the emo-

**TABLE 7.6. Principle Techniques of Validation Therapy**[a]

1. Use non-threatening, factual questions—who, what, where, when, how, but not why.
2. Repeat a key word.
3. Use eye contact and a nurturing voice.
4. Use appropriate touch.
5. Reflect genuine feelings.
6. Link the behavior to universal human needs.
7. Use a vague pronoun when the meaning is not clear.
8. Mirror the person's motions and emotions; move with the person.
9. Do not confront disorientation or contradict disoriented ideas, but do not affirm them, either. Instead, validate feelings.
10. Use nonverbal modalities—music, drawing, movement—to facilitate the expression of feelings.
11. Use reminiscing.

[a] From *The Validation Breakthrough: Simple Techniques for Communicating with People with Alzheimer's-Type Dementia,* by N. Feil, 1993, Baltimore, MD: Health Professions Press. Copyright 1993 by N. Feil. Adapted with permission.

tional content of the confused person's message. The reflection of the person's feelings is so stripped of reality anchoring as to stop just short of entering the person's delusion. It is most typically used with people with moderate to severe Alzheimer's disease, where attempts to orient the person to "objective" reality may yield small rewards for considerable efforts and may provoke needless confrontation. Validation therapy reportedly results in increased emotional understanding and more harmonious relationships. Its goal is not to make the person more objectively functional or oriented. This is an approach more adapted to caregiving than to formal psychotherapy (Case 7.4. Tillie). This general perspective is increasingly getting incorporated into more comprehensive dementia care programs (Jones, 1996; Olsen, Ehrenkrantz, & Hutchings, 1993; Robinson, Spencer, & White, 1989).

*Validation Therapy. Case 7.4. Tillie*[a]. Tillie was an 88-year-old woman in "time confusion" who was found by Gloria, a nurse trained in validation therapy, in the wrong bed. Tillie pointed at Gloria and accused, "You can't have him, you hellstopper. Don't think I don't know convertabodies. Now go away," and she spat at Gloria. Gloria calmed her own fears and observed Tillie. She bent close to her and said in a caring voice, "She was a hellstopper? What did she do to you?" Tillie answered, "She stole my boyfriend. That's what. All the boys. With a convertible. Hellstopper. Stopper." Gloria massaged Tillie's back and asked, "You're angry because she stole your boyfriend?" They talked about the convertible car, and Gloria guided Tillie out of the bed and back to her own floor. Gloria asked, "When you say hellstopper, do you want someone to stop her from hurting you?" Tillie replied, "It's too late. Too late," and cried.

[a] From "Validation Therapy for the Time-Confused," by N. Feil, 1986, *Geriatric Care, 18*(5), 1–2. Copyright 1986 by N. Feil. Adapted with permission.

## SELF-AWARENESS

Work on self-awareness pervades neuropsychotherapy and neurorehabilitation. Overestimation and underestimation of one's own disabilities can result from emotional or motivational needs, emotional states, lack of information, misinformation, impaired executive functions, cognitive impairments, and pre-illness personality characteristics. Distorted self-awareness can be complicated by misperceptions of disability by family members, which may be based on a lack of information and of experience or on their own emotional needs. The exact mix of causes is often difficult to determine and changes over time and with recovery, but it is important to understand for planning interventions.

### *Overestimation of Disability*

Some people with brain illnesses underestimate their own abilities and overestimate or catastrophize about their disabilities. This misperception can come from thought patterns of depression and frustration, impairments in reasoning, and a lack of information about recovery and rehabilitation. It can be a convenient way to maintain a desired dependence or disability role with secondary payoffs of attention from others, relief from burdensome responsibilities, and/or compensatory payments (Cicerone, 1991). Overestimating disability can vary with the time course of the illness (Figures 7.1 and 7.2). This type of person may go through a cycle: try, fail, quit, despair, and develop learned helplessness (Moore & Stambrook, 1995).

*Risks*

Overestimation of disability can be a hidden obstacle to many other rehabilitation goals (Table 7.7).

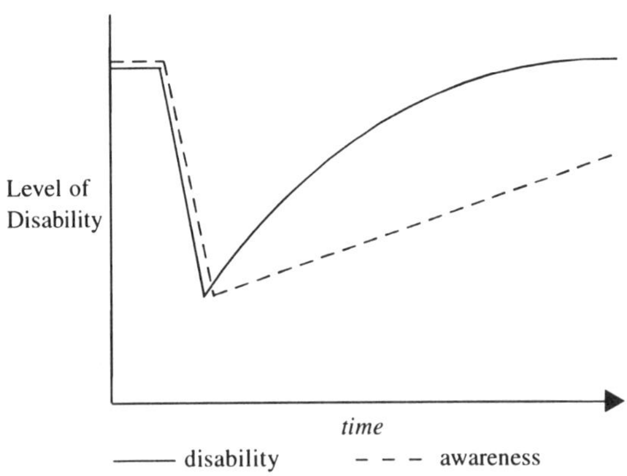


FIGURE 7.1. Awareness versus disability, sudden onset, with depression/catastrophic reaction.

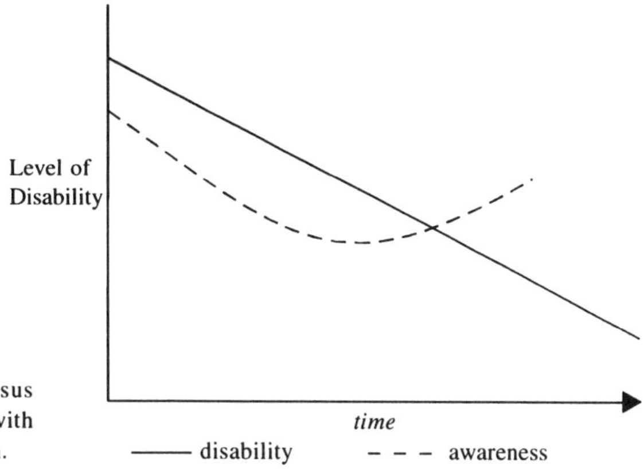


FIGURE 7.2. Awareness versus disability, progressive onset, with depression/catastrophic reaction.

*Techniques*

The choice of techniques for working with overestimation of disability (Table 7.8) depends in part on the causes. Related techniques can be adapted from those for underestimation of disabilities (in the following section), and for overprotection (Chapter 13).

*Mild Illness*

The person with a mild TBI, brain infection, neurotoxicity, or similar condition sometimes faces a peculiar dilemma. She may have no outward sign of a brain disorder, such as motor or speech difficulties or visible scars, so others see her as normal. Yet she knows something is wrong. Perhaps she cannot remember or concentrate as well as she used to, or has bursts of anger she does not understand, or cannot express her thoughts clearly. She may hide her invisible disability from others and be seen as unreliable. Alternately, she may try to convince others that something is wrong and may be seen as a complainer or a hypochondriac. In attempting to convince others (sometimes including unsympathetic medical personnel), she can come to believe that she is more incapacitated than she is.

**TABLE 7.7. Risks of Overestimation of Disability**

| |
|---|
| The pain of depression itself. |
| Lack of rehabilitation effort and decreased recovery. |
| Overprotection by family and decreased recovery. |
| The expense, burden, dependence, embarrassment, and discouragement from unnecessary caretaking services. |
| Disengagement and withdrawal from appropriate activities. |

**TABLE 7.8. Techniques for Working with Overestimation of Disability**

| |
|---|
| Educate the person and the family about the course of recovery and of rehabilitation (see Family Education in Chapter 6, p. 96). |
| Be generous with praise and encouragement (as long as it is accepted as genuine). |
| Focus on short-term, achievable goals. |
| Break down tasks into achievable components. |
| Maximize success experiences. |
| Maintain progress records that are accessible to the person, and review them frequently with the person. |
| Use humor, good-natured goading, and mild competition to get the person to try something. |
| Contract with the person and the family to try selected activities, even if they do not believe they will be successful. |
| Consider evaluation and treatment of depression. |
| When the person has sufficient cognitive abilities, techniques for challenging cognitive errors of depression (Burns, 1981; Hibbard et al., 1987) can be used (regardless of formal diagnosis of depression). |
| When secondary gain is contributing to overestimation of disabilities, those issues need to be addressed directly through neuropsychotherapy, family education, family therapy, or work in a larger social context (see Chapter 13). |

In such circumstances, the symptoms should, of course, be evaluated. Given the known limitations in the sensitivity of neuropsychological tests, the experience of the symptoms should generally be validated and the possibility of continued symptoms should be acknowledged (Cicerone, 1991; Kay, 1992), even in the face of equivocal test results. Reinterpretation and reframing of the significance of the symptoms is often necessary (Mittenberg, Zielinski, & Fichera, 1993). Once symptoms are acknowledged, labeled, and better understood, they often become less frightening and disabling. From that point the focus should be on increasing function and actual activity. Attitudes and beliefs that maintain symptoms and decrease function should be addressed and reframed. Finally, she may need to adjust her self-image and decide how and when to tell others about the symptoms.

### *Underestimation of Disabilities*

Underestimation of disabilities (See Lack of Awareness of Deficits, Chapter 11, p. 233) can come from any combination of the following (Figures 7.3 & 7.4):

1. Direct injury to the neural substrates of self-awareness. This organic lack of awareness of deficits, or anosognosia, may be partial or complete; it may be present for some deficits but not for others (Prigatano & Schacter, 1991), and may vary with how questions are asked (Sherer et al., 1998).
2. Lack of relevant experience following the brain illness that prevents the discovery of the problems.

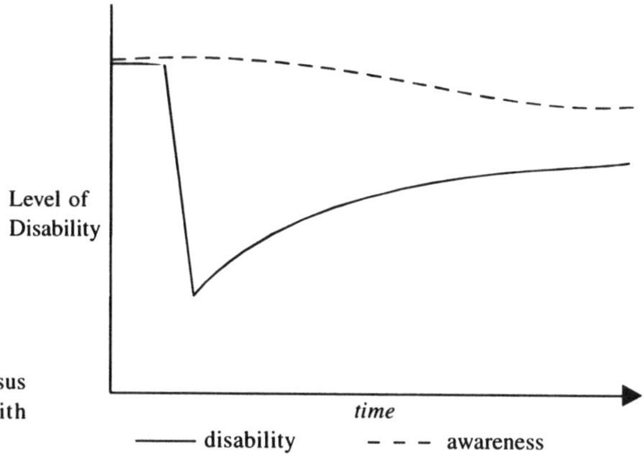


FIGURE 7.3. Awareness versus disability, sudden onset, with anosognosia/denial.

3. Impaired generalization skills preventing the projection of difficulty in one area to another.
4. Psychological denial, a primitive defense mechanism wherein the person simply refuses to accept the reality of the deficit (see Denial, Chapter 9, p. 156).

It is important not to confuse hope with lack of awareness. "I hope to return to work" is different from "I'm ready to return to work," although both might get expressed as "I'm going to go back to work" (Ridley, 1989).

*Risks (Table 7.9)*

The underestimation of disabilities is one of the most common, critical, challenging, and frustrating problems in all of neurorehabilitation and neuropsychotherapy.

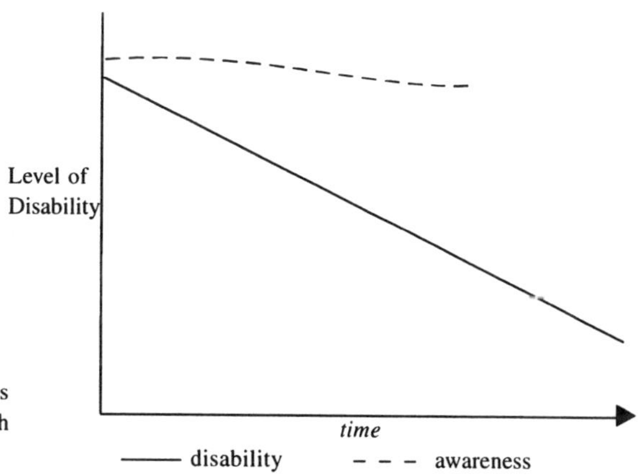


FIGURE 7.4. Awareness versus disability, progressive onset, with anosognosia/denial.

**TABLE 7.9. Major Risks of Underestimation of Disabilities**

| |
|---|
| Safety (when the person attempts something dangerous she is not capable of, e.g., driving, using firearms, using power tools). |
| Interpersonal problems (aggression, broken promises, disinhibited sexual behavior, etc.). |
| Financial losses (loss of work, impulsive spending, failure to pay bills, etc.). |
| Limited recovery due to lack of rehabilitation effort. |

### *Interventions: General Considerations*

*Using the Evaluation to Guide the Intervention.* The first three sources of underestimation of disabilities listed previously are organic and primarily cognitive. When people with only these types of lack of awareness are given information about their deficits they often react with interest, gratitude, indifference, or incredulity, but rarely with anger, anxiety, or distress. Intervention strategies for these forms of lack of awareness can be primarily cognitive. Treatments for anosognosia are described in the following paragraphs. A lack of relevant experience can be addressed by providing relevant experience. Impaired generalization can be improved through cognitive rehabilitation and direct instruction.

Denial, however, is primarily an emotional defense mechanism. When denial is confronted the reaction is usually resistance, anxiety, and escape. Denial needs to be addressed gradually with supportive confrontation while supplying more adaptive replacement defenses (see Denial, Chapter 9, p. 156).

*Distinguishing Knowledge from Action.* Crosson and colleagues (1989) distinguished three levels of self-awareness (Table 7.10). Both interviews and observations are needed to distinguish among these levels. A person's awareness may vary among these levels for different disabilities. For example, she might have anticipatory awareness of her of hemiplegia, but only intellectual awareness of her impaired judgment.

With intellectual awareness (Cases 7.5. R.; 7.6. Cerebra), it is possible to reach a therapeutic alliance for an intervention plan and a strengths and problems

**TABLE 7.10. Three Levels of Awareness of Deficits**[a]

| Level | Examples |
|---|---|
| Intellectual awareness | Can repeat what others have described about deficits<br>Can recognize errors after the fact when they are pointed out |
| Emergent awareness | Can recognize errors as they happen<br>Can attribute errors to brain illness deficits |
| Anticipatory awareness | Can predict difficulties with activities based on awareness of deficits and can initiate compensations<br>Can correct errors as they happen |

[a] Adapted from Crosson, et al., 1989.

*The Selectivity of Anosognosia. Case 7.5. R.*[a]. A successful businesswoman had a right frontal astrocytoma surgically removed. She returned to work a year later with a much lower workload. She had only subtle signs of a deficit on neuropsychological testing but was very disorganized on everyday tasks, rarely arriving at work before 11 a.m. and rarely achieving her goals. In a role play as her own direct supervisor, she was able to give logical recommendations for seeking a disability pension. Yet, although she usually recognized and acknowledged her shortcomings, she continued to insist that she attempt to work at her pre-surgery level.

[a]From "Disturbance of Self-Awareness after Frontal System Damage," by D. Stuss, 1991, in *Awareness of Deficit after Brain Injury: Clinical and Theoretical Issues* (pp. 74–77), edited by G. P. Prigatano and D. L. Schacter, New York: Oxford University Press. Copyright 1991 by Oxford University Press. Adapted with permission.

list, but considerable direct feedback is needed to work on emergent awareness. With emergent awareness, it is possible to begin training compensatory strategies, but work on recognizing risk factors and warning signs of problems (see Chapter 8. p. 138) is still needed. When anticipatory awareness is present, compensatory and restoration strategies can be firmly established and elaborated.

On the other hand, some people verbally deny deficits, but they collaborate with therapies and adjust to disabilities in their actions. Verbal acknowledgement of deficits then becomes a lower priority for intervention.

*Supportive Confrontation.* Underestimation of one's disability calls for supportive confrontation, where the comfort of the therapist's support for the person overcomes the discomfort of confronting the disability. Such education also often confronts psychological denial, so it is important to prioritize interventions according to immediate needs in her life. As long as she is not dangerous, does not jeopardize her future, and is cooperating with rehabilitation, it is best to confront a lack of awareness gradually.

Supportive confrontation must maintain a delicate balance between hope and despair. Reactive depression is an almost inevitable component of coping with the losses of brain illness. It is likely to come in waves of awareness. The task of the neuropsychotherapist is not to prevent such experiences, but to help

*To Know Is Not Enough. Case 7.6. Cerebra.* Cerebra was a neuropsychologist who developed a right frontal tumor and left neglect. Because of her training, she was highly knowledgeable about left neglect, and was well aware that she had it. She reported that when she thought about it consciously she could compensate for her neglect. However, as soon as she got busy or distracted she found herself losing things and bumping into things on the left. Her verbal, academic, and clinical knowledge of her left neglect, although extensive, was not adequate to allow her to compensate for it consistently.

the person to navigate them successfully (see Linge, 1980, and Meltzer, 1983, for moving first-person accounts of this process in psychologists recovering from brain illnesses).

*Struggle.* It is all too easy for caregivers to get locked into a struggle with someone with a brain illness over a lack of awareness of deficits. She may insist on going out alone, driving unsafely, drinking alcohol, or refusing therapies, for example. She may doggedly repeat a single position, getting more and more emotionally and cognitively entrenched. Occasionally such struggles are benign or even productive and result in insight. Usually they are painful and unproductive.

Such protracted struggles are to be avoided when possible. If she is in post-traumatic amnesia, it may be easy to distract her, after which she may forget the issue and cooperate. Later in recovery, distraction or postponement at the beginning of a struggle helps to avoid entrenchment. When feelings cool it may be possible to propose creative solutions or compromises and bring these around to a self-awareness technique (Case 7.7, Juan).

*The Perspective of the Person with the Brain Illness.* Whenever possible, work on awareness proceeds from the perspective of the person with a brain illness to encounter and explore areas of difficulty together with the therapist. It is almost always possible to get her to acknowledge some problem, even if only through projections onto others; for example, "My parents don't understand me," "My husband doesn't love me," or "No one will hire me," and to guide her toward self-awareness in exploring these problems (Case 7.8. Ingrid).

### *Techniques*

*Feedback Tools.* Mirrors, photographs, audiotapes, videotapes, work samples, writing samples, and arts and crafts products are useful feedback tools that can

> *Negotiating Supported Failure. Case 7.7. Juan (fictitious).* Juan was a young man with deficits in attention and in balance from a TBI who lived with his parents. He insisted to his father that he be allowed to walk alone to his friend Amal's house, five blocks away. His father postponed the discussion and aborted rising emotions by saying that they would discuss it with Juan's mother when she got home. His parents said that they did not think he was safe walking alone, although he did. They proposed that he walk to Amal's house with one of them walking a few steps behind him so he could prove to them he could do it safely. Juan objected that they would say he was not safe no matter how he did. They proposed that Amal follow him and judge his safety and Juan accepted. Through this process he discovered that he could not yet negotiate street crossings safely, because Amal had to pull him back from walking in front of a car.

*Who's in Charge Here? Case 7.8. Ingrid (fictitious).* This dialogue illustrates using the perspective of the client to work on anosognosia.

*Neuropsychotherapist*: Ingrid, You have told me that your problem is that your doctor won't let you drive. Why did she say that is?

*I*: Oh, yeah, I remember. She said I have that left neglect, whatever that is.

*N*: Well, here's a handout that describes it. Let's read it together. (In the process of reading Ingrid neglects some of the words on the left side of the page. The neuropsychotherapist points this out, and Ingrid is able to recognize it.)

*N*: Do you remember when you missed some words in your reading? Why do you suppose that was?

*I*: Careless, I guess.

*N*: Let's take a look at the words you missed. You see, they are all here on the left side. That's left neglect. If you're not noticing things on the left side, how do you suppose that might affect your driving? What's on your left when you drive?

*I*: The on-coming traffic. Gee, I guess that would be a problem!

*N*: That's right! Fortunately, there's therapy for left neglect. You'll have to work at it, and I can't promise your doctor will let you drive, but it's worth a try. . . .

In this example the clinician goes from the problem Ingrid perceives—"My doctor won't let me drive"—to the experience of an underlying neuropsychological problem—left neglect—tying that back to Ingrid's problem and to a rehabilitation strategy.

help increase self-awareness (Ellis, 1989) (Case 7.9. J. D.), especially when similar pre-illness materials are available. These are most useful when the person has been implicitly or explicitly prepared for the feedback.

Many people resist being photographed or seeing themselves on tape. This reticence must be accommodated and respected. It may help to record benign activities first to let the person adjust to the experience. Clinicians must always get permission to tape or to photograph someone.

Taping can be used in the absence of a therapist or of another helper in the taping, review, or both, if the person has the appropriate abilities. Videotaping can be used to check on walking, dancing, acting, social presentation, homemaking tasks, work tasks, and so forth. With audiotaping the person can practice talking, making music, interacting with others (Case 7.10. Elvis), and rehearsing events

*Mirror, Mirror, on the Wall. Case 7.9. J. D. (Case 6.1, p. 86, revisited).* J. D. arrived for every therapy session dressed in a suit and tie, apparently trying to continue to dress the part of a lawyer and to recapture his previous role. However, he usually failed in the fine details—his hair was mussed, his tie was askew, his shirt tail was out, his jacket was food-stained, or his fly was unzipped. One part of the therapy session, therefore, was often carried out in front of a mirror.

*And Now, from Studio R. Case 7.10. Elvis.* Elvis was a 17-year-old male seen 8 years after a TBI affecting primarily his right hemisphere. He had good motor, memory, and language recovery and had completed high school with adequate grades, although he had few friends and was only marginally accepted socially (contrasting with good pre-injury socialization). He had significant visual–spatial, social judgement, and musical difficulties and had limited awareness of his impairments. Following graduation there was little structure in his life. He neither studied nor worked and gradually slid into depression, which is why his mother brought him for therapy.

When asked about his future, he said that he did not need to study or work because he was going to be a rock music star. He played a guitar at home, but did not play with anyone else. I asked him to sing. He was too embarrassed to do this, but agreed to tape record himself and bring the recording in. At the next session he "forgot" to bring the tape. During the following session we listened to the tape together. He was terrible. Little was said; it was not necessary. During the following session he talked about getting a part-time job and going back to school, both of which were eventually achieved with considerable direction, structure, and weekly homework. With meaningful activity, his depression lifted and therapy terminated with his successful integration into a disabled students support group at his community college. A year later he called to report his academic successes and plans and to ask for advice regarding a girlfriend whom he met through the support group.

such as leaving a message on a telephone answering machine, public speaking, and saying something emotionally difficult to another person.

*Neuropsychological Tests.* Test results and test readministrations can be used as educational treatment tools. For some people a straightforward discussion of test results compared to a normative sample is adequate. Arguments about validity of tests, qualifications of testers, the meaning of "normal," and so forth are best avoided. Special preparation before testing can help (Case 7.11. Thomas).

Care must be taken in using this approach either to use informal measures, as in Case 7.11, to avoid breaking test protocol, or to note the breaking of protocol in the test report. Reviewing the details of errors on tests of memory, on problem-solving, on information, or on visual construction with the test-taker could invalidate future administrations of those tests.

It can be very effective to give the person a copy or a summary of the neuropsychological report. If this is written clearly, without technical jargon, it can clarify issues and decrease paranoia.

*Self-Awareness Training.* The key to retraining self-judgement is that the person practices making judgments about her abilities both before and after an activity

*Using Tests to Build Awareness. Case 7.11. Thomas (fictitious).*

*Neuropsychologist*: You told me you don't think you have any thinking difficulties from your brain injury. People with brain injuries often have thinking difficulties they are not aware of because the part of the brain responsible for that awareness is injured. I would like to give you some tests of your thinking abilities so you can understand your injury better and so that we can know how to help you better, OK? I will say 4 words I want you to remember. I will ask you for them in 5 minutes. Most people remember all 4. How many do you think you will remember?

*Thomas*: All four.

*N*: OK, we'll write that down, "you think you will remember all 4 words after 5 minutes." Here are the words . . .

[5 minutes later] Here we see you said you thought you would remember all 4 words like most people, but you only remembered one. People with brain injuries are often unaware of their thinking difficulties because the awareness part of the brain is injured. Could this have happened to you?

*T*: I suppose it could have.

*N*: What do you think this little test showed?

*T*: Maybe my memory isn't as good as I think it is?

*N*: Let's write "Memory difficulty" and "Decreased self-awareness" on your strengths and problems list. I imagine you might feel sad and frightened to find you can't do something you thought you could. Is that how you feel?

and gets feedback about her judgments, and not just about her abilities and errors in the activity (Table 7.11, Stage 1). Ideally, this practice will be in the form of errorless learning, particularly in the second and third stages. The second stage uses this procedure and the awareness it has generated to incorporate compensations into functional activities. The third stage weans the person from dependence on the cues of the therapist. This technique is best applied when psychological denial is not high, and after intellectual awareness has begun.

*Games.* W. R. Chittum, Johnson, Chittum, Guercio, and McMorrow (1996) have developed and tested a board game for the direct training of deficit awareness in individuals with severe traumatic brain injuries. They focused progressively on knowledge, on comprehension, and on application and achieved improved awareness, as probed by independent interviewers.

*Self-Monitoring Exercises.* The incident log, feelings journal, and other self-rating inventories can be helpful in making self-observation more overt. Sometimes self-monitoring alone improves self-awareness.

**TABLE 7.11. Self-Awareness Training**

Stage I: Increasing Awareness

This stage begins when a therapy plan and program have been established.

1. Clinician Orients Client to Self-Awareness Training
   The clinician explains that impaired self-awareness is a common consequence of brain illness, referring to the strengths and problems list. In addition to working on the ability to do the specific task, they will be working on improving the client's ability to judge her own performance on the task before and after doing the task. This is part of rehabilitation and is not to punish or shame her.
2. Client Predicts Task Performance
   The clinician prompts with specific questions, quantifying and writing down predictions when necessary.
3. Client A ttempts the Task
   Clinician allows the client to do as much as possible, helping only when necessary.
4. Client Evaluates Her Own Task Performance
   Clinician prompts them with appropriate questions.
5. Client Gets Feedback
   The clinician's feedback is especially about the client's predictions and evaluations as compared to the actual performance. Feedback is not morally judgmental.

Stage II: Compensation

This stage begins when the client has developed some awareness of her disabilities but is not able to initiate compensations.

1. Clinician Orients Client to Self-Awareness Training
2. Client Predicts Task Performance
3. Client Plans Compensation or Strategy
   The clinician cues and assists as necessary.
4. Client Attempts the Task
5. Client Evaluates Her Own Task Performance
6. Client Gets Feedback
7. Client and Clinician Evaluate Compensations
   They plan new compensations if needed.

Stage III. Fading

This stage begins when the client is fairly reliable at judging her task performance and at initiating compensations. The clinician gradually fades use of explicit steps of Stage II (Table 8.7). Depending on the individual and on the activity, cuing may be transferred to a cue card. Evaluation of compensation strategies is the last step to be faded.

*Medical Records.* It can be very useful to review CT scans, EEG reports, emergency room notes, behavior descriptions, examination reports, and so forth with the person and to put copies in the therapy journal. This review can help her to gain perspective and to stress the seriousness of the original illness and the hope of continued recovery. Care must be taken to get the approval of the attending physician and of the authors of the records.

*Educational Materials.* Many good public education materials describing various aspects of brain illnesses are available from advocacy organizations, from support groups, and from other sources, or they can be prepared in advance (DeBoskey, Hecht, & Calub, 1991; Mace & Rabins, 1991). Well-chosen materials that are brief and easy to read can help the person understand that her illness experience is not unique and that there is no conspiracy or personal vendetta to consider her incompetent or in need of restrictions.

*Group Therapy.* Group therapy that truly facilitates interactions among people with brain illnesses (and some support groups) may allow the person to experience the depth of her loss and to realize its manifestations in many different areas of life.

*Supported Failure.* Some people with brain illnesses need to experience failure in the "real world" to realize their limitations and their need for adaptations, compensations, or treatment. Certain life experiences can be encouraged as therapeutic exercises or as homework assignments, if the risks are tolerable. Some can be orchestrated to prevent disaster. If Juan (Case 7.7) steps off a curb unwisely and gets frightened by a car whizzing by while Amal pulls him back, this would be supported failure. Similarly, many rehabilitation programs place people in job stations with a job coach before they risk former jobs or new job opportunities (Parenté, Stapleton, & Wheatley, 1991).

*Real-Life Experiences.* Real-life experience is the best way to improve self-awareness for some people. Passes to home or to the community from the rehabilitation hospital can be crucial. It is best to prepare people with impaired self-awareness for possible difficult experiences on their first passes and upon discharge. Some initially refuse rehabilitation services entirely. The seasoned therapist will avoid rejecting the person for this reason and will leave the door open if the person comes to feel the need for treatment. The following type of parting statement allows someone to save face in a later return for services:

> I do hope you are right, and that you are able to return to work as soon as your arm heals. Many things can happen. Here is my card. I will send you my report. If you find that things are more difficult than you expected for any reason, please call me and come back. We will see how you are doing and what we can do to help.

*"I Told You So."* Confronting a lack of self-awareness is often uncomfortable for clinicians and for family alike. Once the person has come to recognize her limitations, clinicians and family may be tempted to vindicate themselves with expressions of "I told you so." This does little to build a relationship or to advance therapy. It can sometimes be referred to usefully, however, when tackling remaining impaired awareness. For example,

> Do you remember that video of you when you were still in the hospital and you thought you could walk when you couldn't? What was it we called that problem? . . . Lack of awareness, that's right. Thank goodness things aren't that bad anymore and you can walk now. But now you think you are ready to drive and no one else does. Do you think that might be happening again, that lack of awareness?

### *Conclusions*

Disorders of self-awareness are varied, common, and problematic in brain illnesses. It is important to prioritize practical problems caused by disturbed self-awareness and to understand the causes of the impaired self-awareness thoroughly. Interventions can then be fit to these circumstances, combining compensation, restoration, and cognitive and emotional strategies. Even when practical priorities (such as safety, rehabilitation plans, financial issues) are under control, self-awareness remains an important theme in intervention and in the construction of a new self-image.

## *TELLING OTHERS*

Coping with problem emotions and behaviors includes structuring the environment, especially the social environment, to minimize those problems. For example, one may need to explain to others the behavior of the person with a brain illness or may need to ask them to behave a certain way. Caregivers may do this when the person cannot. As the person becomes capable, therapy can focus on developing a "rap" or "script" of what to tell and ask of others. Different raps for different social situations can be written on cue cards and can be practiced in role plays. Learning to tell others about the problem benefits the person in several ways (Table 7.12).

For some people, telling others is natural and may happen spontaneously with a slight suggestion or as therapy homework. For others, it is interpersonally and/or cognitively difficult. The task can be approached with hierarchies of difficulty of who to tell and how to tell them (Table 7.13) that have been worked out

**TABLE 7.12. Benefits to the Person with a Brain Illness in Telling Others about her Problems**

| |
|---|
| "Owning" the problems more deeply and taking responsibility for changing them. |
| Understanding the problems more thoroughly by trying to explain them. |
| Developing the trust of others because they hear an acknowledgement of the problems and an attempt to change. |
| Getting others to understand the problems better so they do not take the problem too personally. |
| Getting others to respond appropriately to problems and to give feedback. |

**TABLE 7.13. Techniques for Telling Others about a Neuropsychological Problem[a]**

| |
|---|
| Send someone a handout about the problem. |
| Give someone a handout about the problem. |
| Write and send a letter to someone about the problem. |
| Write and give a letter to someone about the problem. |
| Read a cue card about the problem on audiotape or on videotape. |
| Explain the problem referring to a cue card on audiotape or on videotape. |
| Explain the problem without a cue card on audiotape or on videotape. |
| Read a cue card about the problem to someone over the phone. |
| Read a cue card about the problem to someone in person. |
| Role-play explaining the problem to someone with the therapist. |
| Role-play explaining the problem to someone in group therapy. |
| Explain the problem to someone, referring to the cue card. |
| Explain the problem to someone without the cue card. |

[a] To be used for constructing a personal hierarchy of difficulty.

in therapy. For some it is easiest to tell family members and most difficult to tell strangers. For others it is reversed. Cultural differences are very important (Case 7.12. Raj).

What and how to tell others should receive attention in any extended intervention, because it touches on other important themes of coping: personal responsibility, self-image, social skills, and community reintegration.

*"You Just Don't Understand!" Case 7.12. Raj (Case 3.1, p. 32, revisited).* A young, Middle Eastern immigrant was seen in outpatient rehabilitation in the United States for a mild TBI that had left him unable to work for 2 years due to cognitive difficulties and to impulsive anger. One of his most persistent problems was explaining his unemployment to his high-achieving, extended family living in the same city whom he saw frequently. His psychologist struggled with him over this for many sessions, pressuring him to tell his extended family what had happened. Eventually he described to the psychologist (and his wife, from the same country, confirmed) that mental disabilities were a source of considerable shame, dishonor, and misunderstanding for families in his culture, and he gave a number of examples from his experience. This goal was dropped from the rehabilitation plan, but trust in the relationship with the psychologist never entirely recovered.

# 8

# Intervention Strategies for Problem Feelings and Behaviors

## From Caregiver Management to Self-Regulation

### *INTRODUCTION*

Feelings and behaviors with sudden onset can become problems following brain illnesses (Table 8.1). Sudden-onset feelings, such as frustration, anxiety, or depression, may be problems mostly for the person with the illness, whereas others may be unaware of them. Problem feelings may lead to behaviors that are problems for others, such as impulsive anger resulting in aggression. Sometimes problem behaviors do not have prominent emotional components, for instance, some impulsiveness, cognitive rigidity, perseveration, reflex crying, and inappropriate laughing and cursing.

Sudden-onset problem feelings and behaviors resulting from brain illnesses have a number of common characteristics and intervention strategies, regardless of whether the problems are reactions to the illness or direct organic changes. These principles may or may not apply to pre-illness problems.

The common characteristics of these problem feelings and behaviors are that they come on suddenly, often unexpectedly. They often also go away suddenly. The reactions are out of proportion to or inappropriate to the circumstances. The person may be surprised at and overwhelmed by their intensity. The feelings and behaviors often make it difficult to function, especially to remember and to employ therapeutic strategies.

Common intervention strategies are to evaluate and to label the problem, to learn to recognize risks and warning signs, and to learn to back off from the

**TABLE 8.1. Problem Feelings and Behaviors with Sudden Onsets that Can Result from Brain Illnesses**

| |
|---|
| Impulsive anger |
| Anxiety and panic |
| Sudden depression |
| Reflex crying |
| Inappropriate laughing |
| Inappropriate cursing |
| Emotional lability |
| Embarrassment |
| Frustration |
| Impulsiveness |
| Excess talking |
| Cognitive rigidity or perseveration |
| Wandering or elopement |
| Sexual acting out |

situation, to calm down, and to try again. Typically this strategy is first employed by caregivers and then is taught to the person with the brain illness. As self-awareness and self-control are regained, the time needed to calm down decreases and becomes more automatic within the situation. This common strategy needs to be individualized to the problem and to the person, as detailed in later chapters.

Techniques of self-management of emotions and of behaviors are skills that everyone learns as they grow up, but these can become impaired by brain illness. Relearning to recognize and to manage problem feelings and behaviors is a task of emotional rehabilitation. People with brain illnesses may be suddenly confronted with changes in their emotional functioning with which they need to learn to cope. Caregivers who help with this emotional rehabilitation can include rehabilitation staff, family, friends, and co-workers.

## *INTERVENTIONS*

### *Identifying Circumstances or Risks*

Identifying the circumstances under which a problem feeling or behavior arises can improve emotional and behavioral control by making it more predictable and less frightening and by permitting the avoidance or the modification of those circumstances or preparation for them. The circumstances can be identified by collecting the stories of a number of the episodes and forming a hypothesis about which circumstances are most important. The hypothesis can be tested by examining future episodes or even by trying to predict or to construct the circumstances that produce the problem. The stories of the episodes can be collected by interview and by using an incident log (see the following sections).

### *Identifying Warning Signs*

Identifying warning signs that a problem emotion or behavior is beginning also helps improve emotional and behavioral control. Warning signs are identified by observation, by interviews, and by collecting stories about episodes. The first list of warning signs may be short and may include part of the problem, such as shouting, cursing, or hitting. Later, more subtle warning signs are discovered, including thoughts, feelings, and fantasies.

### *External Behavioral Control Strategies*

When someone is emerging from a coma, is confused, is disoriented, or is entirely lacking in self-control, or is severely deteriorated from a progressive brain illness, the caregivers have most of the responsibility for managing problem behaviors and feelings. The most important strategies in these stages involve structuring the environment so as to avoid these problems (Burke & Wesolowski, 1988; Howard, 1988; Jacobs, 1993).

#### *Physical Safety*

The environment should be kept free of objects that could be dangerous with the person's problem behaviors, such as weapons, sharp instruments, poisons, fire, electricity, motor vehicles, and breakable things.

#### *Level of Stimulation*

Some people do best when they are kept busy and distracted. Some are restless and need to stay physically active. Others may be hypersensitive to sound, to light, to movement, to touch, or to smells, and can easily become overstimulated. The optimal level of stimulation for someone may vary with fatigue. It can be helpful to explore and manipulate this dimension systematically, with ongoing written records, if necessary.

#### *Social Stimulation*

The person with a brain illness is usually more likely to be calmed by a person familiar to him from before the illness than by strangers or caregivers whom he cannot remember. Sometimes an individual will respond better to people of one gender, age, or type. It can be worthwhile to attend to who works best with him. Many people are overstimulated by a crowd and respond better to just one person or to being left alone. Others fear abandonment or follow social conformity demands when many are present.

*Orientation and Explanation*

Providing frequent orientation information and explanations to the confused person can help to reduce problem behavior. The information given should be relevant to his immediate experience, rather than formal orientation in time and space. In particular, it is important to let him know what is happening and what will happen in the immediate future and why, what is expected of him, and anything that may be unpleasant. For example, for someone in post-traumatic amnesia it would helpful to say

> Hi, I'm Marisol, your nurse. You're in the hospital because you had an accident and hit your head. Are you done with your breakfast? Good, because now it's time for you to go see your physical therapist, Jorge, to learn to walk again. I'll take you in your wheelchair. Are you ready?

That would be preferable to

> Hello, Señora Mora. Today is Wednesday, January 10, 1996. It's 9 a.m. We are in the National Rehabilitation Hospital at Kilometer 5 South in Managua. Are your ready for therapy?

*Validation Therapy*

Some people who are confused will not accept orientation information from others but will insist on their own misperceptions and misunderstandings. Struggles over orientation information are not useful and usually entrench the person in misunderstanding. Validation therapy (Feil, 1993) takes empathy with the confused person's perceptions a step further. Designed for people with Alzheimer's disease, the approach largely abandons attempts at formal reorientation in favor of empathy with the emotional content and reality of what the confused person is expressing (see Table 7.6, p. 121). Confused emotional expressions, verbal and nonverbal, are gently and nonjudgmentally probed with open-ended questions, such as "Who did that?" "Where were you when that happened?" Key words from the person's expressions, even if they are jumbled paraphasias, are repeated. A low, nurturing voice, eye contact, and appropriate touch, such as a hand on the back, are used to express accompaniment (see Case 7.4. Tillie, p. 121).

This may be more effective than conventional reality orientation for dealing with problem behavior and for encouraging appropriate interactions in dementia. It remains to be seen if these techniques are useful in acute brain illness recovery, where there is much more hope for recovering conventional orientation. In such a use, the caregiver would want to push more toward reality orientation and to avoid perpetuating a delusion.

*Adequate Rest*

People who's brains are severely dysfunctional generally need a great deal of rest, and they need it frequently. They may not tolerate more than a few minutes of focused activity or of stimulation. As recovery progresses they may still need quiet rest every hour or so. Even when recovery is apparently complete, many still need an afternoon nap to function adequately. An activity diary that tracks activity in half-hour segments for several days may help pinpoint rest needs and plan an optimal schedule to avoid problem behaviors due to fatigue.

*Managing Incidents*

Even with the best of prevention plans, problem incidents will happen. Management plans (Table 8.2) should be made in advance when possible and should be individualized for the person and the type of problem. Once a plan is chosen, it needs to be evaluated regularly to be sure that it is effective. The plan can later be incorporated into the structure of the "back off, calm down, try again" strategy for learning self-control described in the following material.

The strategy of social cover-up (Table 8.2) is primarily to manage embarrassment. It is the polite trick of supposedly not noticing someone's problem while at the same time fixing it (Martin, 1984), for example, changing the subject to the flowers on the table while wiping the face of the person who is drooling.

A number of strategies are often tried but are rarely helpful. Direct confrontation rarely helps. Meeting anger with anger, with a show of force, or with attempts at physical restraint usually escalates the anger. It usually makes matters worse to tell someone with reflex crying, "Don't cry!" or to tell someone who is embarrassed, "Don't be embarrassed," to laugh at someone who is embarrassed, or who is doing something impulsive, or who has reflex laughing or to insist that someone who is frustrated keep trying. Reprimand is a possible strategy if a firm reprimand, given early in the presentation of a problem by someone whom the person respects, has been shown to help abort a problem incident.

**TABLE 8.2. Strategies for External Management of Incidents of Problem Behaviors (for Use with Individuals with Little Capacity for Self-Control)**

| |
|---|
| Distraction |
| Isolation |
| Reassurance |
| Social cover-up |
| Validation therapy (Table 7.6, p. 121) |
| Changing stimulation |
| Changing the people present |
| Explanation |
| Appropriate touch |
| Reprimand |
| Medication |
| Physical restraint |

### *Medications*

Psychotropic medications have quite different effects on injured brains than on intact ones, because the target organ is damaged. The neuropsychotherapist should make sure that the prescribing physician is acquainted with this specialized field ("Medication Update" section of the *Journal of Head Trauma Rehabilitation*, Gualtieri, 1991). Some antidepressants, anticonvulsants, anxiolytic agents, and other medications can contribute significantly to a program for restoring emotional control. Controlling behavior through chemical sedation should be viewed as a temporary last resort.

### *Physical Restraints*

As a last resort, physical restraints for behavioral control may be considered. Even here, creative environmental manipulation can decrease problem behaviors (Jones, 1996). For example, mattresses on the floor and beanbag chairs can prevent falls without the person feeling physically confined. Electronic warning devices can guard against wandering too far while providing greater freedom of movement within a defined area than possible with physical restraints.

## *"Back Off, Calm Down, Try Again"*

When the person begins to exercise some control over his own behavior, the most important strategy for dealing with incidents of problem emotion or behavior is for the person to back off from the situation, calm down, and return to the situation and continue the activity (adapted from Sonkin & Durphy, 1989). The individualized time out (or relaxing break, regrouping, or break time) can be complex. "Back off, calm down, try again," is a slogan that caregivers and people with brain illnesses can understand, remember, and apply in different circumstances. This procedure is ideally a temporary means toward learning less cumbersome and obtrusive self-control techniques, but when that is not possible, it can be an end in itself. For progressive conditions, it is a strategy that can be taught early, as problems emerge, to have it available later, should problems worsen.

Backing off is not punishment or negative consequences. It is learning self-control. Ideally, it comes before rather than after problem behavior or feelings. The person should feel support in learning self-control, not rejection for failing.

### *Back Off*

The person backing off needs to leave the situation that is stimulating the feeling. If the problem is anger with other people, the person needs to be out of communication with them (out of sight, out of earshot). If the problem is frustration with a task, the person may simply stop trying the task without actually moving. For anxiety, panic, sudden depression, reflex crying, embarrassment, and so forth the person may want to be with someone else when calming down. Backing off may be need to be explained to others, especially for impulsive anger. This explanation can be included on the cue card.

Warning signs are used as indicators of the need to back off. Cues to back off usually come first from caregivers who then fade the cuing as the person learns to recognize the warning signs and to self-cue. Both parties should work toward recognizing warning signs as soon as possible to shorten the calm-down period. Ideally, this technique leads to not needing to back off because the person recognizes warning signs and calms down in context before the feelings get out of hand.

### *Calm Down*

Choosing an approach to calming down is individual and experimental. Many people already use some technique to calm themselves or know what makes them feel relaxed. Others can chose something from Table 8.3. Calm-down strategies may change with learning and with recovery.

How long should the person calm down? Until they are calm and ready to return. Because time away is to be used to learn self-control and not as punishment, the amount of time spent does not depend upon the "severity" of the "offense." If a caregiver is present for the calm-down period, perhaps helping to guide relaxation or cue card use, she may help judge when it is time to return and help teach the person to recognize signs of being calm. Calm-down time spent alone should be for a certain number of minutes based on that person's usual

**TABLE 8.3. Strategies for Self-Calming**

| |
|---|
| Muscle relaxation |
| Deep breathing |
| Calming visual imagery |
| A quiet setting |
| Closing eyes |
| Soft music |
| Physical exercise |
| Meditation |
| Self-hypnosis |
| Prayer |
| Distraction |
| Writing |
| Imagining the presence of a person of respect or authority |
| Medication |

pattern, using a timer if necessary. Later, the person may learn to recognize "calm signs" such as being able to smile, breathing normally, or just "feeling ready." These may be put on the cue card.

### *Incident Log*

In many treatment plans the incident will be recorded in the incident log after the person has calmed down and before he returns to the situation. This step should be on the cue card.

### *Preparing to Return*

Once the person is calm, the plan may include preparations to return to the situation, as noted on the cue card (Table 8.4).

### *Try Again*

Backing off is not an excuse to avoid a situation. The person usually needs to return and to deal with the situation again. If the emotional reaction has been strong, it is best to do something else first. For example, an argument is likely to get rekindled if it is discussed right after calming down. It is better to wait a few hours to discuss the issue again. Some activities, such as a mildly frustrating task or a conversation interrupted by reflex crying, can be resumed immediately. Others—a disagreement over a game, an overreaction to a loud noise—may be appropriately abandoned.

**TABLE 8.4. Possible Preparations for Returning from Backing Off**

| |
|---|
| Affirmations |
| Positive self-statements |
| Prayers |
| Lists of questions to review, for example: |
| Do I need to apologize? |
| Do I need to explain why I left to anyone? |
| What can I do to avoid this next time? |
| Do I need to ask for help? |
| Cognitive strategies, for example: |
| There must be another way to do this. |
| Cut the problem down to size. |
| Check the work. |
| Reframing or cognitive restructuring of self-statements |

### *Self-Statements*

Some problem feelings are made worse by self-defeating thoughts and beliefs, such as "I'll never be able to do this!" "I'll never get any better!" "I'm going to lose it!" "She hates me!" (Burns, 1981, Meichenbaum, 1977; Moore & Stambrook, 1995). Replacing these with more accurate and helpful self-statements can abort episodes of problem feelings; for example, "I can do it if I take my time." "I'm getting better, bit by bit." "I can control myself." "She loves me, even if she is upset with me sometimes." People with amnesia may not learn self-statements easily or remember to use them, so cue cards are often necessary.

Many people with executive function difficulties and adequate language skills can use language to structure their activities; for example, "I'm getting frustrated. I need to leave this alone for a while and calm down. I need to sit down and breathe deeply." Such self-instructions can be read aloud or silently, or can be memorized and spoken aloud or internally. To facilitate the transition to internalized self-control, cue cards should be written in the first person ("I need to rest," instead of "You need to rest."). An exception to this might be early in the treatment of a person who has little faith in himself, but who has much faith in someone else (a rabbi, for example) who could write or authorize the cue card. A religious individual may prefer to write a prayer that would be helpful in calming down or in coping.

### *Cue Cards*

Individualized cue cards for problem emotions and behaviors should include a short list of warning signs, steps to take when backing off, and ways of calming down. They may change as the person progresses; for example, adding or removing warning signs and steps, adding "calm signs," adding instructions to write in the incident log, adding self-talk, and so forth. Cue cards should be short, simple, and in the person's own language. Only essential words and abbreviations should be used.

### *Role Playing*

Recognizing warning signs, backing off, calming down, and returning can be hard to learn and to carry out, especially when one is emotionally aroused. It is also hard for someone with amnesia or with aphasia to learn as a verbal sequence, although it may be learned as an activity through preserved procedural learning.

Back-off routines need to be practiced just as fire drills that help people know what to do automatically when emotionally aroused and not thinking clearly. Back-off routines should be practiced at times when they are not needed, to make the procedures familiar to the person with the brain illness and to everyone who will be around. They can be practiced in the clinic, in therapy, at home, and anywhere that the problem could arise. Practice back-offs are just like real ones except that the person initiating them announces that it is for practice.

### *Practice Crossing the Threshold*

The person with a problem feeling or behavior from a brain illness has a "new" brain and has new thresholds for when feelings and behaviors become problems. He needs to learn where those thresholds are to "recalibrate" control mechanisms. Emotional rehabilitation requires encountering that new threshold many times to know where it is. For this reason, provided no damage is done, frequent, controlled incidents of problem feelings and behaviors are desirable early in the relearning of emotional control. Instead of being seen as discouraging treatment failures, these incidents can be reframed as chances to learn.

Once control techniques have been learned, the system can be "stress tested" by trying progressively more difficult and provocative circumstances. For example, a soccer fan has trouble tolerating the noise and excitement of a real game. Once he has learned to recognize when he is getting overstressed, he has mastered self-control techniques in easy settings, and he has a backup plan of leaving the situation, he can test the system. First he plays a soccer video game, then he watches a game on TV alone, then he watches one with friends. Next he watches a small neighborhood game away from other fans. On successive occasions he slowly works his way into the crowd and tries bigger games.

## *RECORD-KEEPING AND PROCEDURES*

### *Incident Log*

An incident log (Tables 8.5, 8.6, see Table 6.3, p. 93) is useful in understanding the problem initially, in dealing with incidents at the time, and in gauging progress and the success of various strategies. The log may not be needed for

**TABLE 8.5. Sample Incident Log**

| Frustration Incident Log | | | | | | | |
|---|---|---|---|---|---|---|---|
| Date & Time | What Happened? | Circumstances | Level | Warning Signs | Strategies Used | Cues | Who? |
| | | | 1 *Mild*<br>2<br>3 *Mod*<br>4<br>5 *Sev* | 1 *Confused*<br>2 *Errors*<br>3 *Breath*<br>4 *Tense*<br>5 *Cursing* | 1 *Back off*<br>2 *Self talk*<br>3 *Easier task*<br>4 *Get help*<br>5 *Rest* | 1 *Full*<br>2 *Spec dir*<br>3 *NS dir*<br>4 *Spec ob*<br>5 *NS ob*<br>6 *Self* | |

**TABLE 8.6. Example of a Completed Incident Log**

| Frustration Incident Log | | | | | | | |
|---|---|---|---|---|---|---|---|
| Date & Time | What Happened? | Circumstances | Level | Warning Signs | Strategies Used | Cues | Who? |
| | | | 1 *Mild*<br>2<br>3 *Mod*<br>4<br>5 *Sev* | 1 *Confused*<br>2 *Errors*<br>3 *Breath*<br>4 *Tense*<br>5 *Cursing* | 1 *Back off*<br>2 *Self talk*<br>3 *Easier task*<br>4 *Get help*<br>5 *Rest* | 1 *Full*<br>2 *Spec dir*<br>3 *NS dir*<br>4 *Spec ob*<br>5 *NS ob*<br>6 *Self* | |
| 2/20 10A | Broke dish | Kids yelling | 4 | 4,5 | 1,2,5, asked kids to play outside | 6 | Me |
| 2/20 1P | Confused sorting laundry | | 3 | 1,2 | 2,3 | 5 | Me |
| *2/20 5P* | *Burned rice* | *Radio, rushed* | *4* | *1,2,3,4,5* | *1,2,4* | *2* | *John* |

simple or for rapidly resolving problems, but it may be used for complex or for protracted problems. The log can be kept by therapists, by the family, and/or by the person with a brain illness, depending on his level of responsibility. Log sheets can be kept in the memory book, in the therapy journal, or in the medical record.

*Possible Sections of the Log*

*Date and Time: What Happened?* This section contains a brief description of the incident, especially what the person with brain illness felt and did, the environment in which the incident happened, and any necessary background. Special variables of interest may be emphasized, such as the level of fatigue, who was present, or recent activities.

*Level.* In this section, the level of the problem feeling or behavior is rated, usually on a scale of 1 to 5 or 1 to 10. Exemplars of specific points on the scale should be worked out individually.

*Warning Signs.* Behaviors and feelings indicating an incident was coming should be noted here.

*Strategies Used.* The strategies tried and their effects should be noted here.

*Cues.* Cues given by caregivers to the person to take action to avoid a problem should be noted in this section.

*Who?* The initials of the person who filled out the incident should be recorded here.

*Other.* Other variables that could be of particular interest are medications, special medical conditions, use of alcohol or drugs, particular feelings such as jealousy, interpersonal factors, or whatever the therapist or the person thinks may be important.

### *Getting Started*

Together with the person with the brain illness, the therapist identifies the target problem behavior or feeling and fills it in at the top (Table 8.5). They then choose variables to be observed, beginning with just a few variables so the task is not too demanding, and so others can learn how to do it and will actually complete it. As the system gets established, more categories can be added and more information can be gathered.

The space beneath the titles is used to enter exemplars of different levels of a behavior or a feeling, warning signs, strategies, and different levels of cuing. Incidents are recorded either by writing a number or by writing a description. For warning signs, strategies, and cues, more than one number might be written for a given incident. Ideally, all log users would receive training in how to record episodes. It is best to record as many episodes as possible, but an incident log can still be effective even if only the most problematic incidents are recorded.

Levels of the behavior or the feeling, warning signs, and strategies are individualized, but levels of cuing can be standardized on the continuum of responsibility (Table 8.7).

### *Analyzing the Results*

The incident log can be used to look for patterns in the problem incidents. Do they happen at particular times of day, in particular locations, or with particular people? Are they associated with meals, lack of food, fatigue, medicines, and so forth? Which warning signs are most reliable? What types of cues are effective and necessary? Which interventions work best?

When patterns emerge, these can be confirmed by focused record keeping. Patterns can be used to anticipate and to avoid problems and to refine effective strategies. The therapist reviews the incident log regularly with the person, noting progress and setting new goals.

### *Progress Chart*

Progress in dealing with the problem can be charted on scatter graphs (Figure 8.1) as the level of severity, the level of cuing used, or the level of self-control (see next section).

**TABLE 8.7. Levels of Cuing**

1. Full cue—Specific observation and direction:
   "Fred, you are shouting. You need to take a time out."
   "You are grimacing and breathing hard. Go lie down and relax."
   "I see you are about to cry. Look up, take a deep breath."
2. Specific directive cue:
   "Look at your panic card."
   (Caregiver makes an agreed-on "Time Out" hand sign.)
   Caregiver flashes a behavior card saying, "Stop and Think!"
3. Nonspecific directive cue:
   "James, make a good choice."
   "What's the best thing you can do to deal with this?"
   (The caregiver takes a deep breath and looks toward the door.)
4. Specific observational cue:
   "You look red in the face."
   "You're laughing too much."
   Behavioral flashcard: "Talking too much"
5. Non-specific observational cue:
   "What are you doing?"
   "Katie . . ." (Where the cue is conveyed by the tone of voice)
   "What do you notice about what you are saying right now?"
6. Self-cue
   "I'm feeling angry. I'm taking a time out." (Takes a time out.)
   "I'm talking too much. You tell me what you think now."
   "Dear, I'm scared. Could you rub my back and help me calm down?"

### *Progression of Self-Control*

The progression of self-control over problem behaviors and feelings (Table 8.8) follows the continuum of responsibility. Responsibility for the program gradually passes from caregivers to the person with the brain illness. Levels of responsibility (Table 8.8) are zones, not steps or stages. For example, a person could be working at Level 5 but might sometimes function at Level 4 with perhaps an occasional slip to Levels 3 or 2, with a few exceptional episodes at Levels 6 or 7. Not all programs will begin at Level 1 nor will end at Level 10. Also, programs for the same person may be at different levels for different problems; for example, at Level 8 with frustration, but at Level 5 with anger.

As self-control progresses there is a gradual reduction in the back off, calm down, try again procedure. The person becomes more sensitized to risks and to warning signs, initiates backing off sooner, and needs less time to calm down. Calming down becomes more efficient. Physical backing off is replaced with mental backing off. The skills are tried out in increasingly difficult circumstances in the person's zone of recovery, following stress inoculation training (Meichenbaum, 1985, 1992, 1993). Eventually, the person is again able to man-

| Level | 1 | 2 | 3 | 4 | 5 | 6 | 7 |
|---|---|---|---|---|---|---|---|
| 6 | | | x | | x | xxx | xx |
| 5 | | x | xx | xxx | xx | x | |
| 4 | | x | | xxx | xx | | |
| 3 | x | | xx | x | | | |
| 2 | xx | xxx | xxx | | | | |
| 1 | xxx | xx<br>xx | | | | | |

*weeks*

Frustration Progress Chart

FIGURE 8.1. A progress chart. In this example, there were eight episodes of frustration in the third week. Three required a specific, directive cue (Level 2), two required a nonspecific directive cue (Level 3), two required a nonspecific observational cue (Level 5) and one was self-cued (Level 6). In the column for that week there are 3 dots at Level 2, 2 dots at Level 3, 2 dots at Level 5, and 1 dot at Level 6.

age stresses in their context, with the back-off procedure reduced to a pause, a deep breath, and a self-statement. The more elaborate procedure remains available for extraordinary circumstances.

### *Relapse*

Relapse most often comes from overconfidence, when the system is abandoned, or from encountering unusual levels of stress. Reassurance, reframing, and refresher training is usually adequate to deal with the problem (although with some conditions it can be an indication of a return or a worsening of the neurological condition, which may need to be evaluated).

### *Cultural Considerations*

Written record-keeping may not be realistic for some people. Alternatives might include tape recording an incident log or establishing a time each day when the person with the brain illness and a family member review the incidents of the day, with one of them then recounting them to the clinician.

**TABLE 8.8. Progression of Self-Control in Interventions for Problem Behaviors**

| Level | Responsibility | |
|---|---|---|
| | Caregiver | Person with brain illness |
| 1 | Manipulate the environment. Educate others. Identify problems, warning and signs, and strategies. Record incidents in log. | No responsibilities. |
| 2 | Manipulate environment. Give full cues and specific directive cues. Record incidents in log. Begin to educate person with brain illness about problems, signs, strategies, log. | Follow immediate directions, but no carryover expected. |
| 3 | Manipulate environment. Give full cues and specific directive cues. Record incidents in the log and develop a cue card with participation from the person with brain illness. Continue education. | Follow immediate directions with some carryover. Participate in recording incidents in the log and in developing a cue card (developing awareness of the program). |
| 4 | Give specific and nonspecific directive cues. Teach the person with the brain illness about how to manipulate environment to help control his behavior, and his feelings. Record incidents with input from the person with the brain illness. Review progress and strategies with the person with the brain illness. | Back off and practice backing off when cued, partially following cue card. Contribute to recording incidents (begin practice of the program). |
| 5 | Give nonspecific directive cues and specific observational cues. Record episodes cooperatively. Review progress and strategies. | Follow cues and cue cards. Record incidents cooperatively. Begin to structure environment, including partial explanations of problems to others. |
| 6 | Give specific and nonspecific observational cues. Supervise recording incidents. Guide their return to the community. Provide supportive and problem-solving counseling. Review progress and strategies. | Follow cues. Begin to self-cue back-off and practice back-off. Record incidents. Begin to explain the basics of the situation to others with the help of a cue card and the therapy journal. Begin to generalize to the community. |
| 7 | Give nonspecific observational cues. Guide increasing risks and responsibilities in the community. Provide supportive and problem-solving counseling. Review progress and strategies. | Follow cues. Self-cue to use strategies and follow strategies independently with intermittent cue card use. Explain the situation to others and ask for cooperation with minimal help from written materials. Maintain a log. |
| 8 | Provide supportive and problem-solving counseling. Review progress and strategies. | Use strategies independently in the community. Independently explain the situation and ask for cooperation from others in the community. Maintain a log. |

*(continued)*

**TABLE 8.8.** ***(Continued)***

| | | |
|---|---|---|
| 9 | Provide supportive and problem-solving counseling. Review progress and strategies. | Manage the problem independently with little need to explain to others or to use a log, but be able to do so independently if needed. |
| 10 | Offer congratulations and support. | No problem. Fully responsible for behavior. Help others through the process. Reflect on the experience. |

Physical backing-off is impractical or unacceptable for some; for example, people with severe mobility limitations, sole caretakers of small children, or people in prisons or in other settings that they cannot leave. Creativity is needed to find other ways to withdraw from or to be distracted from the provoking stimulus or activity long enough to let the problematic response pass.

## *CONCLUSIONS*

The key to dealing with sudden-onset problematic feelings and behaviors that result from brain illness is to train the person in anticipating, in recognizing, and in preventing episodes. This process often requires considerable cognitive support, social support, and practice with both real and simulated episodes. If the training is to be effective, it must encounter the person in his zone of recovery.

# III

# Specific Problems

# 9

# Psychological Reactions to Illness

Emotional reactions to injury or serious illness include posttraumatic stress disorder (PTSD) and grief reactions with symptoms such as anxiety, depression, anger, denial, guilt, and nightmares. Such reactions are common whether or not the illness includes lesions to the brain. Injury to the brain can also lead to emotional reactions such as frustration, perplexity, obsessions, and compulsions that may be less common as reactions to nonneurological illness. Nevertheless, all of these reactions are understandable from the perspective of the emotional reactions of neurologically intact people to injury and loss.

Sometimes these psychological reactions mimic neurological changes in personality and in emotions. The individual sections that follow describe how to tell specific psychological reactions from confusable neurological changes. Some of the most common combinations of psychological reactions and neurological changes and their interactive effects are also described.

## *GRIEF REACTIONS*

A grief reaction is the usual response to a loss such as the death of a loved one or the loss of a job or a home (Kubler-Ross, 1969) and illnesses such as a TBI (Haynes, 1994), especially if disability results. Grief may include shock, denial, anger, depression, and acceptance. The personality of the person experiencing the loss influences which reactions predominate. For example, chronically angry people tend to have a predominantly angry grief reaction; dysthymic people often have a mostly depressed grief reaction. In people with brain illnesses grief reactions may be slowed and/or distorted by organic dysfunctions such as amnesia and anosognosia.

The shock stage is a brief sense of numbness, disbelief and inability to function. With brain illness this stage may be masked by coma or by amnesia. It is often over by the time the person comes to the attention of mental health providers.

Denial and depression are discussed in separate sections of this chapter. Anger may be directed toward appropriate or toward inappropriate targets. Caregivers and friends can help the person to channel appropriate reactive anger constructively and to ventilate inappropriate anger harmlessly (also see Chapter 10, pp. 194–208).

The state of acceptance involves reconstructing a new life that takes the new reality into account (see the New Person section of Chapter 6, p. 85). This is the work of rehabilitation.

## *DENIAL*

### *Description*

Denial is a primitive mechanism used to defend against a threat to our sense of ourselves such as news of a loss or the realization that we have done something wrong. For example, a child who drops and breaks a glass may say "I didn't do it" or "It just fell." The man who is told that he has terminal cancer may believe that there was an error or may say "It's just a cyst that can be removed." Denial is often the first and a brief reaction to a threat, which is later replaced with more functional defenses.

The person with a brain illness will often deny her problems. She may accuse caregivers of lying to her, of trying to make her look bad, or of restricting her freedom.

### *Similar Neurological Symptoms*

Denial is similar to and often associated with lack of awareness of deficits (anosognosia) in people with brain illnesses (see the Self-Awareness section, Chapter 7, pp. 122–134; the Lack of Awareness of Deficits section, Chapter 11, pp. 233–237). Denial is more likely than anosognosia to produce an emotional reaction when it is confronted. When anosognosia is not mixed with denial, the person may acknowledge a deficit when it is pointed out, but may fail to take it into account in her behavior. Anosognosia is confined to neurological deficits, whereas denial may extend to other areas. For example, the person with anosognosia may not notice her left hemiplegia, but she will acknowledge her broken arm or her heart disease. The person with a brain illness with denial may deny that someone was killed in her accident or may deny her paraplegia. Denial is more likely in people with a history of using denial.

### *Similar Nonneurological Conditions*

Someone may realize she has an impairment but may lie about it and say that she does not have one to get something, such as a driver's license or child custody. What clinicians take for denial may be an expression of optimism or of hope (Ridley, 1989).

### *How to Interview Regarding Denial*

The person with a brain illness will, of course, deny using denial, so her family is more likely to be aware of the problem. However, the family may also deny her problems. Denial is revealed through the interview by comparing observed signs with her description of her condition.

### *How to Observe/Test*

The person's reactions to test failures should be observed as well as differences between what she can do and what she says she can do. Personality tests can reveal denial tendencies; for example, high K and 3 scales on the Minnesota Multiphasic Personality Inventory-II (MMPI-II; Butcher et al., 1989). The person in denial often has a hard time accepting news about her condition.

### *Practical Problems*

The person in denial has difficulty seeing the need for therapy and accepting limitations on her activities. She may try to do unsafe things such as drive or carry a gun. She may be unable to plan effectively for her future.

### *Interventions*

1. The confrontation of denial should be gradual, supportive, nonjudgmental, and prioritized according to practical needs. Here is a brief introduction to an initial confrontation:

> When someone has a major illness it can take a while to realize and accept what has happened. It can be hard to believe what others tell you about your condition. It may be a while before you really understand all the ways it has affected you. I know it's hard, but I'd like to talk with you a little today and again later about some of the ways your illness has affected you. What things have you noticed that most concern you?

2. It is better not to participate actively in someone's denial, because this may confuse her and prolong the denial.

3. Sometimes it is wise to participate passively in the person's denial by postponing telling her all of the truth about her condition. The clinician might tell her as much as she is able to handle at the time and add more later. For example, she (or a denying family member) might be told about her deficits, with no response given when she says she thinks she will recover in a week. A few days later a realistic time course of recovery is discussed. A few days after that it may be time to talk about implications for work, travel, home life, and so forth. Leaving room for realistic hope helps recovery and motivation.
4. In confronting denial, it is important to understand the person's strong feelings. She may need many chances to talk through changing feelings and plans. "I told you so" messages are not helpful, and it is best not to dwell on her earlier positions.
5. Confronting denial requires a good rapport. Sometimes it is best to pick the staff or family member who has the best rapport with the person with the brain illness to do the job.
6. It can be important to coordinate with others. The best supportive, gradual confrontation can be undermined by staff, by program participants, by friends, or by family who actively participate in the person's denial. Well-meaning others sometimes confront denial too directly and stiffen resistance or cause a severe emotional reaction.
7. Denial is often best confronted through experience rather than through discussion. Staff and family members can coordinate "supported failure" experiences where the person tries to do things in the clinic or at home and encounters problems. These experiences can be arranged with adequate supervision and emotional support.
8. Interventions for self-awareness (Chapter 7, pp. 126–134) can be used when denial is combined with anosognosia.

## *DEPRESSION*

### *Description*

Depression is often a normal reaction to brain illness and to other losses and is a part of natural grieving. With brain illness, however, depression can be delayed, and it may not reach its worst until more than a year after the illness, especially when anosognosia slows one's appreciation of the loss and when amnesia slows the realization of the grieving process.

Depression is more likely to be persistently problematic in people with a personal or a family history of depression.

Depression is one of the most common long-term problems in mild (Busch & Alpern, 1998) and severe TBIs (Morton & Wehman, 1995), stroke (Gordon et al., 1991), Alzheimer's disease (Gilley, 1993), and Parkinson's disease (Rao, Huber, & Bornstein, 1992). However, in all neuropsychological conditions there is an important question as to what exactly is depression (see the story of Maria at the beginning of Chapter 1). So many neuropsychological phenomena mimic some aspects of depression (Table 9.1), that it is questionable if depression is a viable concept in persons with significant neuropsychological involvement. In many instances the term masks more than it reveals. To see the extent of this diagnostic problem, consider that someone in a coma meets six of the nine *DSM–IV* (1994) criteria for a major depressive episode (anhedonia, loss of weight, hypersomnia, psychomotor retardation, fatigue, lack of concentration; five symptoms are required for diagnosis, but the person in coma does not meet the exclusion criterion that the symptoms are not due to a general medical condition).

**TABLE 9.1. Symptoms of Depression and Confusable Neuropsychological Symptoms**

| Depression | Brain Illness |
|---|---|
| DSM–IV Symptoms | |
| Mood disturbance | Reflex crying, impaired emotional expression |
| Anhedonia, loss of interest | Impaired initiation, reduced emotional reactivity |
| Loss of appetite and weight | Illness-induced weight loss, weight reduction diet, anosmia, mechanical difficulties with eating, doesn't like hospital food |
| Sleep disturbance | Disturbed sleep due to pain, restlessness, decreased bed mobility, IV tubes, physical restraints, hospital noise, subcortical damage, and so forth. |
| Psychomotor retardation or agitation | Same due to illness |
| Fatigue, decreased energy | Same due to illness |
| Feelings of worthlessness, guilt | Feelings of inadequacy based on reaction to impairments, feelings of guilt due to circumstances of illness or inability to fulfill social roles |
| Loss of concentration, memory | Same due to illness |
| Suicidal thoughts and actions | Black humor from impaired social judgement, self-directed aggression due to impulsive anger |
| Other Frequently Used Symptoms of Depression | |
| Somatic complaints | Multiple serious somatic problems |
| Feelings of helplessness | Genuine incapacity, accurately perceived |
| Tearfulness | Reflex crying, labile emotions |
| Irritability | Impulsive anger, labile emotions |
| Feelings of hopelessness | Impaired planning and anticipation |
| Obsessive rumination | Perseveration |
| Anxiety | Uncertainty about the future due to impaired planning, amnesia (unable to remember being told about the future) |
| Decreased libido | Reduced emotional reactivity, sensory or motor losses interfering with sexual activity |

Along with problems identifying depression symptoms in people with brain illnesses comes the problem of identifying the cause(s) of those symptoms. The *DSM–IV* (1994) distinguishes Major Depressive Disorder from Mood Disorder Due to a General Medical Condition (which includes neurological illnesses and requires that the mood disorder is a direct physiological consequence of the medical condition) and from Adjustment Disorder with Depressed Mood (which may be a reaction to a general medical disorder but not physiologically caused by it). Making these causal distinctions is quite difficult and has not yet been adequately addressed for stroke, for Alzheimer's disease, or for TBIs.

A provisional clinical solution to this dilemma is to regard each depression symptom separately with respect to both etiology and to intervention planning. This does not exclude hypothesizing that an individual's symptom of fatigue, for instance, is due to depression and attempting to treat the fatigue indirectly with psychotherapy or antidepressant medication. However, it also allows for scheduling rest and activity appropriately throughout the day as a direct intervention for fatigue. This symptom-oriented approach helps guard against overlooking and undertreating depression symptoms in people with organic illnesses, and visa versa (Lamberty & Bieliauskas, 1993; Teri & Wagner, 1992).

### *Similar Neurological Symptoms (Table 9.1)*

Lack of initiation (Chapter 11, p. 216) can look like depression, but when activities are suggested the depressed person is likely to resist the activity and to predict failure, whereas the person who merely lacks initiation is likely to go along with the activity and may enjoy it.

Reflex crying (Chapter 10, p. 184) can look like depression, but careful questioning about the person's mood, hopes, plans, and so forth may reveal that she is not depressed. (Caution: some people with reflex crying will at first answer that they are depressed, inferring that they must be because they are crying.)

Impaired emotional expressiveness (Chapter 10, p. 181) can look like depression whether or not the person with the brain illness is actually depressed. Testing emotional expressiveness directly can help to make the differentiation.

Depression is less likely, or may occur late, in the person with anosognosia or with amnesia. It is more likely with frustration, fatigue, perplexity, and impaired language expression. It is more likely with mild than with severe impairments in memory and in attention.

Impaired concentration and memory are symptoms of both brain illness and of depression. The person with a brain illness is more likely to be distractible; the depressed person is more likely to have difficulty maintaining mental effort. Depressed people are usually aware or hyperaware of memory and of attention difficulties, whereas people with brain illnesses may not be. Memory difficulties of depression are typically attention and encoding impairments, whereas brain illnesses often produce consolidation and storage deficits as well (Gass & Russell, 1986; King, Cox, Lyness, & Caine, 1995; Lamberty & Bieliauskas, 1993).

The memory deficit of depression is not known to be modality- or material-specific. The memory deficit of brain illnesses may be modality- or material-specific, most likely involving the modality in which other impairments are present. For example, a person with a stroke with mild word-finding deficits but with intact visual-spatial skills may also be impaired in verbal but not in visual-spatial learning. Perseveration and confabulation are common in brain illness but not in depression.

### *Similar Nonneurological Conditions (Table 9.1)*

Depression can be a reaction to nonneurological losses, as well. Some people with brain illnesses will have a history of mood disorder, and their depression may not be related to their brain illness. Weight loss, a lack of energy, loss of sex drive, and sleep disturbance can all be direct consequences of the debilitation of major illness and of prolonged hospitalization. Sleep can be disturbed by pain, by physical limitations, by equipment such as casts and IV lines, or by a noisy hospital environment.

### *Neuroanatomy*

Some investigators (e.g., Robinson, 1987) believe that depression is more likely with a left hemisphere lesion (particularly a left frontal lesion with expressive aphasia) than with a right hemisphere lesion. Others (e.g., Gordon et al., 1991) believe that there are no significant hemispheric differences. The discrepancy may arise from finding hemispheric differences early after stroke before lack of awareness has recovered or from methodological difficulties in measuring depression.

### *How to Interview*

The state of the art in interviewing people with brain illnesses for depression is the *Structured Assessment of Depression in Brain Damaged Individuals (SADBD,* Gordon et al., 1991, see Appendix B). Even so, the SADBD has its limitations, and its authors stressed the need to weigh aphasia, emotional communication impairments, and lack of awareness in considering which sources of information to rely on.

Questions should be open-ended. Table 9.1 can be useful in exploring symptoms to determine whether they are due to depression or to medical conditions. In the person who is severely aphasic, visual analogue mood scales (Nyenhuis et al., 1997) may be needed (see Figure 9.1 and Appendix B). With amnesia, aphasia, or anosognosia, family members (or nurses) may provide information about disturbances of sleep and of appetite, weight loss, lack of energy, loss of sex drive, loss of interest, and indications of suicidal preoccupation.

### *How to Observe/Test*

Questions of depression versus brain illness (or both) often call for conventional personality testing and neuropsychological assessment. The differential diagnostic issues are many and complex and depend on the specific neurological conditions suspected. They are questions for a neuropsychologist or for an interdisciplinary team and are beyond the scope of this book.

When the question is whether or not depression is also present with a known brain illness, precautions need to be followed (Table 9.2) with conventional depression and personality tests. The SADBD (Gordon et al., 1991) is a structured clinical interview that incorporates adapted versions of the *Hamilton Rating Scale for Depression* (Hamilton, 1960) and the *Beck Depression Inventory* (Beck et al., 1961). Hamilton and Beck items are probed to rule out medical causes of these symptoms. Self-report is compared to external observer ratings to evaluate awareness (see Appendix B). The *Post-Stroke Depression Rating Scale* (Gainotti et al., 1997) is a 10-item, semistructured interview that covers emotional changes common in stroke (see Appendix B). *The Cornell Scale for Depression and Dementia* (Alexopoulos, Abrams, Young, & Shamoian, 1988) and the *Dementia Mood As-*

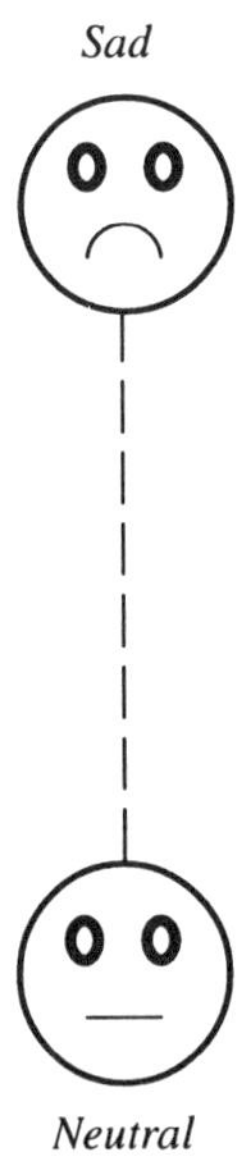


FIGURE 9.1. An example of a visual mood scale item.

**TABLE 9.2. Barriers and Solutions to Depression Testing in People with Brain Illnesses[a]**

| Barrier | Solution |
|---|---|
| 1. Somatic complaints are not good discriminators of depression in seriously medically ill populations | Minimize weighting of somatic symptoms |
| 2. Questions about suicide and sexuality can be jarring and/or inappropriate for medically ill and for older institutionalized populations | Reinterpret or abandon such items |
| 3. Intrapsychic items are underrepresented | Include more intrapsychic items regarding worthlessness, hopelessness, helplessness |
| 4. Older individuals often resist evaluation when not self-referred | Begin with somatic complaints before covering intrapsychic symptoms |
| 5. Depression inventories are depressing to take | Include inquiries about positive affective experiences |
| 6. Depression inventories are cognitively demanding | Administer orally in yes/no format, simplifying content as needed. Rating by an observer. |

[a] From "Issues in the Diagnosis and Cognitive Therapy of Depression in Brain-Damaged Individuals," by M. R. Hibbard, W. A. Gordon, S. Egelko, and K. Langer, in *Cognitive Therapy: Applications in Psychiatric and Medical Settings* (pp. 183–198) edited by A. Freeman & V. Greenwood, 1987, New York: Human Sciences. Copyright 1987 by Human Sciences Press. Adapted with permission.

*sessment Scale* (Sunderland et al., 1988) are based on clinicians ratings and take organic changes into account (Appendix B).

Observations and interviews regarding reflex crying and testing of emotional communication (see Chapter 10, pp. 182, 185) should be incorporated into most depression evaluations in neuropsychological populations, particularly for stroke.

### *Practical Problems*

Grief is a necessary process in emotional coping and growth, but prolonged depression is unnecessary and intrinsically undesirable. Depression holds risks for suicide, lack of motivation for rehabilitation, slow healing and rehabilitation due to poor nutrition and fatigue, loss of function through immobilization, unfulfilled social roles, and premature death.

### *Interventions*

Given the problems associated with diagnosing depression with brain illnesses, a symptom-oriented approach to treatment is important. Rather than assuming that generic treatment for depression (medication, psychotherapy) will address any and all symptoms of depression (see Table 9.1) present in a given individual, each problematic symptom is addressed individually. In this way, if sleep disturbance is due to a noisy roommate, or if a feeling of helplessness springs from caregiver neglect, these problems are less likely to get overlooked, improperly medicated, or dismissed as depression. Of course, treatment for depression may also be appropriate.

1. Educating the person about the course of recovery is often helpful. Some depression can be relieved by mobilizing hope for recovery. Letting her know that depression is a normal stage of grief that almost everyone needs to pass through can also help.
2. For people with anosognosia who are not depressed, predicting possible depression as they improve can help them and their families. If and when depression comes it is less of a shock and a worry, and it can be interpreted as a sign of recovering awareness.
3. Communicating empathy and understanding and guiding family members to do the same can help, particularly for people with impaired communication of language or of feelings. With aphasia, tone of voice, touch, facial expression, and time and attention given may take on more importance. With impaired emotional communication, reflex crying, and lack of initiation, words may become more important for accurate communication of feelings.
4. Standard psychotherapeutic techniques for grief and for depression can be applied to people with brain illnesses who are cognitively able to use them, sometimes with adaptations (Table 9.3).
5. Many antidepressant medications lower the seizure threshold, interact with other medications, have unpleasant side effects, are contraindicated with some medical conditions, and can sometimes make cognitive symptoms worse. Nevertheless, they play an important role in treating depressed people with brain illnesses under some circumstances (Table 9.4). People with brain illnesses often respond well to low doses (Gualtieri, 1991).
6. It is important to keep the person active within the limits of her abilities. This may require confrontation, structuring, cajoling, or pressuring at first. A hierarchy of activities constructed according to the zone of recuperation may help overcome fatigue, embarrassment, anxiety, frustration, and so forth.
7. In educating the family about coping with delayed depression, it can help to relate it to the depressive feelings that they themselves probably went through when the person became ill.
8. Therapy tasks and goals should be structured to maximize success experiences. For example, if the person walks 25 feet in therapy, the goal for the next day may again be 25 feet (rather than 40) with praise for that and for any more she does.
9. It is usually better to avoid comparisons to other people with brain illnesses. Although some people may successfully ward off depression by saying, "I'm lucky I'm not as badly off as X," such comparisons imposed from the outside often backfire.

**TABLE 9.3. Modifications in Cognitive Psychotherapy for Treating Depressed People with Brain Illnesses[a]**

1. Cognitive functioning moderates the treatment strategies used. The more severe the impairment the more behavioral as contrasted with cognitive techniques should be used.
2. Cognitive remediation enhances the person's ability to benefit from psychotherapy.
3. New learning and generalization may be difficult for people with brain illnesses.
4. Awareness of depressive symptomatology moderates therapeutic strategy. Education is needed for lack of awareness of depression. When depression is minimized, behavioral strategies are needed initially while the idea of cognitive distortions contributing to depressed mood is introduced.
5. Mourning is an important component of treatment. The losses that may need to be mourned include change of personality and losses of abilities, of future plans, of social roles, of lifestyle, and of income. With traumatic injury there may be a loss of loved ones injured or killed in the same accident or assault.
6. Premorbid personality, lifestyle, and interests provide a context for understanding current behavior. A person's adjustment may depend more on how much she has changed than on her absolute current condition. Goals and activities should aim at approximating pre-injury life style and preferences if possible.
7. Understanding the discrepancy between actual and perceived losses is essential to treatment. The discrepancy may vary over time and from one domain to another (e.g., cognition vs. motor functioning, vs. social functioning vs. emotions).
8. Reinforcing even small therapeutic gains improves mood.
9. Emphasis on the collaborative therapeutic relationship facilitates a working alliance. Even when therapists need to provide structure, the person with the brain illness should always have choices and authority regarding her own feelings and life history. Her dignity and independence should be respected. Therapy should be empowering.
10. Session flexibility is essential to accommodate disabilities and life changes. Follow-up after formal therapy ends is often needed to maintain gains.
11. Fluctuations in medical status affect the course of treatment. Therapists need to be flexible in accommodating medical changes and to be alert to mental changes that could signal the need for medical intervention.
12. The distortions of family members must be addressed in therapy.
13. Family members' mourning must be addressed.
14. Family members are important therapeutic helpers.

[a] From "Cognitive Therapy and the Treatment of Poststroke Depression," by M. R. Hibbard, S. E. Grober, W. A. Gordon, E. G. Aletta, and A. Freeman, 1990, *Topics in Geriatric Rehabilitation, 5*(3), 43–55. Copyright 1990 by Aspen Publishers. Adapted with permission.

**TABLE 9.4. Indications Favoring the Use of Antidepressant Medications in Depressed People with Brain Illnesses**

Sleep and appetite disturbances are prominent.

There is a significant chronic pain problem.

The person with a brain illness is too depressed or too cognitively impaired to be accessible to psychotherapy.

There is a significant history of depression from before the brain illness.

The depression is severe and persistent.

The person with a brain illness believes in medications and is wary of psychotherapy.

## ANXIETY

### Description

Signs of moderate to severe anxiety or panic include fast, shallow breathing; rapid heartbeat; sweating; dry mouth; trembling; and feelings of weakness--the "fight or flight" reaction of autonomic nervous system arousal. Less severe symptoms include unreasonably avoiding some situations, difficulty concentrating, difficulty falling asleep, agitation, extra movements, tension, gastrointestinal symptoms, muscle pain, and so forth. Anxiety is one of the most common persistent symptoms following a TBI (Morton & Wehman, 1995).

### Similar Neurological Symptoms

Difficulty concentrating can be either a direct consequence of brain illness or a symptom of anxiety. If it is organic it is likely to fluctuate with fatigue, whereas if it is from anxiety it will fluctuate with anxiety. Of course, both may be present. Disorders of the autonomic nervous system can produce symptoms of anxiety, sometimes without the accompanying emotional state.

### Similar Nonneurological Conditions

The person with a brain illness could have a pre-illness anxiety disorder. Anxiety may be related to events other than the brain illness itself. For example, it may be part of a PTSD.

### Associated Symptoms

Cognitive impairments may interact with anxiety. For example, a person who cannot remember what she has been told about what will happen may be anxious about the uncertainty of the future. She may also have emotional memories of stressful experiences, even if she cannot remember the events themselves (Layton & Wardi-Zonna, 1994; McMillan, 1991). Anxiety also results from discovering deficits and from being uncertain about what other deficits may be present (see the Perplexity section that follows, p. 168).

People with sensory intolerance (see the Hyperaesthesia section, Chapter 12, p. 257) may be constantly startled or overloaded by their environment and may become anxious. Anxiety can be a component of the agitation in emerging from a coma or from post-traumatic amnesia. Depression, frustration, fatigability, and perplexity are common with anxiety. Repeated failure may exacerbate anxiety.

Usually anxiety and reduced emotional reactivity do not occur together. The person with planning impairments will usually have difficulty thinking of the future, including worrying about it. Sometimes a person with an anxiety disorder will become relieved of anxiety through brain illness and may even become inappropriately unconcerned.

### *Neuroanatomy*

No particular lesion is associated with anxiety, but anxiety is less likely with frontal and with right hemisphere lesions.

### *How to Interview Regarding Anxiety*

The person with a brain illness is more likely to be aware of anxiety than the family, except that people with amnesia may not remember their anxiety. Interview questions should include subjective worry and also physiological signs such as rapid heartbeat and breathing, easy startling, sweating, avoidance, and so forth.

### *How to Observe/Test*

Anxiety can be observed in nervous movements, in rigid responses, in tense postures, in hyperventilation, in startle responses, and in hypervigilance. If it is suspected that anxiety is interfering on tests of attention, it can be useful to manipulate the conditions to change the anxiety and then repeat the test. For example, one could use a different examiner, change the instructions, or conduct relaxation training just before the test. Conventional personality tests usually measure anxiety.

### *Practical Problems*

High levels of anxiety are intrinsically undesirable, and can interfere with all activities. People with anxiety problems may increasingly restrict their lives and become isolated and avoidant. Anxiety can also lead to other problematic reactions such as anger, shouting, and impulsive behavior. Phobic anxiety interferes with specific activities associated with certain locations or stimuli. Anxiety can interfere with a valid assessment of thinking abilities. However, mild anxiety enhances performance at many activities and may be desirable and even sought out (e.g., amusement park rides, horror movies, high-risk sports).

### *Interventions*

1. Educating the person with a brain illness about what to expect from her condition can help to reduce fear and anxiety. This must be done at a pace that the person with a brain illness is ready to hear so as not to induce more anxiety.
2. Encouraging the person with a brain illness to say what it is she is afraid of can also help.

3. Reducing overstimulation may also be helpful.
4. A daily routine and structure can help to make events more predictable and less anxiety-provoking.
5. Providing orienting information, explanations, and preparation for change and for transition may also help to make events feel more predictable and less anxiety-provoking.
6. Structuring daily activities so as to minimize failure and maximize success may also be helpful.
7. Medications such as benzodiazepines and antipsychotics should be used with great care and only when clearly indicated. With brain illnesses these sometimes sedate and add to confusion and to amnesia (Gualtieri, 1991). Antidepressants and buspirone are less problematic. Brief, repeatable, quantifiable tests of concentration and memory can be used before and after medication to help evaluate whether the medication is interfering with thinking.
8. Standard psychotherapeutic techniques for anxiety and for phobias can be applied where appropriate and when the person is capable. These include systematic desensitization, cognitive techniques such as affirmations, and psychoanalytic approaches. Relaxation training can be applied even with severe amnesia because it may be learned through preserved procedural learning, and it can be supplemented with memory compensations such as relaxation tapes. Systematic desensitization may need to work through gradually introducing the person into actual anxiety-producing situations rather than through fantasy if imagery capacities are impaired.
9. The techniques in Chapter 8 can also be applied, including identifying risks and warning signs; the strategy of back off, calm down, try again; and cue cards for anxiety (Table 7.5a, p. 113).
10. Because of the risk of increasing isolation, withdrawal, and overprotection with chronic anxiety, stress inoculation (Meichenbaum, 1985, 1992, 1993) may be needed.

## *PERPLEXITY*

### *Description*

Perplexity is a feeling of uncertainty or of insecurity resulting from the discovery that one's mind and body are unexpectedly unreliable (Lezak, 1978). It implies a good awareness of deficits, and so is more common with mild than with severe impairments. Often the person feels that she is going crazy. She may complain, "I forget things I never used to forget. I get confused in the middle of doing things that I know I know how to do. I'm clumsy in ways I never was. I can't rely on my memory anymore."

### *Similar Nonneurological Conditions*

PTSD, borderline personality disorder, anxiety disorders, and the onset of schizophrenia may include the symptom of perplexity. These conditions are best differentiated by the history of their time course and by other distinctive symptoms of those disorders.

### *Associated Symptoms*

Anxiety, frustration, fatigue, and mild attention and memory difficulties are the most common symptoms associated with perplexity. A person who is frankly confused may or may not also be perplexed, depending on her awareness of her confusion.

### *How to Interview*

The person will be more aware of this problem than will the family. Interview questions should focus on the fear of going crazy and on feelings of uncertainty and of insecurity.

### *How to Observe/Test*

As perplexity is not necessarily directly observable, it is more likely to emerge from the interview. People experiencing perplexity may show expressions of bewilderment or may stop in the middle of activities and may seem puzzled or overwhelmed.

### *Practical Problems*

Perplexity may produce an adjustment disorder with withdrawal from many activities for fear of failure and may contribute to reactive depression.

### *Interventions*

Reassurance, education, and support groups are the main interventions. The main message is as follows:

> Because of your brain illness you may feel perplexed. You may feel uncertain or insecure because you find that your mind and your body are not reliable. You may make mistakes, drop things, or forget things that you normally would not. You may be afraid that you are going crazy, even though you are not. This is a common and normal reaction. It is likely to be slightly worse when you are tired, anxious, and frustrated. It will go away with time and as you understand better what things do and don't give you problems. It often helps to talk with someone who understands.

## *FRUSTRATION*

### *Description*

Impairments in skills such as memory, attention, language, executive functions, or motor skills that affect a broad range of activities can make frustration a pervasive experience.

### *Similar Neurological Symptoms*

People with increased emotional reactivity, with labile emotions, with irritability, or with impulsive anger become frustrated more easily and intensely than those with simple reactive frustration. People with reflex crying may appear to be more frustrated than they are.

### *Similar Nonneurological Conditions*

People who were high achievers prior to their illnesses are somewhat more likely to become frustrated by their symptoms.

### *Associated Symptoms*

Frustration is more common with good awareness or overestimation of deficits than with anosognosia. It is particularly common and poignant with expressive aphasia. Frustration often increases with recovery from anosognosia. Frustration may be intensified by poor memory, poor planning, and poor problem solving, because the frustrating experience may be unrestrained by memory of successes or by visions of alternative solutions. In other words, with less mental access to the past and the future, frustration overwhelms present awareness.

### *Neuroanatomy*

Frustration can be present with any neurological or neuropsychological difficulty, but it seems to be particularly strong with left frontal lesions.

### *How to Interview Regarding Frustration*

The person who gets frustrated is likely to be somewhat more aware of it than family members, unless she also has a significant memory impairment. Interview questions can focus directly on frustration and on giving up.

### *How to Observe/Test*

Signs of anger, excuses, or withdrawal on difficult tasks may indicate frustration. It is often useful to ask the person to continue trying a difficult task to observe her frustration tolerance; that is, if she gives up easily, if she pushes herself too hard and overreacts, or if she has an appropriate balance in the amount and in the ways that she pushes herself.

### *Practical Problems*

Frustration can produce anger, depression, and withdrawal. It may limit recovery. Frustration can make it harder to think and to act to find solutions to problems.

### *Interventions*

1. The person needs to be told that frustration is a common and normal reaction to brain illness. Support groups can help to normalize the experience.
2. The person who gives up too easily can often benefit from encouragement, from affirmations, and from setting small goals to maximize success experiences. If these are unsuccessful, it may be necessary to consider the person's personality structure, motivators, family situation, and understanding of the disorder and of rehabilitation.
3. The person who pushes too hard and has overwhelming emotional reactions needs to be educated about the process of rehabilitation, the balance of appropriate challenges, and the zone of recovery. Effort and motivation should be recognized, while noting that new skills of monitoring frustration levels, pacing, and using help and rest appropriately are needed for maximal efficiency.

   The following type of message is often useful:

> I am glad to see you are strongly motivated to get better. That drive served you well before your injury and will be a big help now. But now you also need to learn other skills to adapt to your injury to use that drive for its best effect. You need to learn to recognize when frustration is getting in your way. Then you can prevent it, get the rest you need, and still accomplish what you want more efficiently. You also need to learn not to try things you are not ready for.
>
> A little frustration is good. You need to struggle some with things that are now difficult in order to learn how to do them and how to handle frustration. Too much help can prevent this necessary recovery process. But too much frustration is bad. When you can't continue trying because of being overwhelmed by frustration, it is time for someone else to help. The best help usually lets you calm down enough to discover how to do it, rather than having it done for you.

> Choose your challenges. Helpers should do the things that are impossible for you and should try to find ways to make other activities challenging but possible. For example, because you can't use your right arm it's more practical to have someone cut up your food for you, but you don't need to be spoon-fed, even though your left hand is more awkward in getting food to your mouth and you do spill sometimes. You can help with cooking, setting and clearing the table, and washing.

4. The techniques in Chapter 8 can be applied to frustration.

## *EMBARRASSMENT*

### *Description*

Embarrassment or shame is a common reaction to neurological disabilities. This may be embarrassment about the condition that resulted in the disability (e.g., drunken driving, assault, sexually transmitted disease), about the fact of being disabled, or about the behavior that results. Particularly embarrassing conditions include loss of bowel or bladder control, drooling, reflex crying, seizures, automatic cursing, emotional lability, language impairments, and memory impairments. Embarrassment can be particularly poignant for people who appear normal, because abnormal behavior then seems to require explanation.

### *Related and Associated Symptoms*

Embarrassment is often associated with frustration, with depression and with social withdrawal. The degree of embarrassment and the situations that prove embarrassing are largely a function of pre-illness personality, context, and culture.

### *How to Interview Regarding Embarrassment*

The person with a brain illness usually experiences the embarrassment most acutely. With anosognosia,the family may be more embarrassed. Interview questions should focus on situations and on people that provoke embarrassment, beliefs that support embarrassment, and activities that are avoided because of it.

### *How to Observe/Test*

Embarrassment may be less evident in the clinic than in public. If possible, the person should be observed in social situations, especially with strangers and especially where the disability becomes evident.

### *Practical Problems*

Embarrassment can produce social withdrawal and depression.

### *Interventions*

1. Education of the person and the family can do much to prevent or minimize embarrassment. Counseling can include exploring feelings about the disabilities, problem-solving strategies for encounters with others, writing scripts or cue cards for explaining the disability to others, and role playing feared encounters.

2. Role models of others living successfully with similar disabilities can be provided through stories, through historical or contemporary examples, through pairing with someone else with that disability, and through support groups.

3. Planning gradually more risky encounters with others can be part of a social desensitization therapy plan for persons disabled by their shame. The person can be given assignments for particular activities and encounters and can report back to therapy to debrief the therapist after each one.

4. Direct community interventions can include educating classrooms, workplaces, institutions, and so forth about embarrassing behaviors and about how to react to them.

## *CATASTROPHIC REACTION*

Goldstein (1952) coined the term "catastrophic reaction" to describe the reaction of people with brain illnesses when overwhelmed by frustration, anxiety, stimulation, and/or confrontation of their deficits. The term has been used in many ways since then and has lost precision (Ruckdeschel-Hibbard, Gordon, & Diller, 1986), but still retains usefulness. It suggests someone who, through confronting failure, "hits her limit" and is overwhelmed by her own losses and her incompetence. The resulting disinhibited or labile behavior could be tears, aggression, precipitous withdrawal, panic, escape, catatonia, and so forth. The experience often cannot be neatly characterized as frustration, embarrassment, anxiety, and so forth, but is a combination of these.

The concept is useful in that it permits talking about complex experiences, feelings, and behavior without prejudging or categorizing them too narrowly, but it is vague and does not need elaborating here. The major interventions for catastrophic reactions are those in Chapter 8, as well as for the contributing components described in this and in the following chapters.

## *POST-TRAUMATIC STRESS DISORDER (PTSD)*

### *Description*

PTSD is the normal or exaggerated emotional response to a traumatic event such as a battle experience or a life-threatening illness or accident (*DSM–IV*, 1994). There are three types of posttraumatic stress symptoms:

1. Re-experiencing the trauma through recurrent, intrusive memories, nightmares, flashbacks, or intense distress at stimuli resembling the trauma.
2. Avoidance of reminders of the trauma and/or general numbing of emotional responsiveness, such as avoiding activities, situations, thoughts, or feelings associated with the trauma; psychogenic amnesia for parts of the trauma; markedly decreased interest in significant activities; and detachment from others, flattened affect, and so forth.
3. Persistent increased arousal, such as difficulty falling or staying asleep, irritability, difficulty concentrating, hypervigilance, or exaggerated startle response. When the reaction is of short duration, the stressor is not life-threatening, or full PTSD criteria are not met, the diagnosis may be Acute Stress Disorder or Adjustment Reaction (*DSM–IV*, 1994).

### *Similar Neurological Symptoms*

Many of the features of PTSD are easily confused with symptoms of brain illness, especially a minor TBI (Table 9.5). Because TBI and emotional trauma often occur together, it can be difficult to know how to attribute and to treat these symptoms.

#### *Intrusive, Recurrent Memories*

Recurrent, intrusive, distressing memories, thoughts, and images related to the trauma are common in PTSD. People with brain illnesses may have perseverative thoughts and questions, especially with anterograde amnesia, but these are more annoying than distressing and do not relate exclusively to the trauma.

#### *Nightmares*

Nightmares, particularly related to the trauma, are a common symptom of PTSD, but they are uncommon with brain illness and so are useful in differential diagnosis. When present with brain illness, they were most likely also present prior to the illness or due to conditions that also produce hallucinations.

**TABLE 9.5. Potentially Confusable Symptoms: Post-Traumatic Stress Disorder (PTSD) versus Traumatic Brain Injury (TBI)**

| PTSD | TBI |
|---|---|
| Intrusive, recurrent memories of the event | Perseveration, variable content |
| Flashbacks | Disorientation, confusion (not specific to an event) |
| Intense distress on exposure to reminders | Emotional lability, reflex crying |
| Avoidance of reminders | Impaired initiation |
| Amnesia for the event | Organic amnesia |
| Decreased interest in activities | Lack of initiation, reduced emotional responsiveness |
| Feelings of detachment | Reduced emotional responsiveness, lack of empathy from concrete thinking |
| Restricted range of affect | Reduced emotional responsiveness, impaired emotional expressiveness |
| Sense of foreshortened future | Impaired planning |
| Insomnia | Disturbed sleep due to pain, restlessness, decreased bed mobility, IV tubes, physical restraints, subcortical damage |
| Irritability | Impulsive anger |
| Attention difficulties, especially concentration | Attention difficulties, including distractibility |
| Hypervigilance | Distractibility |
| Exaggerated startle response | Distractibility, emotional lability |

*Flashbacks*

Flashbacks are times when the person temporarily seems to reexperience the traumatic event. A soldier may hear a car backfire and jump into a ditch, thinking she is back in combat. An electric shock torture victim may flee when electrocardiogram electrodes are applied. These experiences are usually very emotional and relate directly to the trauma. By contrast, the disorientation of the person with a brain injury may be unemotional. Her idea of where she is will usually relate to immediate stimuli but not necessarily to traumatic events. For example, a brain-injured woman, recognizing that she is in a hospital, may assume that she is there to have a baby.

*Amnesia*

In general, people with neurological amnesia for a traumatic event (they cannot remember it due to a brain injury) are not likely to have a PTSD for that event (Sbordone & Liter, 1995), although they could have a PTSD for stressful events that they remember from before or from after the injury. They may have a grief reaction for their losses. Those with psychological amnesia for the event (they do not remember it because they have repressed or suppressed the memory) will usually have a PTSD. It is possible to have both a PTSD and a brain injury from the same event; for example, those with gunshot wounds to the head often do not lose consciousness and recall the entire trauma. Also, PTSD symptoms can occur in minor TBIs with organic amnesia for the trauma (Hickling, Gillen, Blanchard, Buckley, & Taylor, 1998; Layton & Wardi-Zonna, 1994; McMillan, 1991). Symptoms include avoidance of stimuli associated with the trauma for which there is no conscious memory. These symptoms have been attributed to learning via classical conditioning which is dissociated from declarative memory.

*Withdrawal*

The person with a PTSD withdraws out of phobic fear, depression, or a lost sense of purpose. The person with a brain injury may withdraw for these reasons or because of embarrassment, sensory intolerance, or impaired initiation.

*Sense of Futurelessness*

The person with a PTSD may complain of a philosophical sense of despair, as if there is no point in living, nothing dependable, or nothing to look forward to. The person with organically impaired planning simply fails to think about the future, or thinks about the future inadequately. She either does not complain about it or complains of inability to plan.

*Insomnia*

See the discussion of insomnia under Depression, this chapter.

*Irritability*

The irritability of a PTSD is more likely to arise in the context of events that relate to the trauma, whereas the anger, impulsiveness, frustration, and catastrophic reactions of brain illness are more likely to relate to the disabilities.

*Lack of Concentration*

The person with a PTSD may have difficulty concentrating because of an obsession with the trauma. The person with a brain illness is more likely to be distractible and to perform poorly on attention tests. The person with a PTSD may complain of concentration difficulties and may or may not perform normally on attention tests. Cognitive deficits on neuropsychological tests have been found in PTSDs (Gil, Calev, Greenberg, & Kugelmass, 1990; Raskin, 1997; Yehuda et al., 1995), although the finding is controversial (Zalewski, Thompson, & Gottesman, 1994).

*Hypervigilance*

The person with PTSD may startle easily and may react with fear, especially to stimuli that relate to the trauma; for example, the sound of gunfire, screams, or smoke. There may be a phobic or an obsessive-compulsive quality to her reactions. The connection to the trauma may not be obvious, but it can usually be discovered by redescribing the trauma or by talking about the situation that produced the startle. She may also constantly check out little sounds, as if always on sentry duty. This may disturb her sleep.

The distractibility of brain illness is not specific to the trauma. It can involve any stimulus, such as music, conversation, or objects that are lying around. It may be specific to one sensory modality. Distractibility usually does not produce a marked emotional reaction, except possibly frustration, irritability, or startle. The person may find it particularly difficult to return to her task and to remember what she was doing.

*Guilt*

Guilt about being the survivor or about things done or not done during the trauma is a common part of a PTSD. It is less usual with a brain illness, and when it is present it usually was a prominent part of the person's personality before the brain condition.

### *How to Interview Regarding PTSD*

The person with a PTSD is more likely to be aware of it than are family members. Occasionally a family member may recognize a connection between an intrusive thought, a nightmare, or an avoidance behavior and the trauma of which the person with a PTSD is not aware. The interview should focus on a description of the trauma as well as an exploration of criterion symptoms.

### *How to Observe/Test*

Watch for startle reactions and for signs of fear, anxiety, and avoidance. Some personality tests such as the MMPI-II have PTSD scales. There are specific tests and structured interviews for PTSD (Allen, 1994). Traumatic material can often be seen on projective tests.

### *Practical Problems*

Nightmares, intrusive thoughts, and flashbacks can be quite distressing and painful. Avoidance behaviors can severely restrict the person's participation in life. Hypervigilance, depression, guilt, and withdrawal can be exhausting and disabling. Substance abuse is a significant risk.

### *Interventions*

1. Less severe post-traumatic stress experiences are often dealt with by talking them through as many times as needed in a safe, nonjudgmental, supportive environment. The person describes the event in as much detail as she can. More detail and feelings come with repetition. She should be encouraged to cry, to tremble, to shout, or to laugh without inhibition. This need not be with a professional but can be with family, a friend, a group, or others with similar experiences. She may need to tell several different people.
2. Severe or persistent symptoms such as diagnosed PTSD, Acute Stress Disorder, or Adjustment Reaction often require formal therapy (Herman, 1992). It can take a long time to establish the needed therapeutic trust. The person may not be ready to retell and reexperience the trauma for weeks, for months, or for years, or she may need to repeat it many times for months. Visits to the site of the trauma, to funerals, or to partial recreations of the experience can be useful in stimulating processing of the trauma, provided that the person feels safe and in charge of the experience. Group therapy with people with similar experiences may be needed.
3. Antidepressant or antianxiety medications may be needed for severe, for disabling, or for persistent symptoms.
4. Some hypervigilant and phobic features can be treated through systematic desensitization (Shapiro, 1989) or with other behavioral techniques (Boudewyns, Hyer, Woods, Harrison, & McCranie, 1990).

## *PERSONAL REFORMATION*

### *Description*

Some people who experience a brain illness take it as an opportunity to reform their lives (Case 9.1. Gigi). The brush with death gives some a reason to reflect philosophically or religiously and to reprioritize their life goals. Some abandon habits that have lead to the illness, such as alcoholism, smoking, violence, or risk-taking. Some decide to be of service or to place more value on their family, their faith, or their community. Others decide that life is short and that they will try to enjoy it more (in responsible or in self-destructive ways).

### *How to Interview Regarding Personal Reformation*

Personal reformation may emerge in questioning about the general impact of the illness, about future plans, or about religious beliefs.

*Prognosis? Case 9.1. Gigi.* A 29-year-old, ninth-grade educated, former bartender and topless dancer was referred for possible treatment 1 year after a severe TBI. She had a brainstem hemorrhage and had been in a coma for a month. She had a moderate left hemiplegia and walked with a cane. She had a seizure disorder that was controlled by medication. She had gained weight and was moderately obese. Her language was crude and blunt, but she was respectful and consistent in her requests for help.

She had been physically and sexually abused by her stepfather and she left home at 14 to escape him. She had given one child up for adoption and had given another to the custody of his father. She had a history of alcohol and of polydrug abuse. She had been the victim of multiple abusive relationships. She came to sessions with her boyfriend who was himself disabled with a back injury. She frequently cancelled, rescheduled, or failed to appear for sessions, citing transportation difficulties and problems with neighbors in their public housing apartment.

Her major complaint was problems with rapidly fluctuating emotions, especially sudden depression with suicidal ideation and the urge to use drugs. She reported that she had been clean and sober since the accident and intended to stay that way. Besides her boyfriend, her other source of support was a man 20 years her senior who was 3000 miles away. Her goals were to stabilize her emotions, to return to work and to driving, and to re-establish contact with her son. On testing she had mild to moderate impairments in memory with other functions intact.

She had brief cognitive rehabilitation to consolidate and to improve her memory compensation system and physical therapy to improve her walking. She had brief neuropsychotherapy involving a cue card (Table 7.5b, p. 114) for recognizing and coping with depression. She rapidly learned to apply this successfully. Referrals for substance abuse support groups and brain injury support groups were politely declined, but she accepted a referral to the state vocational rehabilitation agency.

Three years later Gigi called for a follow-up appointment, mostly for reassurance that she was not mentally retarded. She had been working steadily in a protected setting where there were mentally retarded people present. She came in with the same boyfriend. She was still clean and sober and free of depression and was still carrying the cue card, although it had long since been memorized. She was using the same memory book system with which she had finished treatment. She had returned to driving and had established a relationship with her son.

This case is an extreme example of someone who's life was turned around by an injury. A modest investment of therapy in an individual with a severe injury from a rehabilitation team flexible enough to accommodate her situation and help her toward her goals resulted in a very favorable outcome. Prejudices concerning her history could easily have prevented this result.

### *Practical Problems*

Some naive or overly ambitious individuals may attempt unrealistic life changes and may then become depressed or regressed when they fail at these. Some may overindulge.

### *Interventions*

The therapist can guide the person inclined toward personal reformation in exploring values and in choosing realistic, healthy, rewarding channels for her new energy. She may be directed toward a spiritual counselor or toward another person whom she respects.

# 10

# Organic Emotional Changes

Brain illness can affect the intensity of emotional experience and the ability to communicate emotions. These functions may be diminished or increased (see Table 2.2, p. 28), and these changes may be seen in combination. Brain illness can also disinhibit the expression of experienced emotion. Cognitive impairments may change how events are interpreted and the types of emotions experienced.

## *EMOTIONAL COMMUNICATION: IMPAIRED EMOTIONAL EXPRESSIVENESS AND COMPREHENSION*

### *Description*

People with impaired emotional expressiveness may have a flat or a monotone voice, little facial expression, few gestures, and little emotional expression in conversation. Underlying feeling states may or may not be intact. Some people may lose their ability to understand other's emotions from their tone of voice, from facial expressions, from body language, and so forth. They may take sarcasm, irony, or jokes literally. They may misunderstand situations and may have poor empathy (Borod, 1992; Ross, 1981, 1993).

### *Similar Neurological Symptoms*

Lack of initiation looks similar to, and is sometimes associated with, impaired emotional expression. Lack of emotional responsiveness, lack of initiation, impaired empathy, labile emotions, and disinhibition can all make a person appear insensitive to or unable to comprehend the emotions of others. Each of these areas must be assessed separately.

### *Similar Nonneurological Conditions*

Depression, PTSD, catatonia, and depersonalization can reduce emotional expressions. PTSD and depression may or may not accompany impaired emotional expression and must be assessed separately. Catatonia and depersonalization are usually more distinctive. Poor social skills and sensory impairments can result in poor emotional comprehension.

### *Associated Symptoms*

Impaired expression and comprehension of emotions are associated with each other and with impaired awareness of deficits, with indifference, and with reflex crying. Impaired singing and Parkinson's disease are both associated with impaired emotional expression. Visual-spatial impairments and impaired music perception are associated with impaired emotional comprehension.

### *Neuroanatomy*

Impaired emotional expression is most common with right frontal lesions, especially the inferior, posterior, lateral portion (the right Broca's area, Borod, 1992; Ross, 1981; 1993), subcortical or peripheral lesions producing dysarthrias, and lesions of the basal ganglia, for example, in Parkinson's Disease (Blonder, R. E. Gur, & Gur, 1989). Impaired emotional comprehension is most common with lesions in the right parietal and temporal lobes (Borod, 1992; Ross, 1981, 1993).

### *How to Interview Regarding Impaired Emotional Communication*

The family is more likely than the person with the deficit to be aware of this problem. Inquiries should be made regarding a flat voice, a change in voice, a perception of depression, not caring about people, misunderstandings, a change in sense of humor, and lack of empathy.

### *How to Observe/Test*

The examiner should listen for flat voice, especially when discussing emotional topics, and should watch facial expressions. The person can also be asked to judge how others feel or to explain what is happening on a television show, especially a soap opera.

Emotional comprehension can be directly tested by stating a neutral sentence with different moods, such as happy, sad, angry, questioning, and teasing, and by asking the person to identify the mood or feeling (Ross, 1981, 1993).

Emotional expression can then be tested by asking the person to say that sentence expressing each of those moods. If he is hesitant to do this or does not understand the directions well, then he should be asked to imitate the examiner in emotional expressions. It is also important to probe his awareness of the quality of his performance.

*The Victoria Emotion Recognition Test* (Mountain & Spreen, 1993) and *The Emotional Perception Test* (Cognisyst, n.d., see Appendix B) give standardized, systematic probing of emotional comprehension abilities.

### *Practical Problems*

Those around the person may misunderstand his emotional state. Family relations may become strained.

### *Interventions*

1. In the education of the person and the family about the problem, it should be made clear that he is not depressed (if he is not), and that the lessened ability to communicate emotions is not his fault but the fault of the brain lesion.
2. For Expression Difficulties: When it is important for them to know, those around the person should ask him how he is feeling, and this should be modeled for them. They should attend to the content of the answer rather than to the expression. The person should be encouraged to put his feelings into words as a compensatory strategy. If he is aware enough, he can learn to tell those around him about the nature of his problem.
3. Audiotape, videotape, and mirrors can be used for feedback, especially if emotional comprehension is well preserved.
4. Speech therapy and group therapy can focus on improving emotional expression. "Drama coaching" can use others to give feedback about how he sounds and looks.
5. For Comprehension Difficulties: His family should be instructed in stating feelings to him explicitly as a compensation, rather than relying on tone of voice and so forth. This should be modeled for them. He should be encouraged to pay greater attention to expressions of feelings, to ask how people are feeling, and to consider alternate interpretations if he is confused by what someone says.
6. Group therapy with emphasis on emotional communication skills may help. Another strategy might be to view a videotape of a television show, stopping it frequently to ask the person what feelings are being expressed by the characters.

## *REFLEX CRYING AND LAUGHING*

### *Description*

Reflex crying is involuntary crying that can result from brain illness (Shaibani, Sabbagh, & Doody, 1994). Typically the person cries very easily, even when not feeling particularly upset (Case 10.1. A.L.S., Lieberman & Benson, 1977; Ross & Stewart, 1987). The crying comes on suddenly during emotional events or topics regardless of their intensity. The crying has a stereotyped appearance that can be recognized with experience; the face appears to "melt." Sobbing and other vocalization is uncommon.

This is sometimes called "emotional lability," "labile mood," "labile affect," or "pseudobulbar affect." The term reflex crying is preferred because it is usually crying and expressions that fluctuate widely, not actual mood or emotions, and the term is better accepted by people with reflex crying and by their families (Judd & Stoffel, 1989).

Reflex smiling and laughing may be present with or without reflex crying (Black, 1982; Zeilig, Drubach, Katz-Zeilig, & Karatinos, 1996). Reflex laughing and smiling have the same characteristics as reflex crying except the trigger is usually something amusing.

*Report from the Land of ALS. Case 10.1a*[a]. *A. L. S.* A 55-year-old woman with amyotrophic lateral sclerosis (ALS) wrote the following in her "Reports From the Land of ALS."

One effect of ALS is that certain emotional breaks seem to be ineffectual. I have already experienced some of this, been aware while it was happening that I was not as upset or as sad as my crying would imply, nor as uproariously amused as my uncontrollable laughter would indicate. Such episodes of laughter and tears may have slight connection with my actual frame of mind or the feeling which is actually mine at the time. In fact, I usually become very frustrated and angry at my inability to put a halt to such ridiculous behavior!

I begin to smile, but the smile becomes an exaggerated grin, which attaches itself, fixedly, to my face and I have to use all my powers of concentration to remove the embarrassing grimace. If I yield to the impulse, it becomes the onset to equally uncontrollable giggles, which in turn so embarrass me, that I become angry, humiliated, and subject to uncontrollable tears—it is a vicious, see-sawing circle!

*Thank You, and Now for My Next Act. Case 10.1b. Support Group.* I introduced myself to a stroke support group by saying, "You may know my name from an article in your newsletter called 'Reflex Crying.'" Instantly, two men burst into tears—and the article wasn't that great!

[a] From "Control of Emotional Expression in Pseudobulbar Palsy: A Personal Experience," by A. Lieberman, and D. F. Benson, 1977, *Archives of Neurology, 34,* 717–719. Copyright 1977 by American Medical Association. Reprinted with permission.

*Similar Neurological Symptoms*

The person with labile emotions will have rapid fluctuations in his actual mood, not just in the expression of feelings.

*Similar Nonneurological Conditions*

Depression and the labile moods of PTSD and histrionic and borderline personality disorders may involve frequent crying, but the mood is congruent with the crying, and the crying is not stereotyped. Depression, reflex crying, PTSD, and personality disorders must each be assessed separately.

*Associated Symptoms*

Reflex crying and laughing are associated with impaired emotional communication and with motor impairments.

*Neuroanatomy*

Reflex crying is most common with strokes. The motor system is almost always involved, but the cortex need not be. It can also occur with multiple sclerosis, amyotrophic lateral sclerosis, head trauma, tumors, and other localized lesions. Reflex laughing is more common with a TBI (Zeilig, et al., 1996).

*How to Interview Regarding Reflex Crying*

The crying person and the family alike will be aware of the crying, but the crier is more likely to understand that the crying is abnormal. The interview should focus on changes in crying, on feelings while crying, on embarrassment, on misunderstanding, and how the person would like to be treated when crying. Depression should be explored. Because increased crying may be seen in 60% of an inpatient stroke population (Judd & Stoffel, 1989), it is prudent to screen for reflex crying in such populations.

*How to Observe/Test*

One should gently touch on emotional topics such as family when interviewing. If the person cries, he should be asked if he feels like crying and if he feels sad and upset or if the crying is out of character for him. Any particular episode of crying may or may not be genuine, reflex, or somewhere in between. The condition can be rated on the Pathological Laughter and Crying Scale (Robinson et al., 1993).

*Practical Problems*

Risks include misunderstanding and miscommunication with family and with others, embarrassment, social withdrawal, and inappropriate treatment for depression. Reflex laughing can be taken for a lack of caring or for disrespect.

*Interventions*

1. When the person is not crying, he should be asked how he would like to be treated when he cries. Common preferences are as follows:
   - Treat it as an inconvenience, as other facial reflexes such as sneezing or hiccups. Continue the conversation as if it is a minor annoyance that will go away.
   - Some people prefer to be left alone.
   - With genuine crying or crying full of emotion, it is usually helpful to use empathy, understanding, and sometimes touch. This may increase crying, but that may help the person feel better.

   Most usually the person with severe reflex crying would like it to be ignored, whereas the person with mild reflex crying would like it to be treated like genuine crying.
2. When the person is crying, it may help to ask how he feels to find out if the episode is genuine crying, reflex crying, or in between and to know how to deal with him at that time.
3. It is better not to look away in embarrassed silence or to leave, unless that is what the person tells you that he prefers.
4. He should not be told not to cry. His feelings should not be minimized by saying things like "There, there, it will be all right, it's not that bad."
5. Some people can be trained to stop the crying by distracting themselves by looking at the ceiling, by taking deep breaths, by conversation, by activities, or by thinking of other things.
6. The person's crying pattern and how he wants to be treated when crying should be taught to his family through instruction and modeling. They need to know that he does not always mean to be crying; that the crying can be real, reflex, or in between, and that he is not necessarily depressed.
7. The person should be helped to find a way to explain the crying to others and should be encouraged to practice the explanation using a cue card, if needed (see Table 7.5f, p. 117). If this is not possible, the family may need to give others explanations, or written educational materials (e.g., Judd, n.d.). Problem-solving counseling and stroke support groups can address how to stay socially active in spite of the crying.

8. For the person with a severe reflex crying or laughing problem who is interested in treatment with a medication, antidepressants (Robinson et al., 1993; Schiffer, Cash, & Herndon, 1983) or levodopa (Udaka, Yamao, Nagata, Nakamura, & Kameyama, 1984) may help. If the medication is going to help, the effect will be within the first day or two and does not require the full 3-week trial.
9. Education for reflex laughing is similar to that for reflex crying except that other people tend to laugh along with the person with the laughing problem. This generally stimulates him more and everyone may soon become uncomfortable. Others must learn not to laugh along when it is not appropriate. Looking down and wiping his own face can help the laugher to stop laughing.

## *AUTOMATIC CURSING*

### *Description*

People with severe aphasia and people with Tourette's syndrome (Devinsky, Bear, Moya, & Berowitz, 1993) may curse when they do not intend to. Sometimes they will curse when trying to say other things. It does not always seem to be directed or angry cursing. They are usually aware of it and are often embarrassed by it.

### *Similar Neurological Symptoms*

Directed, voluntary cursing congruent with the circumstances may appear in someone who is disinhibited due to a brain illness.

### *Similar Nonneurological Conditions*

Normal cursing is usually voluntary and intended.

### *Associated Symptoms*

Automatic cursing can occur with severe nonfluent or global aphasia. It does not seem to reflect preaphasia cursing habits.

Tourette's syndrome is congenital and usually first appears in childhood. It includes abnormal movements, tics, and other involuntary behaviors. There is often partial control over the cursing and tics; they frequently can be inhibited for minutes or hours, but later emerge compulsively.

### *Neuroanatomy*

Severe aphasia usually results from large, central left hemisphere lesions. In people with aphasia, automatic cursing may be due to the preserved emotional language of the right hemisphere. The neuroanatomy of Tourette's syndrome is uncertain.

### *How to Interview Regarding Automatic Cursing*

The interviewer should ask if there has been a change in cursing, whether it is intended, and whether it is embarrassing or problematic.

### *How to Observe/Test*

In the person with aphasia, automatic cursing can most often be observed with attempts to speak. It should be noted if the cursing is appropriate to the context, if facial expression and other actions are consistent with cursing, if he is aware of the cursing, and if he is embarrassed or distressed by it.

If Tourette's syndrome is diagnosed, it will be important to observe the cursing in various social contexts, the degree of control that can be exercised, and the presence of other tics.

### *Practical Problems*

Risks of automatic cursing are embarrassment and social alienation and isolation.

### *Interventions*

1. It is particularly important to inform the family and the community that the cursing is involuntary, due to the brain lesion, and that the person does not really mean it. It can help to note that it can happen to anyone, and has been observed in ministers, priests, and so forth. It is not due to his personality.
2. For the person with aphasia, avoiding frustrating attempts to communicate in potentially embarrassing situations can help.
3. If social embarrassment and isolation are major problems, it may help to role play dealing with the problem in public, possibly with a family member. Humor may help; for example, a husband might explain to friends, "Did I ever tell you she used to be a sailor?" Cue cards, letters of explanation, and aphasia support groups can also help.
4. If the problem is so persistent and disabling that education is insufficient to deal with it, then the techniques in Chapter 8 may be applied.

5. People with Tourette's syndrome may learn to inhibit cursing in public and then release it in private. Support groups and medication (haloperidol) may help. An analysis of the situations of cursing (see Chapter 8, p. 146) may allow greater control.

## *COMPENSATORY EXAGGERATED EMOTIONAL EXPRESSIONS*

Some people with aphasia use pantomime and exaggerated expression of emotion to compensate, at least in part, for impaired language expression. Such expressiveness is generally voluntary, helpful, and nonproblematic.

## *EMOTIONAL REACTIVITY: IMPAIRED REACTIVITY*

### *Description*

People with brain illnesses sometimes react less emotionally than they did before their illness and than other people do. They may feel happy, angry, sad, afraid, sexually excited, and so forth, less easily, less frequently, less intensely, or not at all (Blumer & Benson, 1975; Prigatano, 1992; Stuss & Benson, 1986; Stuss, Gow, & Hetherington, 1992). They may appear indifferent to the world. Others may see them as automata or as robots. They may be able to identify what situations used to or ought to arouse which emotions but they simply no longer feel them (Case 10.2. Ludwig).

### *Similar Neurological Symptoms*

Some people appear indifferent because they cannot initiate but have normal reactions when external initiation is provided. People who are impaired only in expressing emotions appear indifferent but may report normal internal reactions. The person with concrete thinking may not respond to emotions of others due to a lack of empathy but may have egocentric emotional reactions.

### *Similar Nonneurological Symptoms*

Lack of emotional responsiveness is characteristic of depression, PTSD, or a repressive personality style. In depression and in PTSD, however, there may be increased sadness, distress, and anxiety. In some cultures, extreme emotional control or repression is a valued sign of masculinity, of high culture, or of objectivity.

*Where Is Inspiration Localized? Case 10.2. Ludwig (Judd, 1988).* Ludwig was a 51-year-old, right-handed professor of music and a composer who 10 years previously had right frontoparietal and temporal strokes with left hemiplegia. He reported that following the strokes he no longer listened to music for enjoyment as frequently as he used to, and he said that he no longer had significant emotional experiences from listening to music, although he had no difficulty in remembering his emotional responses to pieces in the past. Also, his musical composition since the stroke had been quite limited, despite efforts. One reason he cited was that he was no longer able to create the emotional milieu or atmosphere he felt to be a prerequisite to composing. This was a very important factor for him but was difficult for him to define or describe. It involved the ability to recall vividly a series of scenes, situations, or moods and use those recollections to generate a coherent piece of music. He compensated for this loss, in part, by writing a textbook of music theory in which he composed the (correct but emotionally sterile) examples.

### *Associated Symptoms*

Reduced emotional responsiveness is sometimes associated with impaired emotional expression, impaired initiation, impersistence, and attentional difficulties. Reduced and excessive emotional responsiveness can coexist; brief outbursts may punctuate long periods of indifference.

### *Neuroanatomy*

Lack of emotional responsiveness is most often seen with lesions to the dorsolateral frontal cortex, the basal ganglia, or the limbic system (Blumer & Benson, 1975; Prigatano, 1992; Stuss & Benson, 1986; Stuss, Gow, & Hetherington, 1992). It is common in Alzheimer's and in Parkinson's diseases.

### *How to Interview Regarding Emotional Reactivity*

Family members, especially spouses, are more likely to complain spontaneously about this problem than the person affected, although the person may complain of reduced libido.

### *How to Observe and Test*

Someone who shows little reaction when others do, or when a reaction might be expected, especially when with their family, can be suspected of having this condition. It is usually necessary to confirm the impression with information about pre-illness emotional responsiveness.

*The Frontal Lobe Personality Scale* (Grace, Malloy, & Stout, 1996), *The Head Injury Family Interview* (Kay et al., 1995), *The Neuropsychology Behavior and Affect Profile* (Nelson et al., 1989), *The Behavior Change Inventory* (Hartlage, 1991), *The Neuropsychiatric Inventory* (Cummings, 1997), and *The Neurobehavioral Rating Scale* (Levin et al., 1987) all evaluate reduced emotional responsiveness (see Appendix B).

### *Practical Problems*

Reduced emotional responsiveness can reduce motivation, disrupt relationships, and make life less enjoyable. It may be an improvement in some who were previously overly emotional.

### *Interventions*

1. Education about this condition can help family members not to take it too personally. Problem-solving counseling can help them to figure out ways to cope with it.
2. Perhaps because these individuals rarely complain about their loss, there is little in the literature about how to restore emotional responsiveness. The following is an untried theoretical suggestion. A series of experiences can be arranged designed to stimulate emotional responses, based on the person's history. The accompanying person can encourage the experience and expression of emotion. These experiences could include the following:
   - Motion pictures of various genres (comedy, romantic, horror, action, erotic), especially those known to have provoked responses in the person in the past
   - Exhilarating amusement park rides (if there are no medical contraindications such as vestibular or cardiac problems)
   - Visits to live sporting events, live theater, concerts, and so forth, sitting close to the action
   - Going to weddings, funerals, parties, and so forth.;
   - Visiting people and locations emotionally significant to the person in the past—former homes, places of worship, graveyards
   - Review family photo albums, movies, videos, etc. When emotions are experienced, the activity could be repeated, possibly with variation, at a later date. The event could also be explored to find what aspects of it were stimulating.

## *LABILE EMOTIONS*

### *Description*

People with brain illnesses sometimes react more emotionally than they did before their illness and than other people do. They may feel happy, angry, sad, afraid, disgusted, and so forth. more easily and more rapidly, and the feeling may go away more rapidly (Prigatano, 1992). The reactions may be quite out of proportion to the events that provoke them, and the events may be trivial in nature. The reactions may be out of character for the person.

### *Similar Neurological Symptoms*

Labile emotions can be confused with reflex crying, with reflex laughing, and with automatic cursing. In those conditions the person appears emotionally labile but does not feel that way. Labile emotions can result from temporary toxicity (e.g., drunkenness).

### *Similar Nonneurological Symptoms*

Labile emotions are common in people with intact brains during extreme emotional stress or fatigue. Similarly, in a person with a brain illness they can be a reaction to the illness experience rather than to a direct organic change. In that case the reactions are likely to be in character and connected to significant events. They can be features of PTSD, of histrionic and borderline personalities, of a bipolar disorder, and of schizophrenia.

### *Associated Symptoms*

Labile emotions are often seen with disinhibition. People with impairments in memory and in planning have little reference to the past or to the future to modulate their experiences. They may overreact, as if the present is their entire reality. Labile emotions may occasionally accompany temporal lobe epilepsy.

### *Neuroanatomy*

Labile emotions are particularly common with orbital frontal lobe damage and may be seen occasionally with irritative (seizure focus) lesions in the limbic system. They can also be present in diffuse injuries, in degenerative illnesses, and as a stage of recovery from moderate and from severe traumatic brain injuries.

### *How to Interview Regarding Labile Emotions*

Both the family and the person with the brain illness are likely to be aware of these changes. The interview should focus on changes in emotions, on feelings of being emotionally out of control, on things done in periods of emotionality, on circumstances of the reactions, and on major concerns about the emotionality.

### *How to Observe/Test*

The person should be observed at times that may be emotional, such as when meeting with the family, when getting frustrated on tests, or when talking about his illness or about the future. He can be questioned about emotional reactions afterward. All of the general neuropsychological personality assessment tools in Appendix B (p. 327) address labile emotions.

### *Practical Problems*

Labile emotions can be exhausting for the caregivers and for the person with the brain illness alike. Negative emotions that serve no purpose in helping the person to adjust are simply unnecessary pain. The family may react to labile emotions with panic, guilt, anger, and so forth. Less severe emotional lability can be a disruption to social relationships and an embarrassment. People with emotional lability may think they are going crazy or may lose self-confidence due to their lost self-control. Occasionally slightly more labile emotions may be a positive personality change (Ranseen, 1990).

### *Interventions*

1. Interventions should be planned only for those labile emotions perceived to be problematic.
2. Regardless of whether lability is neurogenic or psychogenic in nature, those around the person should generally be respectful of and empathetic with the emotions felt, particularly in the early stages of the problem. At the same time they should do their best to remain calm and to avoid reacting with similar intensity, which would be likely to amplify the reaction. Reassurance, orientation, and explanation are often helpful. In some circumstances it is helpful to listen to the feelings; at other times it may be better to distract the person. The appropriate strategy can be determined by trial and error.
3. When it has been determined that the labile emotions are organic and are not a psychological reaction to loss, it becomes important to interpret it this way to the person with the brain illness and to the family. Deep psychological analysis seeking childhood roots of the emotional reactions usually will not be helpful.
4. The circumstances of the problematic lability should be analyzed. When do episodes of lability occur? What helps resolve the situation? Do they

happen more when the person is tired, hungry, in pain, and so forth? Where practical, it is better to try to avoid the states or the situations that produce the problem emotions.

5. Strategies to abort problematic reactions can be helpful. Distraction can help some people, especially those with severe amnesia who rapidly forget what preoccupied them. Other strategies are in Chapter 8.
6. Medications are called for when the problem is persistent, unyielding to behavioral interventions, and disabling. These can include beta blockers, antidepressants, anticonvulsants, anxiolytics, and, rarely, antipsychotics. The medication chosen will depend upon the target symptoms and other medical considerations (Gualtieri, 1991). Antipsychotics and anxiolytics should be used sparingly because they often cloud thinking and interfere with recovery.
7. When neurogenic lability is a persistent problem, even after the person has regained self-control in other areas and when orientation and other cognitive abilities have improved, then a more detailed analysis of the problem is called for from an emotional rehabilitation perspective. Cuing from others, cognitive reframing, self-statements, a feelings journal, and other techniques described in Chapter 8 can be applied.
8. Emotional lability due to an acute psychological reaction to stress will frequently pass relatively rapidly with a structured, supportive, reassuring environment and with supportive counseling.
9. If emotional lability is part of a long-standing personality problem or a psychiatric disorder, then more traditional psychotherapeutic and psychopharmacological approaches can be used. Some individuals resist examination of their personalities, but they may be willing to learn self-control techniques in the context of rehabilitation for their brain illness.

## *IRRITABILITY, IMPULSIVE ANGER, AND AGITATION*

### *Description*

Anger following a brain illness can come from many sources (Table 10.1). The most important source for the clinician to be aware of is the organic impulsive anger (the proposed "organic aggressive syndrome" of S. C. Yudofsky, Silver, and Yudofsky [1989], or Howard's [1988] "'shallow' irritability") that results directly from the brain illness. This can be thought of on a continuum of severity from irritability to impulsive anger to agitation (Silver & Yudofsky, 1994). However, anger often is neither purely neurological nor purely psychological but is a combination of both.

**TABLE 10.1. Sources of Anger following Brain Illnesses**

- Pre-Injury Personality Factors
  - Explosive personality
  - Projection and blaming, chronic complainer
  - Violent lifestyle, culturally sanctioned violence/anger
  - Sociopathy, predatory violence, with or without anger
  - Mania
- Emotional Reaction Factors
  - Legitimate anger at the cause of injury
  - Grief reaction
  - Posttraumatic stress symptoms
  - Frustration
  - Normal, legitimate anger at an appropriate circumstance
- Neuropsychological Factors
  - Increased emotional reactivity
  - Irritability/impulsive anger/agitation
  - Temporal lobe epilepsy personality changes
  - Increased involuntary emotional communication
  - Automatic cursing of aphasia and Tourette's Syndrome
- Cognitive Impairments
  - Confusion
  - Executive function impairments
  - Lack of awareness of deficits
  - Disinhibition
  - Impaired judgment
  - Self-centeredness
  - Delusions
- Medical Factors
  - Pain
  - Fatigue
  - Toxicity
    - Alcohol
    - Stimulants
    - Medications

Agitation is often seen in the early stages of awakening from a coma (Corrigan & Mysiw, 1988). The person is confused and may even be delusional. His striking out is usually in response to physical contact or to a perceived threat. Overstimulation and attempts to restrain often to make it worse. Impulsive anger may persist for a long time, even after mild illnesses. Impulsive anger is most usually part of a disinhibition process.

The distinctive characteristics of impulsive anger (Miller, 1993; Prigatano, 1992; Silver & Yudofsky, 1994; Table 10.2) often allow organic impulsive anger to be distinguished from pre-illness anger patterns. In the words of one man with

**TABLE 10.2. Characteristics of Organic Impulsive Anger[a]**

| | |
|---|---|
| Illness-Related | Begins with brain illness or is made significantly worse by it. |
| Sudden | Episodes of anger come on and go away relatively suddenly, often with long periods of calm in between. |
| Overreactive | Episodes can be in response to minor events, and the feelings and or behavior are out of proportion to the provocation. |
| Unplanned | Episodes are poorly planned and poorly directed. |
| Purposeless | Episodes serve little purpose for the person. |
| Ego-Dystonic | The person having episodes is surprised and embarrassed or distressed by them. |
| Related to Physiological Stress | Made worse by physiological stress such as fatigue, pain, low blood sugar. |

[a] From Miller (1993) and from "Aggressive Disorders," by J. M. Silver and S. C. Yudofsky, in *Neuropsychiatry of Traumatic Brain Injury* (p. 324), edited by J. M. Silver, S. C. Yudofsky, and R. E. Hales, 1994, Washington, DC: American Psychiatric Press, Inc. Copyright 1994 by American Psychiatric Press, Inc. Adapted with permission.

a TBI, "Before the accident, I engaged in hostile behavior when I wanted to and when it served my purpose; now I have no control over when I explode." (Silver and Yudofsky, 1994, p. 324).

### *Similar Neurological Symptoms*

Automatic cursing may be mistaken for anger. Impulsive anger can be a component of labile emotions.

### *Similar Nonneurological Conditions*

Following a brain illness, normal reactive anger may be directed toward the source of the injury, or it may be part of a grief reaction, of PTSD, of frustration, or of other normal anger.

Some problematic anger may predate the neurological illness due to disorders such as mania, schizophrenia, and antisocial, borderline, and narcissistic personality disorders. Some people simply anger easily, or displays of anger and violence may be accepted and encouraged parts of their culture.

### *Associated Symptoms*

Anger may be part of a poor awareness of deficits--the person may get angry about someone else for his failings rather than accepting or admitting to his own disabilities. This can be due to denial, to a lack of awareness of deficits, or to monitoring and judgment deficits. Anger may emerge more when the person is fatigued, in pain, toxic (e.g., from alcohol, cocaine), or when confronted with his deficits. Impulsive anger is more likely in people who are impulsive and uninhibited in other ways as well.

Obsessive anger is one part of personality changes seen in some people with temporal lobe epilepsy, but its characteristics are different from impulsive anger (Weiger & Bear, 1988).

### *Neuroanatomy*

Anger and irritability are common with diffuse brain dysfunction from TBIs, from infections, from dementias, from toxicities, and so forth. Agitation is common for someone emerging from a coma.

Aggressive impulses appear to be generated from nuclei in the hypothalamus, the thalamus, the cingulum, and the amygdala and are regulated or suppressed by the orbital frontal lobes, by the septal nuclei, and by cerebellar structures (Silver & Yudofsky, 1994). Consequently, impulsive anger is especially associated with lesions of the frontal lobes, especially orbital portions. Damage to the anterior temporal lobes and to thalamic and hypothalamic structures has also resulted in aggression in humans and in animals. Anger is associated with irritative lesions or with seizure foci of the amygdala in the anterior medial temporal lobes.

### *How to Interview Regarding Impulsive Anger*

Families are usually more aware of this problem than the person with the brain illness. Evaluation of anger problems is best carried out by a mental health professional due to risks for violence and for substantial harm to others. A "dangerousness" assessment should be a part of any anger evaluation. This book is not an adequate guide to evaluation and treatment of problems of violence, which must include more extensive direct clinical training and awareness of local resources such as police, local laws and practices, emergency room protocols, domestic violence dynamics, involuntary commitment proceedings, locked wards, and so forth. However, many professionals and others can screen and refer individuals for anger problems. Screening should include the presence of anger, violence, threats, the presence of weapons, access to alcohol and drugs, and safety and support for potential victims. Detailed interviewing should examine risk factors, circumstances of anger, types of angry behavior, typical episodes, worst episode, awareness of the problem, previous attempts to control it, and willingness to change. It is particularly important also to interview an informant.

### *How to Observe/Test*

The person with the brain illness should be observed (unobtrusively, if possible) in situations reported to induce anger. It may be instructive to push for performance on a difficult test. The person (or other observers if necessary) can be asked to keep an anger log to determine the frequency, severity, and triggers of the anger (see Chapter 8, p. 146).

The *DSM–IV* (1994) offers objective criteria for diagnosis of a Personality Change Due to a General Medical Condition, Aggressive Type. These criteria are somewhat specific with respect to causality, but do not further differentiate the aggressive behavior. S. C. Yudofsky and associates (1989) have proposed specific criteria for an Organic Aggressive Syndrome.

Many scales in Appendix B (p. 327) include aggression. *The Overt Aggression Scale* (Yudofsky et al., 1986) and *The Agitated Behavior Scale* (Corrigan, 1989; Corrigan & Mysiw, 1988) are useful for rating aggression (not anger) and for measuring changes (Appendix B). *The Head Injury Family Interview* (HI-FI; Kay et al., 1995) is qualitatively rich in its probing of the type and of the time course of affective changes, allowing for interpretation of sources of anger and aggression. *The Behavior Change Inventory* (BCI, Hartlage, 1991) includes several adjectives relevant to anger and allows for cautious interpretation of changes in personality and in sources of anger. *The Rancho los Amigos Scale* (Hagen, 1982) bases its differentiation between Levels 4 and 5 in part on the presence of agitation (Corrigan & Mysiw, 1988). *The Neurobehavioral Rating Scale* (Levin et al., 1987) contains rating items relevant to impulsive anger, such as Disinhibition, Agitation, Hostility/Uncooperativeness, Excitement, and Lability of Mood. It does not differentiate organic from characterological, reactive, or psychiatric characteristics.

The *Hare Psychopathy Checklist* (Gacono & Hutton, 1994) is based primarily on history and so can be used for evaluating pre-illness psychopathy.

Tables 10.3 and 10.4 can help identify the circumstances and signs most likely to be important in anger episodes. Any evaluation for anger difficulties following brain illness should look at all possible and multiple causes (Table 10.1) and should not assume that impulsive anger is the only cause.

### *Practical Problems*

Violence is a significant risk, even in people who were not violent prior to their illnesses. Because of poor planning, such violence can be more destructive than intended. Anger is one of the most significant disruptors of family life and of other social life following brain illness and is a major barrier to a return to work.

### *Interventions*

Treatments for problem anger depend on the factors contributing to the anger. Intervention plans must be individual, based not simply on adding together the treatment for each contributing factor but also on a consideration of other personality and cognitive factors and on the social setting. The main intervention

**TABLE 10.3. Possible Risk Factors Associated with Anger**

| |
|---|
| Stimulation factors |
| Noise level |
| Activity level |
| Unexpected events |
| Lack of structure |
| Personal factors |
| Activity (what is the person with brain illness doing?) |
| Frustration |
| Fear or anxiety |
| Embarrassment, shame, or guilt |
| Discovery or confrontation of impairments |
| Reminders of trauma |
| Interpersonal factors |
| People present |
| Interactions |
| Medical factors |
| Pain |
| Fatigue |
| Hypoglycemia |
| Medications (levels low or high) |
| Alcohol or drugs |

strategies are given in Chapter 8. Following are details specific to irritability, to impulsive anger, and to agitation.

### *Behavioral Management Strategies*

For confused people with minimal responsibility for their actions (e.g., those emerging from a coma or with late dementia), the strategies of caregivers are mostly to prevent or to manage dangerous or objectionable behavior. These strategies include the following:

*Prevention Strategies.* Avoid triggers. Avoid topics, places, and situations that are known to anger the person.

*Make the environment safe.* Eliminate access to alcohol, drugs, potential weapons, and vehicles.

*Regulate the level of stimulation.* Some people need to avoid overstimulation, whereas others may need to be kept busy and distracted with activities they can comprehend. Stimuli and activities for the agitated and confused person who needs distraction include looking through picture books and magazines, listening to music, folding clothes, walking, playing with simple toys and games, engaging in physical exercises, arranging things, riding in a car, playing with pets, and engag-

**TABLE 10.4. Possible Warning Signs of Anger[a]**

| |
|---|
| Speech Signs |
| Difficulty speaking |
| Loud, high voice |
| Strong stresses ("spitting out words") |
| Cursing |
| Name-calling |
| Threats |
| Behavioral Signs |
| Drumming fingers |
| Making fists |
| Squeezing things |
| Appearing confused |
| Increased movement |
| Leaning forward |
| Pointing |
| Pacing |
| Fast movements |
| Bumping into things |
| Moving toward the object of anger |
| Hitting or kicking things |
| Breaking things |
| Throwing things |
| Spitting |
| Threatening people |
| Searching for or picking up weapons |
| Hitting people or animals |
| Kicking people or animals |
| Other forms of violence against people or animals |
| Physiological Signs |
| Fast breathing |
| Fast heart |
| Sweating |
| Overaroused and alert |
| Tense muscles |
| Flushed face |
| Mental Signs |
| Fantasies of doing any of the speech or behavioral signs |
| Negative thoughts about others, such as, "She's a bitch." "I hate him." "Why doesn't he quit bugging me?" |
| Confusion |
| Feelings of frustration |
| Feelings of fear or anxiety |
| Feelings of embarrassment, shame, or guilt |
| Feelings of hurt |

[a] Different people have different signs, and they do not always come in the same order. Some actions on this list do not indicate anger for particular individuals. Some signs are manifestations of anger (behaviors to be avoided) and also warning signs of still more extreme manifestations. For example, shouting may be undesirable, but it may also warn of possible violence.

ing in one-to-one conversation with familiar people about things immediately observable or well known from the past (Jones, 1996; Mace & Rabins, 1991; Reisberg, 1983). Activities and stimuli that are more likely to be confusing and frustrating are complex television shows, group activities and conversations, reading, skilled activities, and talking with unfamiliar people about abstract things not immediately observable. Adequate daily exercise helps control restlessness and agitation.

*Provide an appropriate level of supervision.* Provide the least restrictive, safe environment possible.

*Provide reorientation as needed.* Much of the anger in an agitated, confused, and disoriented individual will result from misperceptions and from misunderstandings of the situation. Staff and family members should provide orientation information, especially concerning the immediate situation. This information should be provided as often as needed, sometimes continually, and especially at transitions from one activity or location to another. For example,

> Mr. Aguila, I'm Maria, your physical therapist. You are in the rehabilitation clinic again today for exercises to help you recover from the auto accident you were in a month ago. Now we're gently going to stretch the muscles in your arm to help it recover. You move your arm this way as far as you can and then I'll help it a little farther. This may hurt a little, but I'm not doing it to hurt you, it's to help your arm get better from your auto accident. Let me know if it hurts.

If the disoriented person disagrees (due to delusions, etc.) the caregiver should neither agree with the delusion nor argue.

*Use physical restrains or medications only as a last resort.* If the previously mentioned techniques fail, physical restraints or medications may be needed. The most common medications for this purpose include the following: anticonvulsants (especially carbamazepine and valproic acid); antidepressants (especially serotonin agonists such as fluoxetine, sertraline, trazodone, and, to some extent, amitriptyline); beta blockers (especially propranolol, nadolol, and pindolol); amantadine; antianxiety medications (especially buspirone and clonazepam); minor tranquilizers (the benzodiazepines); and antipsychotics (these last two groups should be avoided when possible because they have important deleterious cognitive and other effects). When agitation is due to disorientation and to clouded consciousness during emergence from a coma, stimulants (amphetamines) are sometimes effective (Glenn, 1987). The response of injured brains to psychotropic medications is distinct from the response of intact brains to those same medications. Their use in a neuropsychological population requires specialized knowledge (Gualtieri, 1991; Silver & Yudofsky, 1994; Yudofsky, Silver, & Hales, 1990).

*Episode Management.* Finding the safest way to manage episodes of agitation is an experiment with each individual. When the person is confused or has little new learning ability there is little need to worry that a particular strategy may reinforce agitated behavior, because not much learning is likely to take place. Likewise, during post-traumatic amnesia, strategies should not be picked on the basis of trying to teach one behavior or to extinguish another. Possibilities of ways to manage angry outbursts include the following:

*Withdraw.* Leave the person alone for a short time if this can be done safely. As the caregiver leaves, she should tell him briefly what she is doing and why. "You are beginning to get upset. I will leave you alone for a few minutes so you can calm down." For some individuals, one caregiver may remain to help the person calm down.

*Distract.* Change the subject, the focus of activity, or the location. Use a concrete object as a focus when possible.

*Reorient and reassure.* The person should be reminded of where he is, why he is there, and what is going on. Misunderstandings should be clarified. He can be directed toward specific activities aimed at reducing agitation, such as guided relaxation. Reassurance comes from the caregiver remaining calm herself. A good rule of thumb is, "As he goes up, I go down." A calm, reassuring tone of voice can be very powerful in potentially explosive situations.

### *Self-Control Strategies*

With higher levels of orientation, awareness, and memory, self-control strategies can be trained through relaxation, through self-talk, and through cognitive restructuring. The person with a brain illness often needs extra help knowing when and how to apply these techniques. The following strategies allow the person to incorporate these techniques into their context of use.

*Back Off, Calm Down, Try Again.* The main components of this strategy are detailed in Chapter 8 (p. 142). Once the person has left the situation and is calm, the plan may include preparations for returning to the situation, including affirmations, positive self-statements, prayers, lists of questions to review, cognitive restructuring, and reframing self-statements. Questions might include the following: "Do I need to apologize? Do I need to explain why I left to anyone? Do I need to tell anyone my feelings? What can I do to avoid this next time?" The cognitive reframing of self-statements may take these forms: "I don't hate my mother, I'm just angry with her." "He's not a b---, we just disagree." These belong on the cue card.

When the person returns from the back off he may need to explain the back-off or his feelings, apologize, talk through the issue, set a time to talk about an issue, review the episode, and record it in the anger incident log, or resume what he was doing. The choice of what to do depends on the situation. Making the right choice requires social judgment, which may also be impaired. In that case, these judgments can later be reviewed informally with a trusted person or in therapy sessions.

*Cue Cards.* It is usually best to begin the use of the Back Off strategy with a written cue card (Table 10.5a) and with having the person actually leave the situation, especially if memory and anger problems are moderate to severe. Once this technique is learned and applied consistently, the person may make a transition to a mnemonic (Table 10.5b) and to calming down within the situation.

Cue cards can also be used to prepare to stay calm in circumstances that often provoke anger; for example, a man picking up his children from his ex-wife (Table 10.5c), and for telling others about an anger problem (Table 10.5d).

**TABLE 10.5. Sample Anger Cue Cards**

**TABLE 10.5a. Typical Anger Cue Card**

MY ANGER RISKS
- Tired
- Noise, activity, too many people
- Frustrated

MY ANGER SIGNS
- Tight muscles, fists, jaw
- Violent thoughts
- Loud voice
- Fast breathing

TIME OUT
- Say: "I'm feeling angry, I need to take a time out"
- Go outside or bedroom.
- Walk or exercise
- Practice relaxing

PREPARING TO RETURN
- When I can smile I'm ready to go back
- What do I need to say:
  - Apologize?
  - Set time to talk?
  - Ask how they feel?
  - Say what I want?
- Check in

**TABLE 10.5b. Anger Management Program Acronym[a]**

A—Anticipate trigger situations
N—Notice anger signs
G—Go through my anger routine
E—Extract myself from the situation, if all else fails
R—Record how I coped. What can I learn for next time?

[a] Adapted from Novaco, 1975.

**TABLE 10.5c. Cue Card for a Man Picking up His Children from His Ex-Wife**

| |
|---|
| Stay calm. |
| Focus on the kids. |
| Don't let her get to me. |
| If she brings anything up, say, "I'll call you about it." |

**TABLE 10.5d. Cue Card for Telling Others about an Anger Problem**

| |
|---|
| Because of my brain injury, I get angry more easily than I used to. A lot of the time I don't really mean to be angry. I'm learning to control it, so don't worry about it, and please don't take it too personally. If you see me get angry, just give me a chance to calm myself down, or let me walk away. Thanks. |

*Anger Log.* Maintaining the anger log (Table 10.6) helps the person with an anger problem to recognize his own patterns and progress, to own the problem, and to feel responsible for it.

*Role Playing.* Role playing can be used in individual therapy sessions, in group therapy, in a milieu setting such as a hospital or a treatment program, and at home. The most important role play is to practice backing off. Replaying actual

**TABLE 10.6. Sample Anger Journal Format**[a]

| |
|---|
| Date and Time: |
| What Happened? |
| Anger Level (1–10): |
| What did I do? |
| What were my warning signs? |
| What did I feel? |
| Did I back off? |
| What do I need to do now? |
| What can I do better next time? |

[a] See Chapter 8, Incident Log section (p. 146), for discussion.

anger incidents, practicing handling other people's anger, and practicing appropriate assertiveness can also be useful.

*Role Modeling.* In treatment and at home, people with brain illnesses should see staff and family members modeling appropriate ways to deal with their own anger. Staff members should use back-off strategies liberally and explicitly for themselves. A staff with a rigid professional demeanor deprives people with brain illnesses of the opportunity to know how their actions affect other people's feelings.

### *Treating Other Forms of Anger Problems*

*Contributing Cognitive Deficits.* When cognitive or executive function deficits contribute to anger problems, they should be treated as well. Then anger episodes can become another example in work on reasoning, lack of awareness of deficits, impulsiveness, and so forth.

*Executive Function Impairments. Lack of awareness of deficits.* The therapist can train self-awareness with respect to anger by asking the person to predict how many anger episodes he will have over a given interval or whether he will be able to get through a certain event without an anger episode. After an anger episode, the person can be asked to predict what other people will say they felt during the episode to work on empathy skills. These predictions can then be written down and checked out together with the other people. Feedback is then given regarding both the episodes and the judgement process (see Table 7.11, p. 132). Videotapes or audiotapes of actual or role-played anger incidents can be useful.

*Impaired judgment.* Analysis of anger incidents may reveal that poor judgment or misunderstandings were involved. These problems can be tackled cognitively, by retraining strategies for solving social problems and including the strategies in the Preparing to Return section of the Back Off cue card.

*Self-centeredness.* The anger incident log can include a section on "What was the other person feeling?" The anger incident log or the Preparing to Return section of the cue card can contain questions such as, "What would I want if I were the other person?" or "What would be fair in this situation?"

*Perseveration/rigidity/obsession.* When a persistent angry theme or obsession becomes a problem, the person should be directed to write it down to be discussed with the therapist. Staff and family members should seek an agreement with the person to talk about that problem only with the therapist (and with certain others when appropriate). When repetitive questions arise, the answers should be written in the therapy journal, in the memory book, or on a cue card, and the person should be referred to the written answers.

*Medical Factors. Pain and headache.* Possible connections between physical pain and anger episodes can be checked by adding a pain level to the anger incident log. If there is a connection, pain treatments can be added to the Calm Down part of the cue card. It may be possible to avoid risk situations when pain is more intense.

*Fatigue and sleep disturbance.* Connections between fatigue or sleep disturbance and anger episodes can be explored by adding a fatigue level or a Time Since Last Rest or a Last Night's Sleep section to the anger incident log. If there is a connection, the sleep problem can be addressed and rest can be added to the Calm Down part of the cue card. It may be possible to avoid risk situations when the person is fatigued or when they did not get enough sleep.

*Hypoglycemia.* Connections between low blood sugar and anger episodes can be checked by adding a section to the anger incident log for recording time since last eating and what was eaten. If episodes come a few hours after a load of sugar or after many hours of not eating, it may be wise to consult a nutritionist or a physician about tests for hypoglycemia and/or a hypoglycemic diet (small, frequent meals avoiding simple sugars and alcohol).

*Alcohol.* When alcohol contributes to an anger problem the clearest solution is abstinence. Some people need only learn the connection between alcohol and their anger problem or the other problems of alcohol use following brain illness to quit. Others may require more intervention.

*Stimulants.* Stimulants of abuse such as cocaine and high-dose, rapidly acting amphetamines can contribute to anger problems and are best dealt with by abstinence. If stimulants are part of the treatment program but contribute to an anger problem, then the dose or schedule may need to be adjusted. Careful record keeping can help this regulation.

*Medications.* Many classes of medications are associated with irritability and aggression in their use and/or their withdrawal. These include barbiturates, antianxiety medications, opiates and other narcotics, steroids, antidepressants (especially early in treatment), antipsychotics (especially anticholinergic effects), and anticholinergic drugs, including over-the-counter sedatives (Yudofsky, Silver, & Hales, 1990). Careful record keeping with a modified anger log or a medications log can help in regulating medications appropriately with respect to their effects on anger.

*Emotional Reaction Factors. Legitimate anger toward the cause of injury.* The victim of an injury may have considerable legitimate anger toward the cause of the injury such as a drunk driver, an assailant, a negligent corporation, or a government. Such people often need help finding effective and satisfying channels for their anger.

*Grief reaction.* People often try to find reasons for losses in an attempt to control or to prevent future losses. Grief reactions may include displaced anger. People usually work through these reactions by talking out their feelings with a trusted and empathetic person. However, impaired memory or judgment or complicating emotional or personality difficulties can prolong or intensify grief, and psychotherapy may be needed.

*PTSD.* See Chapter 9 (p. 174).

*Frustration.* When frustration contributes to angry reactions, more attention needs to be paid to selecting activities at an appropriate level of challenge. Specific preparation can also be given prior to difficult activities, for example, "Now we are going to try a more difficult exercise. This may be frustrating for you. How will you know if you are getting frustrated? What will you do about it?"

*Normal, legitimate anger toward an appropriate event or circumstance.* People with brain illnesses still have legitimate reasons to get angry. If their legitimate anger is discounted, ignored, or "treated", their anger may, quite appropriately, increase. If they have expressed their anger inappropriately, then their angry behavior should be dealt with separately from their legitimate complaint in a way that does not reinforce inappropriate behavior but which does not ignore the complaint.

*Pre-Illness Personality Factors.* At times, a brain illness can provide a fortuitous opportunity to work on a preexisting anger problem to which a person would not otherwise admit. Beginning an anger management program by addressing the impulsive anger component can help avoid fruitless disagreements about justified anger and blame. Sometimes characterological or reactive anger problems can be dealt with successfully in this way without ever having to use confrontation and insight, or a working alliance can be established that permits addressing deeper problems later. In other words, the therapy gives the message of, "Your brain injury makes you yell and curse when you don't really mean to. We can help you learn to control that so you don't drive away family and friends and lose jobs," rather than, "You've really got a problem with anger. No wonder you're having trouble getting along with people. If you don't shape up you're headed for big trouble."

*Explosive personality.* Therapy is similar for explosive personality anger and brain illness impulsive anger, except that it may also be necessary to examine and to confront beliefs about the expression of anger and to examine the effects that explosive anger has had on the person's life. Assertiveness training may be needed to replace some of the functions that explosive anger served.

*Projection and blaming, chronic complainer, "chip-on-the-shoulder."* Various conventional psychotherapeutic techniques can be used to allow such individuals to see the origins and consequences of their attitudes and to replace them with more responsible and ultimately rewarding attitudes.

*Violent lifestyle or culturally tolerated, sanctioned, or encouraged violence and/or anger.* If clinicians have problems with a participant's angry behavior, they need to consider whether the behavior might be due to his cultural background. Clinicians need to consider carefully the values they themselves bring to treatment and how well they are preparing someone to return to his usual setting. For example, "I statements" and active listening, although useful in therapy, may not be adequate survival skills for life on the streets or in the military.

Multicultural awareness does not mean "anything goes." It is reasonable to expect constraints on behavior in a treatment program for the safety and comfort of participants and of staff members, even if some participants need to act differently outside the program. Loud family arguments may be the norm in some cultures, but they might still disrupt others in an inpatient rehabilitation unit. The constraints of the law should also be respected.

*Sociopathy or predatory violence, with or without anger.* This type of violence usually yields only to firm and substantial external controls (usually the criminal justice system) or to extended psychotherapy backed by external controls. It is a condition to be evaluated and treated by experts.

*Mania.* Mania usually requires treatment with lithium, with carbamazepine, with valproic acid, or with similar drugs. Psychotherapy includes education about the mood cycle and learning to recognize and to cope with it. The neuropsychotherapist may need to coordinate with a specialist to meet the specific needs of the person with brain illness and mania.

### *Integrating the Treatment Plan*

When combinations of factors are responsible for an anger problem (the usual case), the neuropsychotherapist needs to prioritize treatment options. Once a treatment program for impulsive anger is in place, it often establishes enough trust to allow work on emerging factors of emotional reactions or of personality. Violence risk, priority of problems, the relative weights of contributing factors, and the likelihood of treatment effectiveness all need to be taken into account.

## *EMOTIONAL OBSESSIVENESS SOMETIMES ASSOCIATED WITH TEMPORAL LOBE EPILEPSY (TLE)*

### *Description*

Although it is controversial (Treiman, 1991), many investigators and clinicians assert that distinctive personality changes (Table 10.7) can occur with the onset of TLE (or limbic epilepsy or partial complex seizures; Bear & Fedio, 1977; Devinsky & Bear, 1984; Garyfallos, Manos, & Adamopoulou, 1988; Slater & Beard, 1963). These changes appear to occur variably in a small number of people with TLE, especially when the epilepsy goes unrecognized and/or untreated for many years.

These changes are not regarded as direct seizure manifestations, but rather

**TABLE 10.7. Personality Changes Thought to Be Associated with Temporal Lobe Epilepsy[a]**

| |
|---|
| ETHICAL/PHILOSOPHICAL CONCERNS |
| Religiosity |
| Hypermoralism |
| Philosophical interest |
| Sense of personal destiny |
| OBSESSIONAL CHARACTERISTICS |
| Hypergraphia |
| Obsessionalism, compulsive attention to detail |
| Circumstantiality |
| Viscosity, persistence |
| EMOTIONAL CHANGES |
| Emotionality |
| Sadness |
| Guilt |
| Anger |
| Aggression |
| Elation, euphoria |
| Paranoia |
| Dependence |
| Humorlessness, sobriety |
| Altered sexual interest |

[a] From "Quantitative Analysis of Interictal Behavior in Temporal Lobe Epilepsy," by D. Bear and P. Fedio, 1977. *Archives of Neurology, 34,* 455. Copyright 1977 by American Medical Association. Adapted with permission.

as changes in personality resulting from effects of the seizure focus. Subclinical seizure activity may give added emotional significance to some experiences, stimuli, or ideas (Bear, 1979). How such a process works and which experiences or stimuli get so tagged remains a mystery. The personality changes are not necessarily disorders or problems; some claim that they may be responsible for great works of thought and art (see Case 1.2, p. 10, Fyodor; Jones, 1993; LaPlante, 1993).

### *Similar Neurological Symptoms*

The emotional changes of TLE are similar to labile emotions, impulsive anger, and other changes seen with other brain illnesses. Because epilepsy can result from any type of brain illness, it is not surprising that some individuals with epilepsy also have other organic emotional changes. However, whereas organic irritability and impulsive anger usually come and go suddenly (Silver & Yudofsky, 1994), the anger and hostility associated with TLE is described as obsessive and long lasting (Devinsky & Bear, 1984; Weiger & Bear, 1988).

### *Similar Nonneurological Conditions*

Table 10.7 includes symptoms of many psychiatric disorders, as well as nonpathological events such as religious conversion, philosophical preoccupation, and a tendency to write.

### *Associated Symptoms*

Partial complex seizures and related episodes, as well as mild memory loss, are often associated with this condition. Other neuropsychological deficits may be present if there was a neurological illness that caused the epilepsy.

### *Neuroanatomy*

The changes are thought to be associated with epileptic foci in the limbic system, especially the amygdala and the hippocampus.

### *How to Interview Regarding Emotional Obsessiveness*

According to some studies (Bear & Fedio, 1977), the person with a focus in the left temporal lobe is more aware of these symptoms than is his family, whereas with right temporal foci, family members are more aware of the changes than is the person with epilepsy.

This diagnosis should not be made lightly or on the basis of limited evidence such as a single interview or test. Weight should be given to the degree to which changes are spontaneously described by the person and/or by the family member rather than emerging only in response to specific and directed questions. Particular attention should be paid to see whether any identified personality characteristics are actually changes, and whether the changes coincide with the onset of epilepsy.

### *How to Observe/Test*

The conversational style of some of these people can be quite circumstantial. They dwell on a single point excessively. They have great difficulty ending conversations. Their philosophical preoccupations will permeate their conversation. *The Temporal Lobe Epilepsy Personality Inventory* (Bear & Fedio, 1977) is specific for this condition. *The Structured Clinical Interview for Complex Partial Seizure-Like Symptoms* (Roberts et al., 1990) does not address this condition directly, but it does address associated symptoms. *The Washington Psychosocial Seizure Inventory* (Dodrill et al., 1980) and *The Adolescent Psychosocial Seizure Inventory* (Batzel et al., 1991) do not address this condition, but they are excellent for a more global picture of adjustment to seizures. See Appendix B (p. 327).

### *Practical Problems*

These changes can sometimes present problems for interpersonal relations, for family life, for work, and so forth. Some of the changes can also be channeled toward considerable productivity that contributes substantially to society.

### *Interventions*

1. Successful treatment of the seizures with anticonvulsants or possibly with surgery may arrest, but perhaps not reverse the personality changes.
2. The common adjustment and social problems often associated with epilepsy, such as depression, anxiety, social stigma, employment difficulties, and so forth (Dodrill et al., 1980, 1984), should be addressed with education, problem-solving counseling, and advocacy.
3. There are few known psychotherapeutic interventions specifically for this condition. Many principles in this book can be brought to bear on the situation, particularly education about the condition (pp. 31, 96), increasing self-awareness (p. 122), naming the problem (p. 90), an emotional rehabilitation approach, and reconstructing an image of the new person (p. 85). It may be possible to choose which changes are desirable and which ones are not. Reframing techniques can help the person choose which feelings to act on and which ones not to act on. Problematic emotional and behavioral reactions can be approached with the techniques in Chapter 8, particularly identifying risk factors and warning signs and developing plans to avoid the problem. For hypergraphia, circumstantiality, and obsessionalism, the neuropsychotherapist may need to be quite directive in imposing structure on the therapy process.

## *CHANGES IN TYPES OF EMOTIONAL RESPONSES*

When someone has a change in the type (rather than in the intensity) of emotional response he has to a given experience following a brain illness, for example, laughing at someone's distress rather than being sympathetic, it is usually secondary to a cognitive impairment that results in a distorted perception or interpretation of the experience. This could be due to an amnesia that does not permit relating experiences to one another, to impaired judgement or reasoning, to concrete thinking, to impaired language comprehension, to impaired emotional comprehension, and so forth. Some changes in the type of emotional response could be due to post-traumatic stress symptoms or to reactive depression or anxiety. Changes in personal values due to the experience of illness are also possible contributors. Such changes, when problematic, are usually best addressed through cognitive rehabilitation and conventional psychotherapeutic techniques.

# 11

# Executive Functions

## *INTRODUCTION*

### *What Are Executive Functions?*

Executive functions are the abilities needed to control and to regulate organized behavior. They coordinate the execution of cognitive abilities such as attention, memory, language, and visual-spatial reasoning. They stand at the border between personality and cognition. People with executive dysfunctions have difficulty carrying out plans independently and successfully, interacting appropriately with other people, and controlling their emotions. Executive functions are associated with the frontal lobes, which have rich reciprocal connections with the posterior cortex (associated with many major cognitive functions), as well as with the limbic system (strongly associated with the emotions).

Several models of executive functions have been proposed (for example, Cicerone & Giacino, 1992; Shallice, 1988; Stuss & Benson, 1986). The characterization presented here is derived from Lezak (1995), which was chosen because it is accessible and is sufficiently accurate to inform interventions. Lezak described executive functions as having the following four components:

#### *Choosing a Goal*

Goals may be as simple as deciding to eat when one is hungry or as complex as choosing one's life work. Choosing a goal requires recognizing one's own needs, initiating a search for goals, and contemplating the future.

#### *Planning*

Planning requires initiating a planning process, reasoning out the needs of the situation, and sequencing the steps.

*Execution*

Executing a plan requires starting and stopping, inhibiting inappropriate actions, following the sequence of the plan, and monitoring the execution to make sure it is achieving its goal.

*Evaluation*

Evaluation involves identifying and correcting errors and recognizing when the goal has been achieved (or is hopeless).

### *What Are Impairments in Executive Functions?*

Table 11.1 lists the most common descriptors of executive dysfunctions. Some of these concepts are closely related, whereas others are unrelated or are even opposites. Opposites often appear in the same person; for example, a lack of initiation along with impulsivity (Cicerone & Giacino, 1992). Some descriptors seem more cognitive, whereas others seem more like personality characteristics. Those elaborated in this chapter represent the spectrum of the most important executive dysfunctions.

Not all of the descriptors in Table 11.1 are necessarily negative. Organic changes in executive functions are occasionally viewed as positive by others, especially when a shy, introverted person becomes a bit more outgoing and assertive (Ranseen, 1990), or when an aggressive person becomes more mellow and easygoing.

Executive dysfunctions are prominent in Attention Deficit Disorders (Barkley, 1997) in children and in adults.

**TABLE 11.1. Executive Dysfunctions**

| | | |
|---|---|---|
| Decreased self-control | Childish | Inflexible |
| Euphoria | Self-centered | Impaired sequencing |
| Mania | Unempathetic | Grandiose |
| Despontaneity | Concrete | Confabulatory |
| Facetiousness | Lacking abstract attitude | Distractible |
| Disinhibition | Unable to shift attention | Unable to prioritize |
| Impulsiveness | Unable to use feedback | Lacking drive |
| Slowness of thinking | Unable to maintain performance | Restless |
| Poor judgment | Unable to anticipate | Shallow affect |
| Disorganized | Unable to self-monitor | Lethargic |
| Unreliable | Lack of self-reflectiveness | Unrealistic |
| Poor insight | Unconcern | Socially inappropriate |
| Apathetic | Outbursts of irritability | Decreased self-concern |
| Indifferent | Perseverative | Withdrawn |
| Lack of ambition | Impersistent | Extroverted |
| Decreased initiative | Assertive | Stimulus-bound |

### *Evaluation*

Because executive functions share common ground between cognition and personality, they cannot be evaluated adequately from either one of those perspectives alone. Cognitive tests can evaluate some specific aspects of executive functions well, but the very structure (both cognitive and social) of standardized testing compensates for many of the impairments of interest so they are not fully revealed in that context (Lezak, 1995; Malloy, Bihrle, Duffy, & Cimino, 1993). Likewise, treatment programs are often so highly structured that executive dysfunctions may not be evident. For this reason, the evaluation of executive functions must also rely heavily on interviews, observations in unstructured and social contexts, and qualitative observations on testing. Formal instruments of neuropsychological personality assessment also contribute, particularly structured interviews, observer rating scales (Appendix B, p. 327), and the Frontal Lobe Personality Scale (FLOPS; Grace et al., 1996).

Because executive functions have a strong personality component, their impairments can be difficult to distinguish from personality or psychiatric disorders or from cultural characteristics. The primary means of differentiation is in the temporal association between the executive dysfunction and the neurological illness (Case 11.1, Groucho). Other means of differentiation are more specific to particular symptoms, personality features, and circumstances.

### *Interventions*

Executive dysfunctions overlap cognition and personality not only in conceptualization, but also in intervention strategies (Table 11.2, Campbell, Duffy, & Salloway, 1994). Step 4 of this schema does not imply that self-regulation must be trained in the clinic; it can be trained in the community using a natural re-

> *Disinhibition or Sexual Harassment? Case 11.1. Groucho.* A 78-year-old man was admitted to a rehabilitation unit following a right hemisphere stroke. It was soon noticed that he touched, squeezed, and pinched female staff members in private areas at every opportunity and made frequent crude remarks with obscene language. At first this was taken as disinhibition due to his stroke and female staff members learned to stay out of reach as much as possible, confronting him firmly but calmly when necessary. It was later found through interviews with his family that this was not a change in his behavior. They further noted that he had very little respect for women. The head nurse (female) confronted him to no avail. Assigning male nurses and therapists to him was a help, but the situation continued on the ward and in hallways. Finally his physician (male) confronted him and told him that further rehabilitation would not be possible if the behavior continued, whereupon it stopped.

**TABLE 11.2. General Schema for Executive Dysfunction Intervention**

1. Compensate Externally for executive dysfunction through structure (schedules, cues, reminders, written procedures, restricted access to danger).
2. Build Awareness of the nature of the problems.
3. Retrain Self-Regulation (procedures, internal compensations, problem-solving schemata, social skills, self-managed compensations such as alarms and daily planners, etc.).
4. Generalize Self-Regulation training to other settings (home, school, work, community, etc.).
5. Fade External Compensations as relearned self-regulation permits.

covery model with generalization training focusing on transferring self-regulation from one community setting to another. Step 5 may overlap considerably with generalization training. Differences in detail in the implementation of this schema for specific problems may involve the external compensations used, the self-regulation techniques trained, the appropriate settings for generalization training, and the ways of fading cues.

## *IMPAIRED INITIATION (ABULIA)*

### *Description*

Impairment in initiating activity, such as thought, speech, movement, and extended activity, is called *abulia*. Motivation and enjoyment may or may not be intact. In severe cases (akinetic mutism), the person may not start anything at all, including speaking and eating, and may need total care. People with milder abulia may not initiate plans or activities on their own, but they may comply with suggestions and requests of others and participate in activities that others initiate. They may sit passively and do and say very little spontaneously, or they may give brief and unelaborated responses when others speak to them. Abulia may affect enjoyable activities as much as disagreeable chores (see Case 5.4, p. 78, Salvador). Abulia can affect the initiation of plans and/or their being carried out. Some people with abulia "talk a good game," often telling others about their plans but never following through on them. In pure abulia, other cognitive abilities are intact.

Abulia is a philosophical perplexity. We typically assume that if someone wants to do something, they will; that is, that initiation reflects volition. With abulia, however, the two can be dissociated, so someone may have the desire and ability to do something but lack the ability to initate doing it.

### *Similar Neurological Symptoms*

Abulia can be found with other disorders of start-stop mechanisms, such as impulsiveness, perseveration, and impersistence. Abulia is associated with other executive dysfunctions, such as problems with organization, with self-regulation and with monitoring, anosognosia, and concreteness. Abulia often co-occurs with emotional indifference and with impaired emotional communication.

With prospective memory impairments the person does not remember to do something at the appropriate time in the future, rather than being unable to initiate it. A lack of initiation of movement is a prominent characteristic of Parkinson's disease, but the abulia may also extend to thought, to plans, and to speech.

### *Similar Nonneurological Conditions*

Personality characteristics that are easily confused with abulia include passivity, laziness, stubbornness, and a lack of caring about oneself or about others. In these conditions, however, the person may initiate action to avoid or to sabotage undesired activities and may express verbally or otherwise her desire to avoid certain activities. Further, these conditions may be selective—being willing to play basketball but not to wash dishes, for example.

The depressed person is more likely than the person with abulia to complain of poor motivation, lack of pleasure, and low energy, and to resist participation in activities.

*Selective mutism*, in which the affected person does not speak for emotional reasons (sometimes due to emotional trauma), may appear similar to severe abulia, but the lack of initiation may be confined to speech. Someone with catatonic schizophrenia may remain stationary and mute for long periods of time. The person with schizophrenia typically loses all contact with the external world and does not respond to any stimulation, whereas the person with abulia may respond.

### *Neuroanatomy*

Abulia is most commonly associated with diffuse injury, with injury to the frontal lobes, especially the dorsolateral anterior portions (Stuss & Benson, 1986; Stuss et al., 1992), and with lesions in the basal ganglia, especially the caudate nucleus (Bhatia & Marsden, 1994) and the substantia nigra.

### *How to Interview Regarding Lack of Initiation*

The family may be more aware of and frustrated by the abulia than is the affected person, although they may call it laziness. Interview questions should focus on illness-associated changes in spontaneous activities, responses to suggestions and to structure, spontaneity in conversation, the need for direction and for nagging, the use of unstructured time, and on ruling out depression and lowered motivation. Mild abulia may not be evident until the person is left to choose her own activities.

### *How to Observe/Test*

Abulia is often better assessed through interviews and through observations than through formal testing. Testing often provides compensating initiation structure, thus masking the problem. Verbal and nonverbal fluency tests, picture description tasks, and The Tinkertoy Test (Lezak, 1995) are sensitive to some dimensions of abulia, but their relationships to real-life difficulties have not yet been fully explored. The examiner should observe whether the person quits easily or too quickly on tests and whether she seeks novel solutions. The person should be observed during unstructured time and when little stimulation is present. Failure to initiate conversation spontaneously and failure to elaborate on comments or on answers may be noted on interview. The FLOPS (Grace, et al., 1996) Apathy scale measures abulia.

### *Practical Problems*

People with a severe loss of initiation may require total care. People with milder problems frequently require supervision or cuing to get things done. They frustrate caregivers, who must constantly encourage them to be active. They are unlikely to take responsibility for things, and they may not do their share of work unless specifically prompted to do so. They may let problems go instead of fixing them, and this may become a safety risk.

People with abulia tend to have interpersonal problems. They are poor conversationalists and appear unresponsive to others. They may alienate people, especially when others see them as unmotivated, uncaring, or lazy. Others may stop talking with them or suggesting activities because they think they have chosen to be quiet or inactive, or are depressed, or would take offense.

### *Interventions*

1. Compensate Externally: Moderate to severe levels of initiation impairment are commonly addressed in occupational therapy, in cognitive rehabilitation, and in other parts of rehabilitation for functional activities through daily schedules, alarms, "Things To Do" lists, and cued sequences of activities (Sohlberg & Mateer, 1989). Psychotherapists working in rehabilitation need to be thoroughly familiar with compensation techniques for initiation (Table 8.7, p. 149, and Table 11.3; Case 11.2, Dumi), and to coordinate their work with cognitive rehabilitation for higher levels of initiation.
2. Build Awareness: Awareness of abulia can be built through direct education and through comparisons to pre-illness activities. When depression, indifference, or poor motivation are also present, an added message is

**TABLE 11.3. Hierarchy of Initiation Cuing Systems**

| Category | Examples |
|---|---|
| Immediate human cue | A person observes and cues the person with the brain illness (Table 8.7, p. 149) |
| Distant human cue | Telephone call reminder<br>Letter reminder<br>Note left for the person<br>A helper sets an alarm, a timer, or other mechanical reminder |
| Active mechanical cue | Alarm<br>Timer<br>Personal electronic organizer memo or schedule alarm |
| Passive mechanical cue | Written schedule<br>Calendar<br>List of things to do<br>Written sequence of activities |
| Active associated cue | Take pills with meals<br>Check laundry when clock chimes |
| Passive associated cue | Observe that something needs doing (washing, repairing, putting away) and doing it |

needed: "Motivation comes from doing, not from waiting." It may take extra time to build enough therapeutic trust (or to use trust in a family member) to convince the person to try things that she does not feel motivated to do.

Family education should emphasize that a lack of initiation is due to brain illness, not depression, poor motivation, or laziness. It may be necessary to role-model how to get the person to do things without nagging or punishing her. If the family believes they should leave her alone and that she will do something if she wants to, their desires for her independence should be acknowledged, but they should be gently redirected to see that, in this instance, that will not work. Families should be taught that they will need to provide structure to substitute, at first, for her lack of initiation. One useful metaphor is that caregivers provide a "prosthetic initiation," later faded to an "orthotic initiation," and then to independence. Another metaphor is that she is like a car with a dead battery and they need to roll start her each time they want her to do something.

Work on initiation can be complicated by previous struggle and control issues in the family, pre-illness laziness, passive-aggressive attitudes, impaired emotional responsiveness, anxiety, or depression. These may require skillful negotiation or mediation between the person with the illness and other family members regarding appropriate goals. It may be possible to "buy time" with a few common and agreed-on goals, espe-

*Reveille. Case 11.2. Dumi (fictitious).* This example is presented to illustrate general cognitive rehabilitation strategies for a lack of initiation for those unfamiliar with them. It includes transitions to psychosocial functions.

Dumi was a young man with severe initiation difficulties from a TBI. Prior to his injury he had struggled with his parents, especially his mother, over his responsibilities around the house and over his dress. His parents agreed that it would be easiest if his father cued him. His parents set a goal of independent dressing. Dumi resisted at first, but he agreed when reminded that he wanted to look good for "the ladies" and when his parents conceded that he could put his earring on when he was all dressed. The plan that was designed to meet this goal included maximum assistance at first, with gradual withdrawal of help. At the beginning, his father reminded him to get dressed and supervised the process. At that time Dumi had double vision and reading was difficult. Therefore, his father laid the clothes out on his bed in the right sequence for putting them on. When his reading ability recovered, the therapist, his father, and he made a checklist with the steps for dressing written in considerable detail. At first, his father reviewed the checklist with him and checked off each step as it was completed. Then he reduced assistance by asking Dumi to read the checklist alone, complete each step, and check it off. Then items on the list were shortened from, for example, "Select socks, put them on, select shoes, put them on" to "Put on socks and shoes." Then his father supervised from the next room, only occasionally checking or shouting a reminder to keep at it. Eventually, they established a routine sufficiently automatic that the checklist was eliminated.

A later goal was that Dumi would cook a meal each evening. He agreed to this goal when he saw it as a step toward moving out of his parents' home. With some help, he learned to plan menus in advance, write out the steps needed (shopping, assembling ingredients, mixing or cutting up ingredients, etc.) and then made his own checklist to use to help him start each stage. He gradually advanced to conventional shopping lists and cookbooks.

Dumi was hesitant to participate in a communication group, but he agreed to try it once if it would help him "with the ladies." On watching himself on video afterwards, he was able to see that he had not said anything for the entire group unless directly asked, and that "the ladies" present seemed unimpressed. He agreed to a goal of initiating conversation 3 times in 20 minutes. If he had not said anything for 10 minutes, the therapist flashed a "Say something" card. Similar procedures took him through goals of asking questions and responding to other's opinions. Eventually he role-played (on video tape) other social activities such as giving compliments and asking for a date.

cially with things the person wants to do and cannot initiate. Success in working on those goals and on natural recovery may then allow negotiations of more social goals, such as maintaining good family relations.

3. Retrain Self-Regulation: The person with abulia participates in setting goals, in choosing and implementing compensations, and in monitoring

progress. The clinician maintains responsibility for the success of the system and for passing responsibility for compensations to the person with abulia.

Restoring social initiation can follow these same lines. Concrete goals can be practiced through role playing. Initiation in conversation can be trained with group work using cue cards (Case 11.2. Dumi). Training the restoration and the generalization of initiation is helped by linking a schedule to social commitments. The person is more likely to take a walk at 10 a.m. if she has a standing agreement to walk with her neighbor.

4. Generalize Self-Regulation: Once schedules, "Things to do" lists, and similar compensations are in place, these can be reviewed regularly to make sure they are sufficiently inclusive. It is important to include not just chores and tasks, but recreation, social activities, spiritual practices, and so forth.
5. Fade External Compensations: Fading of cuing systems can follow the hierarchies in Tables 8.7 (p. 149) and 11.3. Because everyone uses some initiation cues, these only need to be faded to the point that feels comfortable.
6. Routines and cuing systems should be started early in the course of progressive brain illnesses to maintain function later.
7. The orthotic initiation approach may appear to conflict with standards for patient's rights in chronic care institutions because of the dissociation between volition and initiation. Staff members may need education to recognize when cuing and help with initiation are needed to help someone to do what she wants to do.
8. Preliminary reports (Barrett, 1991; Cowell & Cohen, 1995) suggest that there may be pharmacological treatments for abulia, specifically amantadine, bromocriptine, and lisuride, and possibly tacrine and donepezil.

## *DISINHIBITION*

### *Description*

People with brain illnesses may say or do things that are dangerous, hurtful, silly, socially inappropriate, or foolish. These comments, emotional displays, or actions may be done "without thinking"; that is, the person does not stop and think about the appropriateness or about the consequences before acting.

Disinhibited (impulsive) actions can include stuffing the mouth when eating, crossing the street without looking, grabbing hot pots or hot food without protection, inappropriate flirtation or advances, excessive talking, interrupting, not letting others talk, and not knowing when to end a conversation. In severe cases, the person may grab whatever is in front of her and play with it, break it, or try to eat it. Emotional expression and emotional reactivity can also be disinhibited, producing reflex crying, automatic cursing, emotional lability, irritability, and so forth.

*Similar Neurological Symptoms*

Impaired planning, organizing, monitoring, and judgment can produce rambling, disorganized speech and behavior with impulsive qualities. Someone who is only disinhibited but with intact judgment may feel guilty or embarrassed about her own actions, whereas someone whose judgment is also impaired is unlikely to have regrets. A distractible person may appear to be disinhibited and impulsive, switching attention from one thing to another quickly.

*Similar Nonneurological Conditions*

Disinhibition and impulsivity may be seen in people with antisocial personality disorder, with immaturity, or with mania. These other common disorders can be distinguished from organic disinhibition and impulsivity mainly on the basis of history and of experience with both types of disinhibition. Impulsiveness following brain illness is often pervasive across many types of behavior, whereas personality-based disinhibition tends to be more self-serving and selective. However, because TBIs can be the result of impulsive acts, disinhibition may be both a pre-injury characteristic and a symptom of injury.

People from cultures other than the examiner's may have other ways of organizing conversation or narrative or may have other norms of behavior that may be mistaken for disinhibition.

*Related Symptoms*

Impulsiveness is associated with all of the executive dysfunctions.

*Neuroanatomy*

Disinhibition is commonly seen with frontal lobe disorders, especially orbital frontal lesions (Stuss, et al., 1992) or right hemisphere damage, as well as with diffuse brain illness. It is an acute effect of the neurotoxin alcohol.

*How to Interview Regarding Disinhibition*

Family members are usually more aware of and concerned about problems of disinhibition than are the disinhibited people. Questions can focus on danger, on confidence in leaving the person alone, on embarrassing behaviors, on talkativeness, on emotional responses, on tact, and on getting in trouble.

### *How to Observe/Test*

Impulsiveness is often best observed in unstructured social settings. Impulsivity can be noted on neuropsychological tests, usually as qualitative observations, and especially on problem-solving, vigilance, motor sequence learning, and unstructured tasks. It is also reflected in errors of commission and confabulation. The examiner should observe whether the person is careful and accurate or too fast and careless and if she can control the problem with instructions to slow down and to be more careful. With talkativeness and interruption, it is important to note response to social cues and explicit correction.

### *Practical Problems*

Impulsivity presents risks of accidents, aggression, embarrassment, social offensiveness, sexual vulnerability, and victimization. Interpersonal relationships and work can suffer.

### *Interventions*

1. Compensate Externally: Treating impulsivity is difficult. In extreme cases physical confinement is necessary. In severe cases, compensations for disinhibition include keeping the immediate environment uncluttered, removing dangerous or fragile objects, and restricting access to vehicles, tools, weapons, fire, matches, poisons, medicines, drugs, and alcohol (see Chapter 8).

   When the person with the brain illness is dangerous or offensive, staff and family members should set firm but understanding limits. Appropriate phrases include "I don't want you to touch me like that," "It's not OK to hit," and "Please don't talk like that here." Giggling, smiling, or getting angry in response to inappropriate sexual advances will often encourage them.
2. Build Awareness: It is essential to avoid the politeness with which we often overlook social blunders. Instead, the disinhibited person needs explicit, discrete, understanding and nonjudgmental reeducation about her behavior (see Chapter 8). For example,

   > One problem you have from your brain illness is that you are impulsive. You do things suddenly and without thinking, which causes problems. For instance, just now you came out to greet your cousin when you were only half-dressed. That is not appropriate. We will help you relearn what is appropriate. When you do something impulsive we will tell you, then ask you or tell you what might have been a better thing to do.

   Staff and family members should not laugh at disinhibited behavior, except when the person recognizes her mistake and laughs at herself.

Family members need to know the nature of disinhibition. They may need help anticipating when impulsivity could be a problem, help in structuring external compensations, and emotional support.

3. Retrain Self-Regulation: Training of self-control often begins with activities that are frequently repeated. A routine of reminders or procedures can be developed on cue cards to use in approaching situations where disinhibition is a particular problem. For example, a person who impulsively stands up from a wheelchair might use the 5 L's routine: 1) Lock brakes. 2) Lift foot rests. 3) Line up feet. 4) Lean forward. 5) Lift. A person who talks too much might review these cue card reminders before a gathering: "Don't talk too much. Listen. Don't interrupt."
4. Generalize Self-Regulation: Some people with mild to moderate disinhibition can be taught memorized verbal routines or schema to guide their behavior in various situations. These might first be read from cue cards, later memorized and spoken aloud, and later internalized. Although difficult, it is possible to teach the use and generalization of problem-solving routines such as:
   a. What is the problem?
   b. What is my goal?
   c. What are the ways I can get my goal?
   d. What is the best choice?
   e. Now how do I do it?
   f. (Afterward) Did I do it?

   The person learns to state aloud each question and her answer. Learning to speak one's plans aloud and then internalize that speech is helpful in controlling acquired impulsiveness (Cicerone & Giacino, 1992).

   For people who are reasonably intact cognitively and whose major problem is disinhibition (e.g., someone with localized orbital frontal lobe damage), education about disinhibition and about inappropriate social behavior can be the primary focus of extended neuropsychotherapy. The need for such additional help may also depend on the position and level of responsibility for decision-making held by the person.

   The "Back Off" procedure in Chapter 8 (p. 142) can be modified to "Stop and Think," followed by a generalized problem-solving routine. Possible risk factors and warning signs for impulsive behavior are listed in Table 11.4. If the social dimension of the problem is prominent, there may be cue card instructions to apologize, to ask for help, or to ask if there has been a problem.

   Techniques for controlling social impulsiveness can be further trained through role playing and group exercises, as well as with progressive simulated and real-life stressors and risk factors for disinhibition (Hopewell et al., 1990).

   Disinhibition is usually the greatest problem in the situations that

**TABLE 11.4. Possible Disinhibition Risk Factors, Warning Signs and Strategies (Excluding Emotional Disinhibition)**

| |
|---|
| Risk Factors |
| New, unfamiliar, or rare situations |
| New people |
| Attractive people |
| Busy, active times |
| Emotional excitement |
| Unexpected events |
| Lack of a plan |
| Warning Signs |
| Feelings of confusion |
| Feelings of excitement |
| People acting uncomfortable |
| People trying to leave |
| People telling me not to do something |
| Making mistakes like tripping, breaking something |
| Strategies |
| Stop and think |
| Is this dangerous? |
| What is my plan? |
| What is the best choice? |
| Do I need to ask for help? |
| What would Mom do? |
| What will people think? |

are most unexpected and least frequently encountered. For this reason, the training of generalization of learned routines and Stop and Think procedures needs to go through a graded progression of social and problem-solving risk. Generalization training may need to extend for a long time (perhaps monitored by a family member or a coach rather than a therapist) or it may need to be refreshed on occasion.

5. Fade External Compensations: The fading of external structure and restrictions can be nerve-wracking for families. It may help to develop backup plans, especially for when the person ventures into the community alone. An emergency instruction cue card and rehearsal of its use and a cellular phone or beeper may help.

## *PERSEVERATION*

### *Description*

Perseveration is the unintentional and inappropriate repetition of a sound, a word, a statement, an idea, an action, or an action pattern. It can take several forms (Hotz & Helm-Estabrooks, 1995a, 1995b; Sandson & Albert, 1984):

1. Continuous or motor perseveration is the repeating of simple actions such as overdrawing (drawing the same line many times), putting too many humps on the letter "m" and "n" when writing, repeating letters, stuttering, or adding extra beats when tapping rhythms. The person is unable to stop an ongoing action.
2. Recurrent perseveration refers to repeating a previous response in a new but similar situation. For example, when asked to name "nose, eye, ear, and mouth," a person with aphasia might respond "nose, eye, eye, nose." When asked to draw a square and then asked to draw a circle, she might draw two squares.
3. Stuck-in-set perseveration occurs when a person continues to perform an activity in a way that was appropriate to the previous activity. For example, if asked to say how a dog and cat are alike she might say that they are animals and pets, but then, if asked how they are different, she might perseverate with similarities by saying, "They have fur and tails."
4. Memory perseveration occurs when, after a delay or interference, people repeat something they previously said or did, because they do not realize or are not sure that they have already said or done it. For instance, some memory-impaired people will tell the same stories or jokes over and over to the same people or will ask the same questions. This type of perseveration is rarely included in the literature on perseveration (Hotz & Helm-Estabrooks, 1995a), but it is one of the most common forms complained of clinically (Mace & Rabins, 1991).

   The term perseveration is sometimes used pejoratively to describe behavior that is not quite any of those that were described previously, but might instead be called persistence or preoccupation. For instance, "He's still perseverating on wanting to go home." This type of "perseveration" is even sometimes taught as the "broken record technique" of assertiveness (Hopewell et al., 1990).

### *Similar Neurological Symptoms*

The person who is disinhibited may talk excessively and not stop, but this may be rambling rather than repetitive. People who are restless may pace or repeat actions because they want to be active, not because they cannot stop or change.

### *Similar Nonneurological Conditions*

Mild perseveration is a part of everyday life in people with intact brains (Hotz & Helm-Estabrooks, 1995b). Ritualistic behavior may appear perseverative.

People with obsessions or with compulsions may appear to perseverate in that they are overly focussed on an idea or action, but they usually also have associated anxiety. However, in severe obsessive-compulsive disorder, it appears that there may be an underlying hyperactivity of the cingulate cortex, the thalamus, and the basal ganglia (McGuire et al., 1994; Perani et al., 1995). Also, obsessive-compulsive symptomatology (Max et al., 1995) and ritualistic behaviors (Ames, Cummings, Wirshing, Quinn, & Mahler, 1994) have occasionally been reported as a consequence of brain lesions. A mild amount of obsessive-compulsiveness is an appropriate but inefficient compensation for memory impairments (e.g., the person who frequently checks that she has her keys or that she turned off the stove to be sure she did not forget).

### *Associated Symptoms*

Perseveration is often made worse by fatigue and by task difficulty. It is associated with attention disorders and with other executive dysfunctions. Continuous perseveration is associated with disorders of sequencing, of praxis, and of executive functioning. Recurrent perseveration is associated with disorders in the system that is perseverating; for example, naming perseveration in aphasia or praxic perseveration in apraxia. Stuck-in-set perseveration is associated with disorders of executive functioning, abstract reasoning, and problem solving. Memory perseveration is associated with amnesia.

### *Neuroanatomy*

Continuous perseverations are associated especially with posterior frontal and with right hemisphere lesions. Recurrent perseverations are associated with left posterior lesions. Stuck-in-set perseverations are associated with frontal and with subcortical lesions, especially in the dorsolateral regions. Although perseveration is usually seen following frontal lesions, it has also been seen with temporal, with parietal, and with subcortical lesions (Hotz & Helm-Estabrooks, 1995a).

### *How to Interview Regarding Perseveration*

The affected person will sometimes be aware of her perseveration, but her family is likely to notice it more because it can be annoying to them. Questions can focus on repetition of all sorts, on inflexibility, on speech and writing problems, on difficulty with transitions, and on problem-solving difficulties.

### *How to Observe/Test*

A variety of tasks that involve repetition can be used to assess perseveration. Commonly used tasks include continuous "m-n-m-n" writing, drawing loops, repeating tapped rhythms, naming tests, verbal fluency tasks, drawing, memory recall tests, and abstract reasoning tests (Hotz & Helm-Estabrooks, 1995b).

### *Practical Problems*

People with moderate to severe perseveration may find some activities inefficient or impossible. They will probably be frustrated and embarrassed if they are aware of the problem. Others can be annoyed by inefficiencies and by repeated questions and stories. Stuck-in-set perseveration contributes to concrete thinking and to a lack of empathy.

### *Interventions*

1. Compensate Externally: There are two major compensations for continuous, recurrent, and stuck-in-set perseveration: interruption and pacing. With *interruption*, the activity is stopped and a distracting (and very different) activity or rest intervenes before the person resumes the original action. A variation on the interruption strategy is alternating activities. Changes between dissimilar activities are planned frequently enough to keep perseveration from building up. External interruption compensations involve another person recognizing the perseveration and redirecting the perseverator or using an alarm to signal changes in activity.

   *Pacing* is when the activity is linked to or cued by some other sequence. External compensations using pacing involve another person or external stimulus timing the action, such as stutterers who speak more clearly when paced with a metronome.
2. Build Awareness: Continuous and recurrent perseverations are easy for family and for perseverators to learn to recognize and to understand. They can be described concretely and are easily pointed out.

   Stuck-in-set perseveration is more difficult to describe and point out. Stuck-in-set perseverations are like a car stuck in the mud; the more the driver spins the wheels, the deeper the car digs in. This tendency is especially exasperating in an argument; the more the person repeats her position, the harder it becomes for her to see any alternative. It may require the procedures of Chapter 8; for example, a cue card with "Signs of being stuck," and so forth. External cuing may cause conflict: "I'm not perseverating! You're perseverating!" Careful preparation may be needed to prevent such problems. Informal cuing may help: "Look, we're not getting anywhere. Let's just talk about this later."
3. Retrain Self-Regulation: Training self-interruption or task alternation self-control strategies for continuous or for recurrent perseveration is a rela-

tively straightforward task for cognitive rehabilitation. Self-pacing strategies involve using nonperseverating systems to pace perseverative ones. For instance, some stutterers (perseverative verbal system) can sing (nonperseverative musical system) without stuttering.

Self-interruption for stuck-in-set perseveration can use a variation on the major strategy of Chapter 8: back off, distract, try again (Table 11.5). Self-statements such as "There must be another way to do this," or "But how does he see it?" can be included on the cue card. Problem-solving routines (described previously under Disinhibition) can be used as pacing devices.

4. Generalize Self-Regulation: *Generalization* involves learning to recognize perseveration in other settings and learning to implement interruption and pacing strategies in other settings. This is particularly difficult for implementing general problem-solving strategies.
5. Fade External Compensations: Fading cues is relatively straightforward.
6. With memory perseverations, people can sometimes be taught to recognize when they are repeating. People close to them can learn to give agreed-on subtle cues to let them know that they are being repetitious. For someone who repeats questions, it may be possible to train her to seek the answer to her question in a standard place, such as on a blackboard or in a memory book. Having the person repeat or write the answer may allow them to use procedural learning so the question self-cues the answer. Mace and Rabins (1991) suggested that, at least with people with Alzheimer's disease, addressing the emotional concern behind the question may stop the perseveration better than giving the factual answer. For

**TABLE 11.5. Possible Perseveration Risk Factors, Warning Signs, and Strategies**

| |
|---|
| Risk Factors |
| Fatigue |
| Doing one thing for too long |
| (specific type of activity, such as talking, writing, drawing) |
| Anxiety |
| Lack of structure |
| Problem-solving |
| Warning Signs |
| Repetition |
| People getting annoyed |
| Can't seem to get anywhere |
| Strategies |
| Do something different, then come back |
| Rest |
| Count what I'm doing out loud (or other pacing system) |

example, for someone who repeatedly asked, "When is my mother coming for me?" the answer, "Your mother has been dead for many years" was either upsetting or ignored. The answer, "I will take care of you" worked much better.

## *CONCRETENESS*

### *Description*

Concrete thinkers fail to appreciate the abstract or symbolic qualities of ideas, of comments, or of things (Cicerone & Giacino, 1992; Goldstein, 1952). They are drawn to the most immediate, salient, and tangible features of the environment. They interpret language literally (Case 11.3. Portland); have trouble understanding metaphors, subtlety, and double meanings; and fail to appreciate humor that looks beyond literal meaning.

Concrete thinkers inappropriately generalize solutions from one setting to another. They have difficulty thinking beyond their current thought (stuck-in-set perseveration). They may be unable to abandon failed solutions to a problem; for example, pushing on a door that opens by pulling, then leaving frustrated.

*I Am NOT Concrete, I'm Flesh and Blood. Case 11.3. Portland.* The following approximates an actual Neurology Grand Rounds with a man with a TBI.
*Neurologist*: What is today's date?
*Portland*: May 3, 1976.
*N*: Good, that's right. What city are we in?
*P*: Boston.
*N*: Good. What building are we in?
*P*: The V.A. Hospital.
*N*: Good. What floor are we on?
[Portland looks at the floor and observes that it is made of cement.]
*P*: Concrete.

The following two jokes do not involve people with brain illnesses, but they do illustrate concrete thought.

My young son and I were driving through the town of Concrete, Washington. We saw the sign for the Concrete Laundry. Knowing my fondness for such jokes, my son asked, "Why would people want to bring their cement in here to wash it?"

A carpenter was nailing shingles on the side of a house. His supervisor asked, "Why are you throwing half the nails away?" "Because those stupid nails have the head on the wrong end." "You fool, those nails are for the other side of the house."

Concrete thinkers often cannot see beyond their own perspectives to recognize other people's points of view and needs. They may therefore lack empathy and may seem self-centered and selfish (Eslinger, 1998; Santoro & Spiers, 1994). For example, a couple was being interviewed about the changes in the man following a frontal lobe lesion. His wife cried as she described how he had changed from a loving, attentive husband into someone who didn't have enough sense to come in out of the rain. He was amused by the description and laughed, oblivious to his wife's distress.

Another aspect of concreteness is the tendency to be stimulus-bound. Concrete thinkers may be drawn by a nearby object and may try to use it or to respond to it, regardless of the circumstances. For example, they might eat food that is present even if they have just finished a full meal, drink from a cup even if it is empty, answer aloud questions asked by someone on television or on the radio, open drawers and doors, turn on machines, and so on, like an overly curious child.

### *Similar and Associated Neurological Symptoms*

Concreteness may be mistaken for or accompanied by distractibility or poor planning.

### *Similar Nonneurological Conditions*

Children, people who are mentally retarded, and people with limited or with no education often think concretely. People who do not speak a language well may interpret unfamiliar figures of speech literally. People with antisocial personality disorders are self-centered, selfish, and lack real empathic ability, but they will not think concretely in general.

### *Neuroanatomy*

Concreteness is associated with diffuse injury and particularly with lesions of the frontal lobes.

### *How to Interview Regarding Concrete Thinking*

The family is more likely to be aware of concreteness than is the person with the brain illness. Questions can focus on self-centeredness, on their sense of humor, on miscommunications, on frustration, and on problem-solving difficulties.

### *How to Observe/Test*

There are no tests specific to concrete thinking, rather it is a quality of thought observed in many circumstances. Concreteness may be seen in problem-solving strategies, in reasoning tasks, and in explanations given. Asking the person to explain jokes may be revealing, although there is much individual variation in humor appreciation. Concrete thinkers can also be asked to explain the plots of television shows and the motivations and the reasoning of the characters.

### *Practical Problems*

It may be hard to communicate effectively with concrete thinkers. They may not be able to solve day-to-day problems well. Others may find them selfish and unlikable. Interpersonal relationships can suffer due to a lack of empathy and to childishness.

### *Interventions*

1. Compensate Externally: The interventions described for stuck-in-set perseveration are applicable to the problem-solving aspects of concrete thinking (also, see Table 11.6). Family members and coaches can help the person negotiate social situations and understand abstract language and humor.

**TABLE 11.6. Possible Concreteness Risk Factors, Warning Signs, and Strategies**

| |
|---|
| Risk Factors |
| New or different situation |
| People telling jokes |
| Trying to solve a problem |
| Conflict with someone |
| Change in the routine |
| Warning Signs |
| I understand the words, but I don't really understand |
| People laughing at me |
| People getting annoyed |
| Can't seem to get anywhere |
| Starting to argue |
| Getting anxious |
| Strategies |
| Ask someone to explain |
| Is there another way to do it? |
| Is there another way to understand that? |
| Do something different, then come back |
| Rest |
| What is the other person thinking/feeling? |
| Ask how the other person feels. |

2. Build Awareness: Frustration and interpersonal difficulties can be examined to help the person discover the problem.
3. Retrain Self-Regulation: Restoration of abstraction abilities can be pursued through cognitive rehabilitation exercises for abstract reasoning, analogies, metaphors, figures of speech, poetry, categorizing tasks, and so forth. Confusion or misunderstanding can be used as a cue to ask for clarification or for help or to self-cue with slogans such as "Look for a deeper meaning."

   For people whose concreteness contributes to self-centeredness and the lack of empathy, active listening exercises can help. The person should be encouraged to try to restate what the other person has said, or to try to say what she thinks the other person's perspective might be. Cue cards for active listening and for awareness of others can be used before social encounters.

   Motion pictures and TV shows, especially dramas and soap operas, can be used to work on understanding the perspective of other people. These techniques can also be applied in group exercises and in family counseling or therapy. Where self-centeredness is causing family disruption it may be necessary to negotiate family agreements about how things are to be done, who is to have what privileges, who does what chores, and so forth.
4. Generalize Self-Regulation: Empathy skills can be modified for application across social settings.
5. Fade External Compensations: Because most external compensations are the interventions of other people, these are faded by cue reduction (Table 8.7, p. 149).

## *IMPAIRED MONITORING AND JUDGMENT AND LACK OF AWARENESS OF DEFICITS*

### *Description*

People with brain illnesses may have problems judging the appropriateness and the sensibleness of their thoughts, comments, and actions and in accurately judging the comments and actions of other people, so they misunderstand and misinterpret the intent of other people's behaviors. People with poor monitoring and judgment may be viewed as tactless and socially inappropriate. For example, they might begin a medical visit by asking overly personal questions of the physician or may make inappropriate sexual advances to people they encounter on the bus. They may not be able to make safe judgments and sound decisions. For example, they may drink alcohol even though they have been told not to do so because of medications they are taking.

An important manifestation of poor monitoring and judgment is failure to recognize one's own deficits resulting from the illness, or anosognosia (see Chapter 7). For example, the person may insist that she is ready return to work and may not realize that she cannot handle all the tasks that she used to do. She may even convince her family and co-workers that she is able to work until she fails at the job. She may have a carefree and euphoric attitude not consistent with her circumstances. She may frustrate others by her lack of worrying and concern for her difficulties and her failure to take her impairments into account in her activities.

Anosognosia is not all-or-nothing. Crosson and colleagues (1989) have described three levels of awareness useful for intervention planning (see Table 7.10, p. 126). In milder forms, the person may simply fail to show an expected amount of concern and interest in the disability. In more extreme cases, the person may deny the presence of a physical deficit such as left hemiplegia and may then fall out of bed because she thinks she can stand up.

### *Related and Associated Neurological Symptoms*

Impaired judgment and anosognosia are associated with all of the executive dysfunctions. Anosognosia is also associated with left neglect, with left hemiplegia, and/or with visual-spatial deficits and with fluent aphasia.

### *Similar Nonneurological Conditions*

Certain personality tendencies, in particular a psychopathic lack of concern or a paranoid distrust of others, may result in behavior that is unresponsive to feedback from others. People with schizophrenia or mania may show tactless, inappropriate behavior and may be insensitive to social norms as well. Psychological denial frequently accompanies neurological lack of awareness, particularly in the early months following injury. Usually, psychologically based denial gradually lessens as the person begins to recognize and accept the changes which have occurred as a result of the brain illness (Case 11.4, Ludwig).

### *Neuroanatomy*

Problems with monitoring and with judgment may follow diffuse damage and are particularly associated with damage to the frontal lobes. Anosognosia is associated with frontal lesions, with right hemisphere lesions, and with Wernicke's area lesions.

*Anosognosia, Denial, or Something Else? Case 11.4. Ludwig (Case 10.2, p. 190, revisited).* Ludwig was a 51-year-old, right-handed professor of music and a composer with right frontoparietal and temporal strokes. During his hospitalization he was, at first, unaware of his hemiplegia. Later he acknowledged it, but he attributed it to the sterile atmosphere of the hospital and felt that if he could only touch something living, such as a plant or animal, or even something that had been living, such as a piece of wood, his hand would work again. When this experience failed to produce recuperation, he felt that once he sat down at his piano again, his hand would regain its movements. Only after discharge from the hospital and the failure of this experience did he accept his hemiplegia (Judd, 1988).

### *How to Interview Regarding Monitoring, Judgment, and Lack of Awareness of Deficits*

Families are usually much more aware of monitoring and of judgment problems than are the people experiencing them. Separate interviews can give a more accurate picture of discrepancies in the awareness of difficulties. The person and the family should be asked similar questions about what are the major problems, their safety, about embarrassing episodes, about social relations, about error correction, about problem-solving, and about specific episodes reflecting on judgment skills.

### *How to Observe/Test*

Observations in unstructured social situations are often valuable. The degree of awareness and of self-correction of errors on testing should be noted. The person with a brain illness can be asked to judge the quality of her performance on tasks as a means of assessing her degree of recognition of her deficits. Her awareness of errors and of deficits on interview, during testing, and after tests can be compared to determine if she has intellectual, emergent, or anticipatory awareness (see Table 7.10, p. 130). *The Behavior Change Inventory* (BCI; Hartlage, 1991), The *Head Injury Family Interview* (Kay et al., 1995), *The Neuropsychology Behavior and Affect Profile* (Nelson, Satz, & D'Elia, 1994), *The Frontal Lobe Personality Scale* (Grace et al., 1996), and *The Temporal Lobe Epilepsy Personality Inventory* (Bear & Fedio, 1977; see Appendix B, p. 327) allow for comparisons between self-ratings and informant ratings, which contribute to an impression of anosognosia.

Judgement is often tested with verbally presented situations such as "What would you do if a fire started in the house?" or "What would you do if you saw a young child walking alone near a river bank?" Such questions have the advantage that standard ones are available, and that situations can also be generated that are adapted to the person's background. The disadvantage is that some people with impaired judgment may say the right thing on a test but do the wrong thing in life.

### *Practical Problems*

Impaired judgement and awareness of deficits can produce safety hazards and risks for squandering money or for becoming victimized. Family and social relationships can become very strained. The person may refuse rehabilitation or other care.

### *Interventions*

Interventions for anosognosia are described in Chapter 7 (p. 122).

1. Compensate Externally: Impaired judgment and monitoring may require supervision; restricted access to danger such as vehicles, sharp tools, poisons, fire, and weapons; and restricted access to the community or to money.
2. Build Awareness: Generally, family and staff should give direct and immediate feedback to the person when an inappropriate comment or behavior occurs. The person should be told what the comment or behavior was, why it was inappropriate, and should then be provided with an alternate, appropriate comment or behavior.

   Families are likely to need guidance in anticipating judgment problems, in setting limits appropriately, and in relaxing those limits when appropriate.
3. Retrain Self-Regulation: Judgment is best retrained first in situations that recur regularly. The person can be taught routines for everyday tasks such as housekeeping and how to deal with routine social interactions such as making purchases. It may be necessary to call explicit attention to those aspects of the activity that need to be monitored.

   In addition to naturalistic judgments, judgment can be retrained through individual and group exercises. "What would you do if . . . ?" situations can be invented or drawn from everyday events. They can also involve discussion of news, television dramas, talk shows, novels, and so forth. Questions such as "Why did he . . . ?" "What do you think will happen next?" and "What are her options now?" can stimulate the exercise of judgment.

   In group treatment, the therapist might use actual or invented situations and ask group members to generate appropriate responses, to critique these responses, and to give feedback to each other. For example, the therapist might ask, "What would you do if your mother made a shirt for you that you didn't like?" and then ask other group members to give feedback. Group members should give feedback about each other's behavior in the session, such as eye contact and turn-taking in the conversation.

4. Generalize Self-Regulation: Generalization can be trained to related tasks and interactions. Impaired judgment is usually most problematic with infrequent or unexpected events. The most pragmatic approach to such situations may be to train the person to ask for help. As a transitional stage, it is generally better that the person is constantly asking, "What should I do?" than that she is acting on her poor judgment. Asking for help can then be shaped into practicing judgment with the helper answering, "What do you think you should do?" With practice, the person may come to ask, "I think I should do X, what do you think?" Much of this type of support can be carried out by family and by friends, perhaps with training and guidance from a professional.
5. Fade External Compensations: Because everyone relies on other people's judgment at least occasionally, the pattern of asking for help or for confirmation of decisions can be faded until it reaches a level that feels natural for all participants.

## *IMPAIRED PLANNING AND ORGANIZATION*

### *Description*

People with brain illnesses may have difficulty forming and carrying out plans and organizing activities effectively. They may have difficulty developing an overall picture of a task, identifying all of the necessary steps, and completing all of the steps in the proper order. If interrupted, they may have trouble returning to and continuing the task. They may have trouble changing a plan to accommodate a changed situation.

### *Related and Associated Neurological Symptoms*

Planning and organizational difficulties are associated with all of the executive dysfunctions and attention deficit disorders. People with attention or memory impairments may make good plans but may then forget to carry them out. People who have deficits of planning and of organization may react to their own inefficiency and disorganization with perplexity, frustration, and anger, often expressed impulsively.

### *Similar Nonneurological Conditions*

General personality styles including impulsivity, carelessness, and a nonobsessive approach may produce poor planning and organization. People with hypomanic tendencies are often poorly organized. Those who are rigid and stubborn may have difficulty considering alternatives in planning. People who lack motivation may not make plans. Depressed people may lack the mental energy to make or to carry out plans. Ways of planning and sequencing activities and organizing space and time vary considerably across cultures.

### *Neuroanatomy*

Planning and organizational difficulties are associated with diffuse brain illness and particularly with damage to the frontal lobes. The right frontal lobe has been particularly implicated.

### *How to Interview Regarding Planning Deficits*

The person with the brain illness and her family may not spontaneously report problems in planning and in organizing in those terms. Questions should focus on the results of poor planning and organizing, such as difficulty accomplishing things, rambling speech, being late, abandoned projects, trouble giving directions, disorganized personal space, and so forth. It is important to check if this is a change from before the illness.

### *How to Observe/Test*

Problems in planning and in organizing can be readily observed qualitatively on many tests. Problems such as starting over repeatedly, proceeding haphazardly, failing to correct errors, and changing the approach to the task in the middle suggest poor planning and organization. The final result may be technically correct but it may have been reached inefficiently.

### *Practical Problems*

People with problems planning and organizing may have difficulty getting tasks accomplished or may produce poor-quality work. They may be very inefficient and may require much time even for simple tasks. They may be late and unreliable for work and for appointments. They may be poor communicators because of disorganized speech. Other people may lose patience with them, have difficulty sharing space and tasks with them, or see them as irresponsible, obstructive, or lazy.

*Interventions*

1. Compensate Externally: Compensations include supervision; written routines; a memory book with a schedule, an appointment calendar, and a list of things to do; labeled and color-coded locations for objects; timetables; prioritizing; alarms; filing systems, and pagers (Evans, Emslie, & Wilson, 1998). Supervisors may need to give instructions one step at a time.
2. Build Awareness: Accurately naming the problem and giving multiple, concrete examples can help to focus a recovery plan and reduce misimpressions of laziness.
3. Retrain Self-Regulation: Planning can be directly retrained through exercises. Activities of priority to the person can be selected and she can be asked to plan how she would do them. At first she should speak her plans aloud, or should elaborate them on paper, on computer, or with another modality. When this process is reliable, the speech or other planning can then be internalized (Cicerone & Giacino, 1992). The modality chosen for making plans explicit should be somewhat familiar to the person and should be something that can usefully guide the activity for her. Someone who has learned to sew, for example, by copying someone else may not be able to guide that process verbally very effectively. It may be more effective to lay out the steps spatially by putting the materials or tools on a tabletop in the order in which they will be used.

   The procedures can also be applied to exercises in social planning and organizing. This may be a part of neuropsychotherapy for someone who is encountering misunderstandings and difficulties with others over social commitments. Work may focus on punctuality, on social decision-making, on planning social events, and so on. This is also the type of help that family members and friends may be able to offer with some training and guidance.
4. Generalize Self-Regulation: When enough examples of successful planning have been accumulated, principles and schema can be derived that work for that individual and can then be applied in other realms of functioning.
5. Fade External Compensations: When external compensations have been mastered, those that are efficient and unobtrusive, such as filing systems and daily planners, can be kept in place. Support, supervision, therapy sessions, and cues from others can become less frequent and can cover fewer areas.

## *IMPAIRED COMMUNICATION PRAGMATICS*

### *Description*

Communication pragmatics are the nonlinguistic aspects of conversation (Kennedy & DeRuyter, 1991; McDonald, 1992). Normally, people follow a set of culturally determined rules of appropriate conversation depending on the situation and the social context. They are aware of the obligations and expectations of each conversation. That is, they realize who can say what to whom, in what way, where, when, and by what means.

People with deficits in communication pragmatics may not have aphasia, that is, they may have normal language abilities, with good articulation, grammar, and semantics. However, they are poor communicators. Their pragmatics deficits result from cognitive and executive function impairments. Pragmatics impairments occur in the following areas:

*1. Nonverbal Behavior:*

- Physical proximity to others (too near or too far)
- Touch (too much; too little, such as not shaking hands; wrong kind)
- Postures and gestures
- Eye contact (staring, failing to make eye contact)
- Voice volume (too loud or too soft)
- Voice inflection (monotone, overly expressive, misplaced emphasis)

*2. Turn-Taking:*

- Not allowing others to speak
- Interrupting
- Not responding

*3. Topic Maintenance:*

- Insufficient information (presupposition)
- Too much detail (circumstantiality)
- Irrelevant information (tangentiality)
- Straying from topic (derailing)
- Switching topics without cues

*4. Social Appropriateness:*

- Inappropriate (laughing at things that are not funny, crude language in a genteel context or vice versa)
- Insensitivity to social roles (asking the therapist for a date)

*5. Conversation Repair:*

- Not recognizing or correcting misunderstandings
- Not asking for clarification

*6. Cohesiveness of Narrative:*

- Poor sequencing
- Poor word choice
- Idiosyncratic meanings
- Overly abstract and vague

The following dialogue illustrates several impairments in communication pragmatics:

*Psychologist*: What did you do today, Joe?
*Joe*: Well, I was going to go to the store but my wife didn't come home. I wanted to get one of those new t-shirts. My cousin has one, the one who lives across the state. He works for the beer company there. You know what he likes to do? He likes looking at dirty pictures. We have a cousin ...
*Psychologist*: Joe ...
*Joe*: Over in Jasper who works on a farm. She doesn't go to church. They live in a . . .
*Psychologist*: Joe, Joe . . .
*Joe*: Yes?
*Psychologist*: What does this have to do with what you did today?
*Joe*: I'm getting to that. They live in a little house on the river and they like to go fishing. Their car is almost . . .

Problems with communication pragmatics can also be seen in written and in other forms of communication, particularly in appropriateness, organization of narrative, and presupposition.

### *Related and Associated Symptoms*

Deficits in communication pragmatics are associated with impaired emotional communication, with other executive dysfunctions, and with impaired attention. The person who has memory impairments may forget what she has said and therefore repeat herself or omit important details. The communication difficulties of aphasia may include aspects of pragmatics; for example, fluent aphasics who are unaware of their comprehension impairments may not ask for clarification when they need it.

### *Similar Nonneurological Conditions*

People with schizophrenia may have odd and socially inappropriate ways of communicating. Various types of character disorders may be associated with poor interpersonal communication styles. Mania and depression can also affect some dimensions of pragmatics such as turn-taking, eye contact, theme maintenance, and conversational repair. It is important to distinguish these conditions, because a pragmatic skill deficit is not likely to be remediated by psychotropic medications, for example. There are major cultural differences in what are regarded as appropriate communication pragmatics in all dimensions.

### *Neuroanatomy*

Pragmatic deficits are most commonly seen following diffuse moderate to severe brain injury. Frontal lobe damage is implicated in producing pragmatics problems because these problems are related to underlying executive deficits. Some components of pragmatics are impaired following right hemisphere damage, especially emotional communication.

### *How to Interview Regarding Communication Pragmatics*

Family members may be able to identify that there is something odd or inappropriate about the person's communication, but they may have difficulty describing it. Questions can focus on clear communication, on staying on topic, on interrupting, and on embarrassment.

### *How to Observe/Test*

Many people with pragmatics difficulties do well on formal language tests and in structured conversations. The examiner should allow enough time and lack of structure in the interview to demonstrate any pragmatic deficits that exist. Examiners may find that they are working hard to keep the person from talking too much, to keep her on track, or to get her to talk at all.

The best way to document pragmatic deficits is to observe natural conversations. Video- or audiotaping can aid analysis and feedback and can provide a baseline observation. Free-form written narrative may also be useful. Pragmatics ratings forms can also be used (Kennedy & DeRuyter, 1991; McDonald, 1992). It is important to define and to describe the particular problems seen accurately and concretely to focus the intervention.

### *Practical Problems*

People with pragmatic deficits often have serious social and vocational problems. Their ineffective and often odd style of communicating often causes other people to avoid them; they may become isolated and lonely.

### *Interventions*

1. Compensate Externally: Other participants in the conversation often compensate, in that they will often ask for clarification when they need it, and so on. Others can serve as conversational "coaches" and help to cover up problems or to bring the person back on track. Cue cards, behavioral flash cards, and other signal systems can be used to prepare for or to cope with some situations (see Chapter 7, pp. 113–118, and Cases 7.1, Gabby, and 11.3, Dumi). Written outlines and editing can be used for writing pragmatics.
2. Build Awareness: Pragmatics deficits are readily observed by family members and by others, but they are identified only with difficulty. Education involves sensitizing the person and the family to these unwritten rules of communication and to their violations. Because these behavioral norms are so complex, it is best to prolong the education process and focus on only a few items at a time. Fortunately, these problems are often readily and concretely illustrated, either live or through audiotape, through videotape, or through writing samples. Identifying pragmatics problems as skill deficits can relieve much worry about possible personality problems and can encourage family members to facilitate socialization.
3. Retrain Self-Regulation: Pragmatics can be retrained both formally and informally through identifying and agreeing to concrete goals and by giving appropriate feedback during conversations. This can be done by therapists or by family members.

   Groups are preferred for the formal treatment of pragmatics problems. Individual and group goals should be set for specific conversations, role plays, or group activities. Group members receive feedback from each other, from the therapist, and from videotape on the effectiveness of their communication.
4. Generalize Self-Regulation: Generalization can be practiced through supervised community outings or in other observed settings in the community (job stations, work, travel).
5. Fade External Compensations: Conversation coaches gradually reduce their interventions through cue reduction (see Table 8.7, p. 149).

# 12

# Cognitive and Medical Problems

The assumption of this book is that its readers have medical and cognitive evaluation and rehabilitation services available, and therefore those topics will not be treated here. This chapter is a selective discussion of those cognitive and medical difficulties most likely to provoke major problems of behavior, of emotions, and of adjustment, and the impact that these difficulties have on neuropsychotherapy and related interventions. For discussions of chronic pain and brain illness see Miller (1993).

## *IMPAIRED ATTENTION AND CONCENTRATION*

### *Description*

Attention deficits are some of the most common, disabling, and subjective cognitive impairments resulting from brain illnesses. For the purposes of this book, attention can be divided into capacity and control (Weber, 1990). People with capacity difficulties are slow to process information. They have trouble concentrating and sustaining attention for long periods of time (Case 12.1. Lu Tan) and are susceptible to mental fatigue. Others may perceive them as lazy or as faking.

People with control difficulties may process information at normal speed at times but have difficulty directing their attention. They may have trouble switching from one activity to another, dividing their attention between activities, and managing interruptions and distractions (Case 12.2. Gramps). They may be overly sensitive to noise, to clutter, and to movement. Others may perceive them as being scattered and irresponsible. Many people have both capacity and control difficulties.

*When Less Is More. Case 12.1. Lu Tan.* Lu Tan was a 38-year-old engineer seen for neuropsychotherapy 6 months after a mild TBI without loss of consciousness. Since his accident he hated the drive to work and rarely went out except to work. Prior to the accident he designed 15 plans a day on his computer; post-accident he designed only 2, even though he worked right through his coffee breaks and lunch hour and stayed late. Testing showed attention impairments.

I asked him to take all of his coffee and lunch breaks and to leave work on time. I suggested that every time he felt himself start to get confused he should stand up, walk once around his desk, and sit back down. With these instructions, in the next week he produced 7 plans a day. He started going to work and leaving an hour early. That way he avoided traffic, and the drive became easier. He stopped trying to listen to the radio and to eat breakfast while driving. The first hour of the work day with few people in the office became his most productive.

Lu Tan was an individual whose drive and ambition had served him well to get where he was, but those same characteristics worked against him when he tried to use them to overcome the fatigue and attentional difficulties that came from his head injury. He needed to learn a new way to pace himself.

### *Related and Associated Symptoms*

People who cannot attend well do not take in new information completely and do not learn effectively, so attention deficits contribute to memory deficits. Poor attentional control and distractibility overlap with executive dysfunctions, most notably disinhibition. Hyperaesthesia contributes to distractability (see the

*I Love You All, but One at a Time, Please! Case 12.2. Gramps.* Gramps was a 55-year-old truck driver who was disabled by a mild TBI, by chest trauma, and by cerebral hypoxia resulting from a machinery accident. Testing had revealed significant attention problems that made him an unsafe driver.

Prior to his accident he enjoyed visits from his young grandchildren and coached one grandson's baseball team. Afterwards he found that he no longer enjoyed a horde of grandchildren running through the house. Coaching gave him a headache. He dreaded the grandchildren's visits and hid in the bedroom. He gave up coaching and didn't even go to the games.

Following my recommendations, he talked his problem over with his wife and with their children and had the grandchildren visit one or two at a time. They picked quieter games to play with him and he read to them. At larger family gatherings, he sat on the edge and watched, or he visited with one or two of them at a time in the next room.

He started going to baseball games again with his daughter and sat away from the crowd. They either came late or left early. He started coaching his son one-to-one, then became an assistant coach, drilling either one player at a time or small groups.

Hyperaesthesia section that follows, p. 257). Attention difficulties often worsen markedly with fatigue. Attention difficulties contribute to information overload, catastrophic reactions, frustration, anxiety, and anger. Attentional difficulties are one of the defining characteristics of attention deficit disorder (Barkley, 1997). Some kinds of seizures, especially petit mal, absence, and partial complex seizures, may look like lapses of attention.

### *Similar Nonneurological Conditions*

Many emotional disorders produce difficulties with attention and with concentration, most notably depression, anxiety, obsessive-compulsive disorder, post-traumatic stress disorder, and schizophrenia. It is easy to fake (consciously or otherwise) attention impairments by not trying very hard to focus on a task.

### *Neuroanatomy*

Diffuse brain injuries are the most common causes of attention and concentration problems. Attentional control difficulties are thought to be associated with anterior frontal lobe lesions, whereas attentional capacity impairments may come from metabolic disturbances and from damage to the subcortical reticular activating system. The ability to focus attention on the environment is associated with the superior temporal and inferior parietal cortices and the corpus striatum (Mirsky, Anthony, Duncan, Ahearn, & Kellam, 1991).

### *Practical Problems*

Attention impairments are among the greatest safety risks for driving, operating machinery, cooking, using sharp tools, and so forth. People with poor attention and concentration usually have difficulty with school and with work. They may be seen as lazy, as passive-aggressive, or as malingering. Inattentiveness may seem to others to reflect boredom or a lack of interest, caring, or love. Attention problems also limit the location, the duration, and the form of neuropsychotherapy sessions and of related interventions.

### *Interventions*

1. Safety precautions may need to be taken if the inattentive person is engaging in potentially dangerous activities such as cooking, using sharp tools, or driving.
2. Family education should include avoiding misunderstandings about attention problems and ways in which the family can help out. Becoming aware of attentional limits and of the risks of information overload can often help to avoid anger, frustration, and anxiety.

3. Cognitive rehabilitation programs typically retrain attention using restoration strategies (Sohlberg & Mateer, 1989). Compensation strategies for attention involve lifestyle changes that affect work, socializing, and many other areas. These include the following:
   a. Reduce distractions. Reduce noise from radios, from televisions, and from loud machinery when the person needs to concentrate or to have a conversation. If noise cannot be avoided, the person can use earplugs or music on headphones to drown out distracting sounds. He can close curtains or even close his eyes to shut out stimulation.
   b. Avoid crowds. Shop and drive during the off-hours and in small stores and streets. Visit with people in small numbers and with small children one at a time. Stay at the edge of large gatherings. Do not try to do anything that requires concentration while in a crowd. Take someone along who can act as a guide.
   c. Avoid interruptions. Unplug the phone or use an answering machine or "Do Not Disturb" signs. Ask others not to interrupt.
   d. Do just one thing at a time.
   e. Get adequate sleep and regular physical exercise.
4. People with attentional difficulties may need help learning to recognize the presence of distractors and the need to use attention compensations. They may need to learn how, when, and whom to ask for help in implementing these compensations. They may need to develop assertiveness to ask someone to turn off a radio or to go to a quieter place to talk, for example. They may need to develop socially acceptable ways to take a break (go to the "rest" room, for example).
5. Therapy sessions may need to be in quiet, distraction-free settings. Communication style will need to take attention problems into account (see Chapter 6, p. 87).

## *IMPAIRED MEMORY AND LEARNING*

### *Description*

Memory problems are among the most common consequences of brain illnesses and present some of the greatest technical challenges to neuropsychotherapy and to related interventions. Those who work with people with memory difficulties should learn about the individual's specific memory problems from the neuropsychological assessment, even if these are not the focus of the intervention. Those who work regularly with people with memory impairments need to be well acquainted with basic concepts of amnesia (see Sohlberg & Mateer, 1989; Squire, 1987; or any neuropsychology textbook). The following phenomena are those most relevant to personality, to emotions, and to neuropsychotherapy:

*Anterograde Amnesia*

*Anterograde amnesia*, the inability to learn new information, is the most common and disabling type of memory disorder. The person with pure anterograde amnesia may hold entirely coherent conversations, giving the impression that he will remember the contents, but then forgets what was said as soon as the topic changes. This presents a major challenge to meaningful, ongoing personal relationships and to psychotherapy.

*Retrograde Amnesia*

*Retrograde amnesia* is loss of memory for events preceding an illness. A lost personal history may need to be reconstructed cognitively and integrated emotionally and interpersonally.

*Procedural Memory*

Procedural learning is the ability to learn motor habits or sequential activities such as typing, riding a bicycle, using a machine, cooking something, and so forth. These abilities are often preserved in people with anterograde amnesia. Procedural learning is important in rehabilitation, because people with poor memory can often use procedural learning as a strategy to help acquire habits. Similarly, ways of dealing with specific emotional or behavioral situations may be trained, even if specific strategies or approaches cannot be remembered explicitly.

*Post-Traumatic Amnesia*

The period of time following a brain trauma or an illness during which the person is awake and behaving, but about which he can later recall nothing is called *post-traumatic amnesia*. It is usually followed by gradually recovering anterograde amnesia, so memories will be hazy for the period of emerging from post-traumatic amnesia. Some emotional reactions, especially fears, may be learned during this time by classical conditioning (Layton & Wardi-Zonna, 1994; McMillan, 1991).

*Prospective Memory*

The ability to remember to do something at the appropriate time in the future (watch a television show, check food cooking on the stove, go to an appointment) is called *prospective memory*. Difficulties with prospective memory are common and disabling. They are associated with attention impairments and with anterograde amnesia (Mateer, Sohlberg, & Crinean, 1987). Prospective memory deficits make some appear unreliable, uncaring, and unmotivated. Compensation techniques are needed for therapy homework.

### *Confabulation*

*Confabulation* is the generation of false memories. It is seen in people with both anterograde amnesia and with disinhibition. They will claim to remember things that never happened. Confabulation may range from a plausible but false reconstruction to an outrageous fabrication. People who confabulate are neither hallucinating nor lying. They truly believe their false memories.

## *Related and Associated Symptoms*

Sensory, attention, and organization impairments may prevent new information from being adequately registered, and therefore it will not be remembered later. People with word-finding difficulties resulting from aphasia may say they cannot "remember" words, which is a fair description, but is not usually regarded as a true memory problem in neuropsychology.

## *Similar Nonneurological Conditions*

People who are depressed frequently complain of poor memory, especially older people. Depressed people do worse on memory tests than nondepressed people, mainly because they do not attend well. However, the information they do take in is usually remembered normally. People with the cognitive distortions of depression frequently see their memory as worse than it is.

People with repressive styles may have trouble remembering things, especially emotionally charged events. Rarely, people may develop psychologically based amnesia. This amnesia is usually easily distinguished from organic memory disorder by good performance on new learning tests and from severe amnesia for specific past events or periods of time. Fugue states, in which the affected person adopts an entirely new identity and claims no memory for the former identity, also have psychological origins.

Malingerers may claim to have memory problems to get out of trouble or to avoid something. Testing techniques for detecting malingered amnesia are constantly improving (Binder, 1992, 1993; Rawling & Brooks, 1990).

## *Neuroanatomy*

Major anterograde amnesia is produced by lesions of the limbic system, especially the hippocampus and the dorsal medial nucleus of the thalamus (Squire,

1987). Learning problems resulting from poor attention and organization are associated with diffuse damage or damage to the frontal lobes. Material-specific amnesia is associated with lesions in the part of cortex associated with the material, especially with temporal cortex lesions. For example, lesions producing aphasia also produce difficulties with new verbal learning. Confabulation is associated with the combination of injury to the frontal cortex and limbic system lesions (Stuss, et al., 1992).

### *Interview Considerations*

The person with amnesia is quite likely to be an unreliable historian. An informant should also be interviewed.

### *Practical Problems*

The most obvious practical problems are that people with poor memory tend to forget things easily. They often irritate others with repeated questioning. They may be unsafe; for example, forgetting to turn off the stove, to put out the fire, or to lock the house or the gate when leaving. They have trouble learning new things and may not be able to keep up in school or on the job. They may get lost easily. Social relations suffer when the person with amnesia cannot maintain a sense of continuity in a relationship. People with severe amnesia may lose their sense of self in a temporal and social context.

### *Interventions*

1. Family education and counseling regarding emotional dimensions of amnesia usually includes helping them to grieve the loss of the person they once knew. It includes help in learning to avoid placing blame on the person with amnesia for not remembering things. It is also a help to focus on the positive. Some people with amnesia retain many of their abilities and emotions, and a significant, if somewhat restricted, relationship can continue.
2. If memory difficulties are due to problems with attention or with organization, then cognitive rehabilitation that restores those functions will improve memory as well (Sohlberg & Mateer, 1989).
3. Attempts to restore memory abilities through memory practice have not been very successful (Wilson, 1987). The major cognitive rehabilitation techniques for memory that are currently practiced are compensations such as calendars, notebooks, and other written systems to help organize and keep track of things to remember. A memory notebook with sections for a daily log of events, an appointment and an event calendar, a daily

planner with a "Things To Do" list, and a place for shopping lists, phone numbers, and so forth is a common aid. Electronic personal organizers, computers, and tape recorders are also used. The person may need to be trained extensively in how to use the memory notebook or other compensation system using preserved procedural learning.

4. Families can help by leaving things in the same place at home and keeping routines and schedules that help the person with the brain illness to form habits that do not rely on forming new memories.
5. People with mild to moderate amnesia are often aware of and appropriately concerned about it. Grief work for the memory loss and working on ways to adapt to it are frequent intervention agendas. Cognitive compensations should be amply used during these interventions.
6. People with severe amnesias frequently have only a dim awareness of their problem and are often indifferent toward it. When amnesia is severe, progress in formal psychotherapy will be slow and not very cost effective. Such individuals may achieve some insight in the session, only to forget it by the time they leave. Using memory compensations to deal with specific behavior and emotional problems may be the more realistic approach.
7. One special emotional problem may arise if the person with post-traumatic amnesia was involved in an auto accident in which someone close to him was killed or was seriously injured. When should he be told this news? Unless the person is clearly depressed or showing unmanageable emotional lability, the best time to tell him is soon after he begins to emerge from post-traumatic amnesia. It is usually best if a family member delivers the news, which may be one of the first pieces of information retained. The person with the brain trauma may be emotionally indifferent and may take in the information with little reaction. He will gradually come to grieve as his recovery of emotions and of cognition allows. To delay the news much beyond emergence from post-traumatic amnesia can make an awkward situation where everyone around the person must keep up the same consistent lie. The news may slip out inadvertently. He may wonder why his loved one is not visiting. When he finally finds out, he may resent that he was not told earlier. To tell him prior to emergence from post-traumatic amnesia is generally pointless (Case 12.3. P. T. A.).
8. Memory compensation techniques for working on emotional and on behavioral problems are described in Chapters 6 through 11.

## *LANGUAGE AND SPEECH DISTURBANCES*

### *Description*

Language and speech disturbances are many and varied (see Mateer & Judd, 1993; most neuropsychology and language pathology textbooks). Those working

*When to Tell? Case 12.3. P. T. A.* A young man was hospitalized on an acute rehabilitation service in a state of post-traumatic amnesia from a severe TBI from a motor vehicle accident in which his wife was killed. Although disoriented and unaware of his accident, he frequently asked about his wife. The rehabilitation team, with his family's permission, decided to tell him the news. When he next asked about his wife, a nurse sat down with him and explained that they had both been in an accident and that his wife had been killed. He looked totally shocked and then became very distressed. She was able to distract him with an activity for a while, and he calmed down. Several minutes later he again asked where his wife was. The nurse again explained and he again reacted as if this was the first time he had heard it and became once again distraught. This cycle was repeated several more times before it became clear this process was not helping his orientation and was only provoking needless distress. The news was postponed until he was able to retain it.

with someone with a language or speech problem need to seek appropriate professional advice on how best to communicate with the affected person. The discussion here focuses on the emotional dimensions of aphasia and of speech disturbances.

*Expressive and Global Aphasia*

Expressive aphasia and global aphasia are frequently accompanied by hemiplegia, by an intense awareness of impairments, by depression, by frustration, and by catastrophic reactions. People so affected can derive tremendous emotional relief from working with a neuropsychotherapist who has the skills to communicate with them, to express empathy for their dilemma, and to serve as a "translator" of emotionally significant messages to the family.

*Receptive Aphasia*

People with impaired language comprehension sometimes are unaware of their deficit (Rubens & Garrett, 1991). They often do not have a hemiplegia or other signs that might more obviously indicate illness to them. They usually have verbal memory difficulties for whatever information is comprehended. They may become paranoid, blaming others for not speaking clearly or for not understanding their aphasic and garbled speech. Others may, therefore, act uncertain or fearful in their presence, thereby feeding their paranoia. Working with such people can be very challenging. Nonverbal body language and tone of voice must be used carefully to try to establish trust. For example, it is important to include such people in the conversation by talking to them, by looking at them, and so forth, and by not talking about them in their presence as if they were not there.

*Speech Impairments*

People who have severe dysarthria, a tracheostomy, or another mechanical limitation to speaking may have language abilities intact, and may communicate with writing, with an alphabet board, with an adapted computer, or by other means. Therapists need to become proficient at these means of communication and to empathize with the frustration that such limitations may provoke.

*All Language and Speech Impairments*

Many people who do not understand speech and language impairments tend to patronize people who are impaired. They may talk to adults as if they were children or as if they were hard of hearing. They may talk in their presence as if they were not there or were not listening. They may try to shield them from important family information or from decisions. The therapist's job includes modeling communication for the family and teaching respect and appropriate interactions. The therapist can also write a cue card or a letter with/for the person explaining what he would like others to know and to do about his condition (see Table 7.5f, p. 117, and Case 12.4. Doris's letter).

Many family members are at a loss as to what to do with someone with

*Case 12.4. Doris's Letter.*

To Doris's friends,

Doris had a mild stroke in December, 1993. I am the psychologist who helps her with some of the problems she has had from that stroke. Although she walks well, she still has some mild trouble with her language abilities, especially when she is tired. This makes it hard for her to explain what is going on. That is why she asked me to write this letter to you.

Doris enjoys your company and would like to keep doing things with you. But sometimes she has trouble keeping up with conversation, especially when a lot of people talk fast, and especially when she is tired. So she may just watch and not say anything or even go rest for a little while. When this happens it is not because she is not interested; she just can't participate.

At times she may have trouble finding the words she wants. She may even forget your name. Please don't take this personally; it is due to her stroke. She is very embarrassed by it. If you are very sure of what she is trying to say you can give her the word she is looking for. Otherwise it is better to just give her time to come up with it, or come back to the topic later.

Doris does not have Alzheimer's disease, she is not going crazy, and she is not drunk. But she has had a stroke and she does need your patience and understanding. She is not embarrassed to discuss her stroke, so feel free to ask her questions.

Thank you for your understanding and for being a good friend to Doris.

**TABLE 12.1. Possible Activities for People with Aphasia and Their Families**

| | |
|---|---|
| Music | Crafts |
| Cooking | Sports |
| Eating | Dance |
| Childcare | Sex and affection |
| Travel | Massage |
| Shopping | Religious services |
| Art | Card games |
| Photography | Some board games |
| Looking at pictures | Housework |
| TV and movies (selected) | Gardening |
| Mechanics | Animal care |

aphasia. One important goal in helping such families to adapt is helping them to find meaningful activities they can share (Table 12.1) Nonverbal therapy modalities, such as art and music therapy, can be quite useful for expressing emotions for people with aphasia (Jochims, 1995; Joraski, 1986; Case 12.5, Frank). Using touch to convey understanding and sympathy is often helpful because it is a nonverbal message that can penetrate aphasia.

## *FATIGUE*

### *Description*

People with brain injuries often fatigue easily. If they are aware of their fatigue, they may complain that they feel tired and do not function well. If unaware, they may simply become less efficient after an extended effort. Cognitive and subjective fatigue appear to be distinct from physical fatigue (LaChapelle & Finlayson, 1998). With focal brain injury, a specific impaired cognitive function may fatigue specifically. For example, someone with aphasia may lose his ability

*Our Song. Case 12.5. Frank.* After a long and full work life, a U.S. man had just retired and he and his wife of many years had begun their first trip to Europe, when he had a stroke. Although he was aphasic and unable to speak, while they were still in their hotel room in England waiting for the ambulance to come he hummed to his wife "their song," the love song that had been sung at their wedding and was a theme in their marriage. That poignant and creative way he found to express his love for her at that moment was a great help to them both in sustaining them through the long and difficult road ahead.

to express himself over the course of a few minutes of conversation and then recover the ability after a period of not talking. Although speech is fatigued, he may still be able to draw or to sew normally, just as one arm might get tired from sawing boards, but the other one can still do the job.

Cognitive fatigue can also be general. The person with a brain injury who appears to have recovered well might be able to work for 6 hours normally but may make too many mistakes in the last 2 hours to be able to work effectively for a full 8 hours.

Fatigue can develop in a minute or less, or it can take as long as all day. Rapid fatigue is more common soon after the brain illness. Recovered symptoms may reemerge with infection or with other stressors. For example, someone who had recovered from left neglect may again neglect the left side when he gets the flu.

### *Related and Associated Symptoms*

All the various symptoms of brain illness can be made worse by fatigue. This includes not only impairments, but also new behaviors such as disinhibition, frustration, perseveration, confabulation, and irritability.

### *Similar Nonneurological Conditions*

Fatigue with brain illness is similar to fatigue without brain illness except that it is more severe and more rapid.

### *Neuroanatomy*

Brain injury anywhere can result in increased fatigue. It may be especially prominent with lesions involving the arousal system (the reticular activating system).

### *How to Observe/Test*

The person with the brain illness should be observed during extended effort. It should be noted whether or not performance deteriorates over time. One way to test fatigue is to give a sensitive, repeatable test such as an attention test early in the morning and then repeat the test late in the afternoon. Subjective fatigue scales and objective measures are beginning to be developed (LaChapelle & Finlayson, 1998).

### *Practical Problems*

When fatigue goes unrecognized, the injured person can appear less reliable and competent than he is. The person with fatigue can accomplish less in a day, and he may not be able to do jobs where breaks are not possible. It can sometimes be hard to persuade people or to demonstrate to them that breaks are important or to get them to rest during breaks. They may sometimes believe that, because they are less efficient, they should try harder and skip breaks, to make up for it, but this may only make their inefficiency worse (Case 12.1. Lu Tan).

### *Interventions*

1. Adequate rest should be scheduled into the person's day, such as an afternoon nap and extra sleep at night.
2. The person should be well rested for important business.
3. Return to work should be gradual, beginning with just a few hours a day in the morning and gradually increasing the hours.
4. The person and the family should be educated about the pattern of fatigue. It can be demonstrated if necessary.
5. For people who show fatigue of specific functions, they and their families can be trained to recognize the fatigue and to switch activities. For example, when the speech of the person with aphasia begins to deteriorate, he might switch to a nonverbal activity such as cleaning house, cooking, gardening, and so forth.
6. The person with the brain illness or his family should be trained to recognize the earliest signs of fatigue as a signal for rest. Alternately, the therapist can figure out how long it takes for fatigue to set in and can plan breaks for shorter intervals. Therapists can experiment to discover how long a rest is needed to restore functioning. For some people, especially those at both extremes of motivation, it is necessary to emphasize that rest is not an excuse to be lazy. The person needs to be persistent and to keep coming back to what he is working on, but he also needs to take breaks to stay efficient. High achievers need to be told that old habits of pushing themselves to work will probably push them into frustration and confusion instead of into achievement.
7. Although it may be useful to push the person to perform longer, more rapidly, and more efficiently in therapy, it is not useful to push him to perform in a work setting unless errors can be easily corrected. Thus, pacing for recovery is distinct from pacing for efficiency.
8. A program of gradually increasing daily physical exercise can help reduce the mental fatigue that accompanies brain illness.

## *HYPERAESTHESIA*

### *Description*

Brain illnesses can make some people intolerant to sensory stimulation (hyperaesthesia), which may affect all sensory modalities or some more than others.

There may or may not be an increased startle reaction. The reaction may be worse when the stimulation is unexpected (startling to the first but not the second ring of the telephone) or when it is beyond their own control (tolerating the noise of one's own hammering but not of someone else's or tolerating the vestibular stimulation of driving but not of riding in a car). Hyperaesthesia is common in mild TBIs (Bohnen, Twijnstra, Kroeze, & Jolles, 1991) and in later stages of Alzheimer's disease (Fisher, Murray, & Bundy, 1991), and may be present in other neurological conditions as well.

### *Related and Associated Symptoms*

Hyperaesthesia contributes to distractability and may be described in that way. It may be responsible for social withdrawal. It may produce irritability. Vestibular disorders can produce selective intolerance of movement. Pain can produce intolerance of specific types and locations of physical stimulation.

### *Similar Nonneurological Conditions*

Exaggerated startle is present in PTSD, in drug and alcohol withdrawal, and in some forms of schizophrenia (Howard & Ford, 1992).

### *Neuroanatomy*

The lower pontine reticular formation appears to be responsible for the startle reflex (Vidailhet, Rothwell, Thompson, Lees, & Marsden, 1992). The lesions responsible for hyperaesthesia are uncertain.

### *How to Observe/Test*

Interviewers should inquire about sensitivity to noise, to light, and to movement. Reports of distractability, irritability, anxiety, and withdrawal should be explored for a possible hyperaesthesia basis. The person's reaction to unexpected noises, bright lights, and busy environments can be observed.

### *Practical Problems*

Distractability, irritability, anxiety, and social withdrawal, even to the point of agoraphobia, are risks of hyperaesthesia. The individual may have difficulty coping with busy, fast environments and may overstimulate easily.

*Interventions*

1. Clear identification of the problem and of its specifics in the given individual (sensory modalities affected, severity, degree of startle, importance of prediction and control of the stimulation) is important for accurate education that can help the person and the family to understand and to manage the problem. For example, rather than avoiding places with bright lights, sunglasses might be used.
2. Many of the cognitive compensations for attention described earlier in this chapter apply to hyperaesthesia.
3. Benzodiazepines have been suggested for the treatment of exaggerated startle (Nigro & Lim, 1992). Animal studies suggest that tricyclic antidepressants may be helpful, whereas serotonin agonists and amphetamines may make matters worse (Kokkinidis & McCarter, 1990).

# IV

# The Social Dimension

Neurorehabilitation has descended from an acute medical care model in which a passive, dependent patient's impairments are evaluated and "fixed" by a physician-directed team. That model has been refined and reformed, in part through a consumer movement seeking more control for the customer, who may be the government, the insurance company, the employer, the referring physician, the person with the brain illness, or the family. These different customers have different agendas.

Rehabilitation, whether of a medical, a consumer, or another model, does not, cannot, and should not deal with the entire life journey of the person who is living with the effects of a brain illness. This book is about interventions for problems and properly stops where interventions end. However, the point of intervention is not simply to eliminate problems but to facilitate the person's getting on with life, however possible, including reintegrating into the community. It is society's choice and responsibility to provide appropriate spaces for all of its members with opportunities for personal fulfillment. The rehabilitation establishment cannot itself provide many of those spaces for people with brain illnesses or force people into them, but it can and should advocate for opening up such spaces in the community through education, role modeling, facilitating disabilities rights groups, legal advocacy, and direct action. Part IV addresses preparing such places and dealing with problem emotions and behaviors of brain illness in a social context.

Even getting on with life, returning to old roles in the family and community, and/or finding new ones is not the entire journey. It is not enough to put the illness behind oneself as if it never happened. The person who experienced it and her family need to find meaning in the experience. It can be a hellish experience; it is not surprising to find some direction in making sense of it from someone who has been through hell on earth. Victor Frankl (1963, as cited in Sachs, 1985) developed an existential psychotherapy based on his experiences in World War II concentration camps. He proposes that people find meaning in life through what they give to the world (creations, service, love), what they take from the world (experiences, encounters, love), and how they face adversity. Instead of simply putting the experience behind ("I had pain and loss. I had problems and dealt with them. I lost a year, but I want to forget about that and go on."), people need to make sense of it and integrate it into their life stories ("A terrible thing happened, as can happen to anyone. I faced it with all the strength I could. I found strengths and weaknesses I did not know I had. I found people who understood and helped me, others who fell by the wayside, and others I have been able to help. I have grown from this experience. I am using that knowledge to make the world a better place. This experience is now part of who I am.").

In an alternate view, Prigatano (1991) noted that life goals based on values of personal intelligence, beauty, and winning (potent in U.S. culture) are likely to be unfruitful and frustrating for the person with a significant brain injury. He pessimistically suggested that psychotherapy can do little to help people with these goals. (Others may be more optimistic that psychotherapy can help people reassess and shift values.) Prigatano suggested, instead, that work, love, and play are values within the grasp of many people with brain injuries.

The intervenor, especially the professional clinician, may not be able to go this entire journey with the person dealing with a brain illness. Psychotherapy to help someone find meaning in their illness may not be justifiable to an insurance company or to a clinical director as reducing symptomatology, disability, or as resource utilization. However, the intervenor can prepare the traveler for the journey and point the way.

# 13

# The Family

### *EFFECTS OF BRAIN ILLNESSES ON THE FAMILY*

Brain illnesses cause tremendous, long-lasting, and usually increasing burdens on families (Kay & Cavallo, 1994; Livingston & Brooks, 1988; Vitaliano et al., 1989). Burden is most closely related to personality and behavior changes in the person with the brain injury, secondarily related to cognitive changes, and least related to physical changes. Burden depends on an interaction between pre-illness personality, the type of personality change present, and the personalities, roles, and resources of specific family members (Brooks, 1991; Livingston & Brooks; Mintz, Van Horn, & Levine, 1995). A primitive but useful model of these relationships (Vitaliano et al., 1989) is the following:

$$\text{Distress} = \frac{\text{Exposure to stressors} + \text{Vulnerability}}{\text{Psychological resources} + \text{Social resources}}$$

In this equation stressors would include behavioral and other changes in the person with the brain illness. The major strains experienced by families include emotional distress, especially depression and anxiety; illness and psychosomatic disorders; interpersonal conflicts; financial stresses; and role changes.

Most research has focused on problems that arise after a brain illness, typically using populations of convenience that have been obtained from clinical settings or support groups. This may select for families with more problems and/or for those more likely to seek help. Very little research has been done to identify how families cope successfully with brain illnesses (Ridley, 1989), although Leaf (1993) reported that faith, family and friends, and clinical services, in that order, were the resources identified as most important by families in head injury support groups in the Midwest United States. Sachs (1985) has even suggested that head injury can be a growth experience for families.

### *Time Course of Illness*

Major implications of the time course of brain illness for interventions with the person are given in Chapter 2.

#### *Sudden Onset of Brain Illness, Gradual Recuperation*

*Grief.* Earlier models of stages of grief (Kubler-Ross, 1969; Lezak, 1986) have been replaced by a cyclical model that recognizes that reactions (Table 13.1) will recur and mix rather than occur sequentially (Kasowski, 1994; Kay & Cavallo, 1994; Rape, Busch, & Slavin, 1992). A brain illness with sudden onset, unlike a death, often has an uncertain prognosis that unfolds over a period of years. Because losses need not be mourned until they are certain, because many deficits and their life consequences only gradually become apparent, because recovery has frequent ups and downs, and because different family members experience the changes differently, the reactions of grieving are very variable. Rosenthal and Muir (1983) called this "mobile mourning." Family burden following a TBI increases over time (Kay & Cavallo, 1994; Livingston & Brooks, 1988). The passing of life's milestones can renew grief or "chronic sorrow" (Olshansky, 1966). For example, as classmates graduate, marry, and have children, the parents of a brain-injured child who does not do these things may grieve anew. Wedding anniversaries may become bittersweet for the spouse of an injured partner.

*Roles.* Many family roles change suddenly with the onset of an acute brain illness. Most of the roles of the person with the brain illness are lost, and many must be filled by other family members. Many of these will gradually revert to the injured member as recovery progresses. New roles of managing medical care and of caregiving may need to be filled.

Particularly difficult role losses to cope with are those of authority, competence, and peacekeeper, especially when there is no one to take them over. There may be family turmoil as members scramble to claim or to avoid available roles. As support from rehabilitation services and from extended family and friends fades away, and possibly as core family members flee the situation, remaining

**TABLE 13.1. Family Grief Reactions to Acute Brain Illness**

| |
|---|
| Shock, numbness, confusion, anxiety |
| Relief, denial, unrealistic expectations, hope |
| Acknowledgment of permanent deficits and emotional turmoil |
| Bargaining |
| Anger, bitterness |
| Mourning, depression, feeling trapped, guilt, working through |
| Acceptance, adjustment, emotional disengagement |

family members may become burdened with still more roles. As the injured member recovers, others may be hesitant to give up newly gained roles, causing additional stresses.

In addition, as recovery plateaus and the family tries to reestablish equilibrium, new roles may have to be sought for the person with the illness (Hallett, Zasler, Maurer, & Cash, 1994). How is she going to spend her time? What will she contribute to the family? For what can she be expected to be responsible?

*The New Family.* It is not only the person with the brain illness who must ultimately construct a new self-image (Chapter 6, "The New Person"), but also the family. Each at their own pace, family members gradually arrive at a new image of their family member and of where they each fit in the family (Figures 13.1, 13.2). A situation initially seen as temporary becomes more or less permanent. Family members try to salvage postponed dreams and to adjust the balance between their own needs and those of the family, especially those of the injured member. Social isolation often affects the entire family. The family readjusts not only its internal dynamics but also its relationships with the outside world. Friends, acquaintances, and activities are dropped; new spheres of social contact of rehabilitation, support groups, sheltered activities, and perhaps lawyers are added. The issue of what to tell others about the illness and about its consequences becomes important for the entire family.

Serio, Kreutzer, and Witol (1997), using the Family Needs Questionnaire, identified the needs of family members after a severe TBI in the family as health information, emotional support, instrumental support, professional support, the support network, and involvement with care.

Sachs (1985) suggested that help for families can go beyond support to allowing family members to salvage meaning from the experience. For example, families may cherish the way they have faced adversity, help other families through

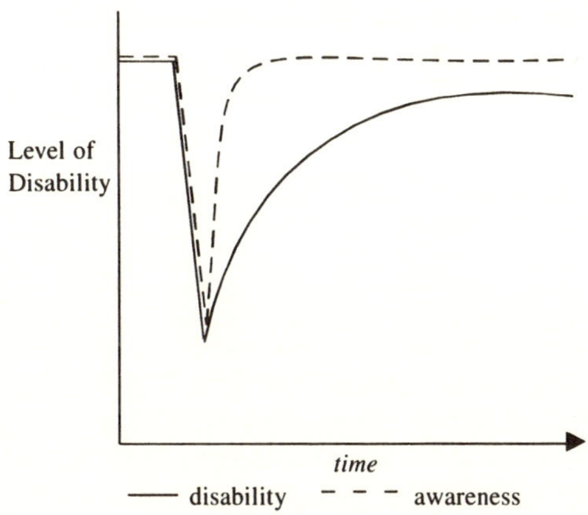


FIGURE 13.1. Typical family awareness of disability, sudden onset. Compare to Figures 7.2 (p. 108) and 7.4 (p. 111).

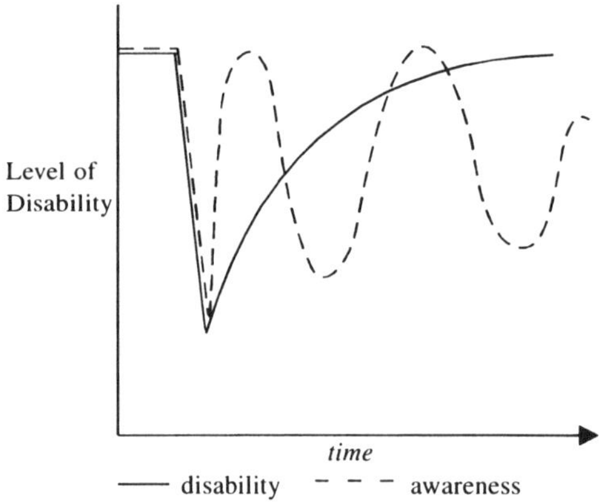


FIGURE 13.2. Family awareness of disability, sudden onset, less stable family member and/or mixed signs or messages. Compare to Figures 7.2 (p. 108) and 7.4 (p. 111).

the experience via support groups, or get involved in brain injury prevention work, in legal reform, or in another social service related to the experience.

*Feelings toward the Person with the Illness.* Blame, guilt, resentment, pity, embarrassment, love, rejection, anger, and sympathy are all common feelings toward the person with the illness. These personal feelings can be complicated by personality, emotional, and behavioral changes in the person with the illness and by how those changes are understood. To know how to feel, the family member may need to know how much to regard the person's behavior as intentional and how much to see it as an organic consequence of the illness.

It is common and appropriate in the early phases of recovery to protect the person with the illness from negative feelings. Later, however, as the person recovers, it can be difficult for some family members to realize that they can again express feelings toward her. "I really couldn't trust that I had my wife back again until I could get mad at her when I needed to." How best to express those feelings will depend on the family's history of emotional communication, the emotions to be expressed, and the condition of the person with the illness. Someone with increased emotional reactivity may need to be shielded. Someone with reduced emotional reactivity, impaired emotional comprehension, or impaired empathy may do better if emotions are frequently and directly expressed and are even exaggerated.

### *Progressive Onset of Brain Illness*

*Grief.* The family's grief for the person with a progressive brain illness is usually less dramatic than with sudden onset illness, but it is no less painful. Denial is common at the outset, because progressive conditions usually begin in barely noticeable ways—a slight tremor here, a lost word there. Different family mem-

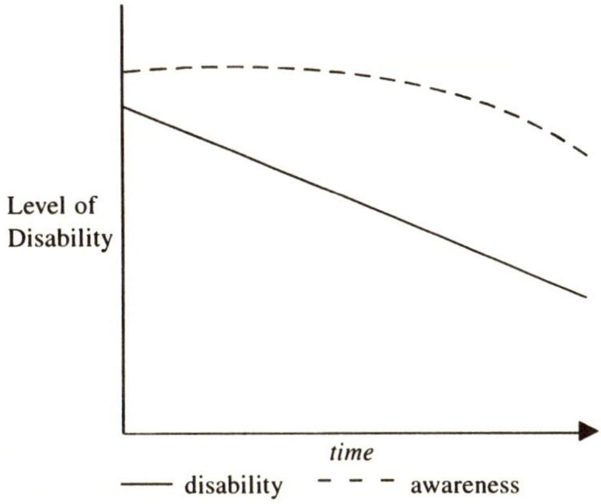


FIGURE 13.3. Typical family awareness of disability, progressive onset. Compare to Figures 7.3 (p. 109) and 7.5 (p. 113).

bers rarely conclude at the same time that something is wrong (Figures 13.3 and 13.4), and so some struggle over this is common. There may be shock, anger, anxiety, and so forth at the time of the diagnosis, but grief comes in recurrent waves. Life's milestones and the appearance of new symptoms are markers. Specific losses are rarely very dramatic, because there is usually enough variability in the person's abilities to hope that the activity can continue a little longer. A spouse is unlikely to realize, for example, "That was the last time we will make love," because there could always be another lucid time next week. Only when that lucid time does not come for months will the loss finally be acknowledged.

*Roles.* Roles change gradually with progressive illness. The clinician or another concerned person can help the person and the family look forward a few months and prepare for coming changes. If, for instance, the caregiving spouse has never

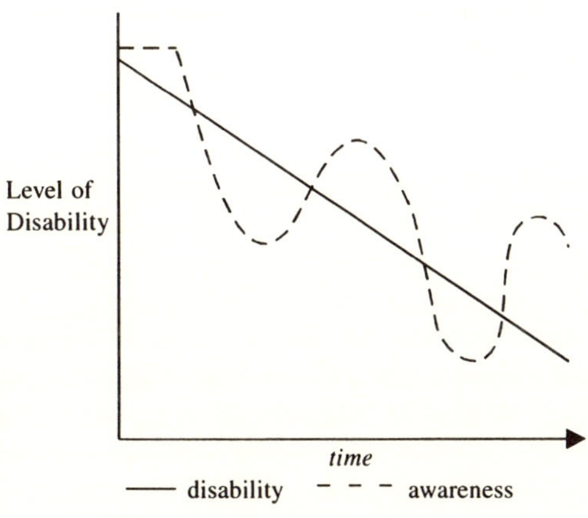


FIGURE 13.4. Family awareness of disability, progressive onset, less stable family member and/or mixed signs or messages. Compare to Figures 7.3 (p. 109) and 7.5 (p. 113).

managed finances, driven a car, or called cousin Jim, it is better to learn these skills before the person with Alzheimer's disease is no longer able. If these transitions are difficult for the person with the illness, it may help to agree on criteria in advance or to find ways for her to save face and to give up roles gradually.

With reduced abilities, new roles and pastimes need to be found. Finding ways to maintain meaningful contact with family members and to contribute to the family is a creative challenge (Table 13.2; Sheridan, 1987; Zgola, 1987). This is often aided by support groups and adult day care centers (Dowling, 1995; Jones, 1996; Mace & Rabins, 1991; Reisberg, 1983).

*The Changing Family.* The family of someone with a progressive brain illness is also in a state of transition. With a time course of 5 to 20 years, such as with Alzheimer's disease, Parkinson's disease, multi-infarct dementia, Huntington's disease, less malignant brain tumors, and some multiple sclerosis, this transition may be no more radical than that which comes with children growing up. The family may come to accept caregiving as part of the family routine. The attitude may be one of "Life will be like this for a while. We will learn to live with it, to keep our own friendships going and our interests alive, and to function as a family in this state." The intervenor can help the family to arrive at this attitude, and to anticipate and to choose those adjustments that make such a steady state possible.

If the disease is more rapid, from a few months to a few years, such as with Jacob-Creutzfeldt disease, rapid multiple sclerosis, and more malignant brain tumors, then more frequent disruptions, crises, shocks, and losses can be expected. Once the diagnosis and prognosis are accepted, the family may think of the illness as a crisis and of caregiving as a temporary disruption. The attitude in this case is more one of "We can let everything go while we deal with this, because it is only temporary. Once it is over we will pick up where we left off, adjust, and go on from there." This attitude may be adequate if the time course is truly short, but if the process drags on, such a family may wind up in a more chronic state of crisis and have little left to pick up when it is over. The intervenor can watch for signs of strain and burnout in the family and can try to prevent such a disaster.

Regardless of the velocity of the illness, a major role for intervenors is to help the family to keep looking ahead so they do not simply wait to react to a series of crises. At some point the person's death will be contemplated. Some people fear thinking about this because they do not want to face the pain or because they believe that in thinking about it, they will wish for it and thereby hasten it or will become impatient for it. Others may face it easily and wish for it openly. Some advance thinking and feeling is advisable for almost everyone, both in preparing to deal with the death and to go on with life afterward. There are almost always important aspects that cannot be anticipated, but some advance thinking may help prevent a crisis.

**TABLE 13.2. Possible Activities for the Person in the Second Stage of Alzheimer's Disease[a]**

- Listening to and singing along with music
- Playing rhythm instruments
- Gardening
- Playing with and caring for children
- Working as an assisted volunteer (childcare center, animal shelter, soup kitchen, nursing home)
- Walking
- Looking at magazines, picture books, and photo albums
- Watching TV and movies with slow action and uncomplicated plots
- Doing simple chores or parts of chores
  - Folding laundry
  - Setting the table
  - Washing dishes
  - Preparing food
  - Dusting
  - Sweeping
  - Vacuuming
- Reminiscing
- Attending religious services
- People watching
- Watching boats
- Visiting the zoo
- Visiting museums
- Visits with friends
- Recording family stories (with help)
- Playing simple board and card games
- Sanding wood and painting
- Using a child's workbench
- Using watercolors
- Getting a massage
- Playing slow moving sports
  - Bowling
  - Shuffleboard
  - Swimming
  - Dancing
  - Darts
  - Catch with a bean bag or balloon
  - Pool
- Appreciating sunsets, flowers, smells, tastes, textures
- Engaging in any overlearned skill or hobby
- Animal care

[a] 2–10 years, severe memory impairment, impoverished but intelligible language, indifferent, apathetic, poor constructions and calculations

*Feelings toward the Person with the Illness.* With the diagnosis of a progressive brain illness, some family members rethink their feelings toward that person over the past few years, when behaviors thought to be intentional may have been due to the illness. Some family members may need to be directed to make such re-evaluations to find some peace and to adapt to the new realities. Many will need help (re)interpreting current and new behaviors. The caregiving role can provoke strong feelings that may change with the stage of the disease and that are often best shared in support groups.

Many family members want to deal with unfinished business in their relationship with the person. Adult children of someone with Alzheimer's disease, for example, may feel that they have never expressed their love, gratitude, apologies, resentment, or anger in the way in which they would have liked. They may have questions about their past or secrets that they need to share. An outside observer can help clarify those feelings, clarify what would bring satisfaction in dealing with those feelings, figure out if the person with the illness can participate in such a process and what its impact might be, and figure out how that might best be carried out given the person's illness.

### *Illnesses of Intermittent Time Course*

*Grief and Other Reactions.* With conditions with intermittent time course, grief is generally not a major family issue except around the time of diagnosis or if the condition is also progressive (such as multiple sclerosis). A family picnic spoiled by a migraine or by a seizure, for example, is not a major loss if there is hope that it can be done another time. For a few families, grief may be important; for example, in cultures strongly prejudiced against epilepsy.

*Roles.* Intermittent conditions may result in intermittent role dysfunction, leading to disruption and uncertainty for the entire family. The uncertainty sometimes makes the entire family revolve around the illness and around efforts to prevent or to conceal episodes.

*Feelings toward the Person with the Illness.* Families may believe that the person has control over the episodes and uses them to manipulate or does not try hard enough to control them. Alternately, they may believe that things they do trigger episodes. Feelings of blame, shame, resentment, and guilt may result. The truth of these beliefs needs to be carefully investigated and the results must be communicated sensitively.

Shame and fear of discrimination may result in the condition becoming a family secret (Woodward, 1993). Overprotection, family isolation, and abandonment by some members can result. This type of adjustment needs to be carefully considered within its context (see Case 7.12, p. 135, Raj). In parts of Africa, for instance, epilepsy is very commonly a family secret, often with justification because of prevalent discrimination and myths (Devlieger, Piachaud, Leung, & George, 1994).

### *Common Family Roles*

Regardless of specific kin relationships, one effect of brain illness is common to almost all family systems. The members feel that they are giving much more to the family and to the person with the illness and that they are getting much less out of the family, especially attention from other members, than before the illness. There may be intensified competition among some family members for the attention of others. What really usually happens is that everyone gives more to the person with the illness and has less to give to others, while the person with the illness takes most of the attention and gives little back.

#### *Spouses and Partners*

The spouse or the partner of the person with the brain illness, whether married or not, straight or gay (all hereafter referred to as "spouse"), is probably the family member who bears the greatest burden (Kay & Cavallo, 1994; Lezak, 1988). With a significant impairment, the spouse at once loses a partner to share life's burdens and gains a tremendous and usually unfamiliar, unexpected, and unfair burden of caregiving. If the illness has changed the person from loving and supportive to indifferent, aggressive, demanding, or resentful, the spouse may find he is married to someone whom he no longer loves or is attracted to. Particularly in younger couples, this creates a pull towards divorce once the situation is clearly stable or deteriorating. An opposite pull may come from guilt, from caregiving obligations, and from pressures from friends and from extended family, especially in-laws.

With someone who is severely disabled, the spouse may be in a social limbo of being nonmarried (Zeigler, 1987). He effectively does not have a wife to share life's joys and woes, but he is not single and free to seek another partner. As a "married widower," grief for the loss of the person he married may not be socially sanctioned or may be repressed. Well-meaning friends may make unhelpful remarks such as "At least you still have your wife." He may be uncomfortable going out socially with his wife, alone, or with someone else and so stays home. Similarly, friends may not want to invite his wife but feel that it would be impolite to exclude her and so they invite neither. He may be tempted to seek solace in another relationship while still a caregiver, risking secrecy, guilt, and jealousy.

Many spouses must quit their jobs to become caregivers. There usually are extra financial strains, household responsibilities, and resources needed in dealing with rehabilitation. Often spouses must care for the extra emotional needs of children who are learning to cope with the effective loss of one parent. If the injured person has become self-centered, there may be overt competition with the children for the spouse's attention. A common reaction is "My wife and I used to have three children before the accident, but now I feel like I'm alone with four." Some spouses eventually adjust to a severely disabled partner through a detached caregiver role, no longer expecting or hoping for a true marital relationship (Lezak, 1988).

*Divorce.* The greatest strains from TBIs are felt by young spouses with small children and financial hardships (Moore, Stambrook & Peters, 1993), and divorce is common. Older spouses, more likely to have a partner with a stroke or with dementia, often accept caregiving in spite of substantial burden (Gallo, 1990).

The divorce decision is emotionally and practically complex and may depend on accurate prognostic information. The therapist who feels divided loyalties or a strong investment in one decision or another may need to refer the spouse to someone else for help with the decision but may still need to supply prognostic information.

*Sexuality.* Sexual problems resulting from brain illness involve not only problems with intercourse but also with interpersonal relationships and with self-image. Primary problems are specific organic dysfunctions, such as hormone disorders resulting from hypothalamic or anterior pituitary damage or from other causes (Zasler, 1988); sensory, motor, and movement disorders; medication effects; and effects of substance abuse. In theory, apraxia can affect sexual skills, as well, but this has been studied little to date. Presumably, the approach described under Sexual Rehabilitation as follows would be worth trying.

Secondary problems are psychosocial sexual dysfunctions. These include most pre-illness sexual dysfunctions, neuropsychological effects of the illness, and effects of social circumstances (Table 13.3). Many are not specifically sexual problems and can be addressed through education and through counseling or through other interventions not requiring specialized sex therapy. Most do require a knowledge of brain illnesses and of their general effects, however. The PLISSIT model for levels of intervention for sexual problems (Table 13.4) can help in choosing an appropriate level of evaluation and of intervention according to staff skills available and the needs and commitment of the person with the brain illness. Sexual ignorance and misinformation are so widespread that basic sex education is fundamental to any significant intervention for sexual problems.

Assessment for sexual problems must be flexible to suit the circumstances. Many people will not volunteer that a sexual problem is present. Inquiry about sexual functioning is routine in any thorough rehabilitation or mental health evaluation. Even with less comprehensive services, sexuality should be included in education about the illness. However, because sexuality is so private, full collaboration with a probing evaluation is not a prerequisite for intervention. A de-

**TABLE 13.3. Secondary (Psychosocial) Causes of Sexual Dysfunction after TBI[a]**

| |
|---|
| Substance abuse |
| Absent or unwilling partner |
| Pre-illness relationship or sexual difficulty |
| Economics, transportation, housing |
| Limited definition of sexuality |
| Lack of information |
| History of sexual abuse |
| Unresolved sexual orientation |
| Impaired self-awareness |
| Impaired social skills |
| Sexual disinhibition or perseveration |
| Lack of initiation |
| Impaired empathy |
| Changes in emotional reactions or in communication |
| Aphasia |
| Apraxia |
| Fatigue |
| Headache |
| Depression |
| Anxiety |
| Guilt |
| Anger |
| Lowered self-esteem |

[a]From "Sexuality and Sexual Dysfunction," by E. R. Griffith, S. Cole, and T. M. Cole, in *Rehabilitation of the Adult and Child with Traumatic Brain Injury, Edition 2* (pp. 206–224), edited by M. Rosenthal, E. R. Griffity, J. R. Bond, and J. D. Miller, 1990, Philadelphia: F. A. Davis. Copyright 1990 by F. A. Davis Publishding Co.; and from Lefebvre (1988). Adapted with permission.

tailed inquisition is not necessary to offer general sex education, social skills and dating skills training, or counseling for values clarification, for example. If a problem explicitly concerns sexual activity, or if an intervention is to be at the Specific Suggestion or Intensive Therapy level of the PLISSIT Model, an in-depth evaluation is necessitated. Suspected primary dysfunctions should be evaluated by a physician. Secondary causes can be evaluated through the Sexual Assessment Planning model (Table 13.5). In addition to information from a general psychological or a rehabilitation assessment, this evaluation includes a sexual history of partners, practices, and problems, which presumably also gets at beliefs and values. When histories of sexual abuse or substance abuse (Lefebvre, 1988, 1990) are ruled our or dealt with, the nature of the present difficulty is explored with each partner separately and as a couple, or with just one partner, if necessary. For whom is it a problem? What is an acceptable outcome for each? How are feelings about the relationship overall? What are the sexual education needs?

Lefebvre (1988, 1990) also presented the following useful guidelines for less experienced practitioners:

**TABLE 13.4. The PLISSIT Model of Levels of Intervention for Sexual Problems[a]**

| Level | | Intervention | Training needed |
|---|---|---|---|
| P | Permission Giving | Communicate willingness to discuss private, intimate matters | Most professionals, some nonprofessionals |
| LI | Limited Information | Sex education, brain illness education | Most professionals, some nonprofessionals |
| SS | Specific Suggestion | Individualized counseling | Counseling and diagnostic skills |
| IT | Intensive Therapy | Directed intervention to change the situation | Specialized training |

[a] From "Sexuality and Dysfunction," by E. R. Griffith, S. Cole, and T. M. Cole, in *Rehabilitation of the Adult and Child with Traumatic Brain Injury, Edition 2* (pp. 206–224), edited by M. Rosenthal, E. R. Griffity, J. R. Bond, and J. D. Miller, 1990 Philadelphia: F. A. Davis. Copyright 1990 by F. A. Davis Publishing Co. Reprinted with permission.

**TABLE 13.5. Sexual Assessment Planning: Areas to Be Assessed[a]**

Practioner's Role
- Values of the practitioner and of the person with brain illness (and partner, if relevant)
- Responsibilities of the practitioner and of the person with brain illness (and partner, if relevant)
- Areas of conflict and their resolution

Cognition
- Educational and intellectual levels
- Cognitive deficits
- Competence

Motivation
- What does the person want from a (the) relationship?
- What does the person feel she has to offer another?
- How broad are the motivational factors in the relationship?

Interpersonal History
- Family background and support system
- Physical and sexual abuse
- Number and quality of previous relationships
- Violence, substance abuse, criminal behavior

Sex History
- Partners
- Practices
- Problems
- Previous treatment
- Reason for consultation

Social History
- Current organized use of time
- The person's perspective on how the world treats her
- Circumstances of the illness
- The person's control over her own life
- Living situation
- Transportation

Vocational History
- Work history before and after illness
- Financial status

[a] From Lefebvre (1988); and from "Sexual Assessment Planning," by K. A. Lefebvre, 1990, *Journal of Head Trauma Rehabilitation, 5*(2), 30. Copyright 1990 by Aspen Publishers. Adapted with permission.

1. People rarely tell you the truth the first time.
2. Not all patients are nice people.
3. Not all patients are like you.
4. It is not up to you to fix every problem.
5. Except for masturbation and fantasy, most sexual behavior occurs in a social context.
6. Most sexual problems are less related to sex than to other problems.

Effective sexuality counseling requires that counselors are well educated about sexuality, comfortable talking about it, well aware of their own values and issues, and able to deal nonjudgmentally with a variety of people and practices.

This section discusses sexuality and brain illness in established couples. Other aspects are discussed in Chapter 14 (pp. 304–309).

*Hypersexuality.* Some people become sexually disinhibited with brain illness. Mild disinhibition may result in more frequent and persistent interest in sex with their partner. In some relationships this is an improvement; in some it is a problem. Strategies for coping with problematic interest include reframing the spouse's perception of the behavior and their attitude toward it, negotiating, setting aside special times, setting firm limits, ignoring it, distraction, redirection, training the person in self-control, substituting acceptable behavior, avoiding circumstances that trigger the behavior, and maintaining a written log of sexual relations. With greater disinhibition, sexual behavior may be directed outside the couple. The spouse may be jealous or embarrassed. Jealousy (or mock jealousy) can be used as a motivator to reduce the behavior (see Chapter 14).

*Hyposexuality.* A more common effect of brain illness is a loss of sexual interest. For some spouses this is an improvement or a relief. Others grieve the loss but are also grateful because they are no longer interested in sex with their altered partner. Often hyposexuality is a frustration for the spouse.

The partner may attempt sex but get distracted. Eliminating bedroom distractions, retraining attention, and/or using amphetamines to improve attention may help. The spouse may experiment with what activities and stimuli help maintain attention. Impaired initiation may reduce sexual activity in an individual who is interested and capable, especially if the spouse does not usually initiate sex. The most practical solution may be for the spouse to learn to initiate. The person with reduced emotional responsiveness may show less interest in sex. One strategy is to maximize what is or has been sexually exciting for that person.

Reduced libido is also a symptom of depression. If this is the case, treatment for depression may eliminate the problem.

*Unattractiveness.* Spouses may find their partner with a brain illness newly unattractive for a variety of reasons. The partner may lack empathy and may be insensitive to the spouse's feelings and needs. In this case, sex may be used quite directly as a motivator in training empathy (see Chapter 11, "Concreteness," p. 230), possibly including classic sexual therapy techniques and exercises such as pleasuring (Masters & Johnson, 1970). This must be done with care, so the spouse does not feel obligated to comply with unwanted sex just because some exercises have been completed or because therapeutic criteria have been achieved. For this reason, it is often better for a therapist to present this motivation than for a spouse. For instance, a therapist might say,

> So you tell me that your problem is that Enrique isn't interested in sex with you now. Why do you suppose that might be? Do you think you might ask him? . . . You did? What did he say? . . . That sounds like what we called 'Lack of empathy' here on your strengths and problems list. So perhaps if we worked on that, eventually he might become interested again, don't you think? Let's look again at the strategies we have for that.

Both increases and decreases in emotional responsiveness or communication may be unattractive or frightening to some spouses. Educating the spouse along with practice and experience in new ways of communicating may reduce this. For instance, it may take desensitizing to reflex crying for a spouse to accept crying during sex. It may take accommodation for a spouse to accept that a partner is still interested in sex but is not enthused.

Physically changed appearance, hemiplegia, movement disorders, loss of sensation, drooling, incontinence, and so forth may be a "turn-off" for some spouses. These reactions may yield to accommodation and desensitization, aided by exploring feelings and values in each partner and helping them to reframe reactions.

Aphasia or other communication impairments may lead to misunderstanding or to detachment. Improving communication and exploring feelings may help to overcome this barrier. Others find sex more satisfying because it helps compensate for impaired verbal communication, as the song in Case 12.5 (Frank, p. 255).

The person with the brain illness may feel unattractive, embarrassed, or low in self-esteem and, therefore, uninterested in sex. There may be fear of failure or performance anxiety. Individual and couples work may help to clarify what is important and to arrive at a new understanding.

*Sexual rehabilitation.* Sexual activities are not simply reflexes or instincts. They are skills that may be impaired by brain illness. Regaining them requires practice, repetition, and patience, as with other skills. Unlike some other skills, they generally also require a willing partner and good communication. It can help to predict failure early in rehabilitation as follows:

> With this injury there have been many things you have not been able to do well at first, but with practice you have learned to do them. Making love (use the person's preferred term) may be like that, too. For most people, it doesn't go well the first few times they try after an injury like yours. That's OK. Don't give up and don't be discouraged. It will take practice, like any other skill, to get it back. You won't mind practicing, will you?

If the prediction is wrong and it goes well, nothing is lost. The couple can think smugly, "We sure showed up those doctors." If the prediction is right, there will be less anxiety about it and the door is open to further discussion.

It is frequently necessary to begin with improving communication about sex and with exploring feelings about the illness. It can then be suggested to couples that they take it slowly, beginning with caresses, hugs, kisses, massage, and so forth, discovering what they now like, how those things make them feel, and what is now possible. This lets them explore changes in physical sensation and in motor abilities and their feelings about them. It gives direction for rehabilitation of those skills. Where rejection, reduced feelings of attraction, or even repulsion are present, this may permit desensitization or solutions to the problem. Finally, starting slowly in this way takes the focus off of sexual intercourse and leaves open the possibility of finding alternate sexual expressions, if needed. Working through a sexual problem can lead to deeper emotional intimacy because of the feelings communicated, even if the sex itself is reduced or is less "mechanically successful."

Detailed information concerning sexuality and specific disabilities is found in The American Heart Association of Wisconsin (1988), Comfort (1978), Griffith and Lemberg (1993), *Journal of Head Trauma Rehabilitation* (1990), Renshaw (1978), Schover (1986), the newsletter *Sexuality Update* by The National Task Force on Sexuality and Disability of the American Congress of Rehabilitation Medicine, and the journal *Sexuality and Disability*.

### *Parents*

Although being a family member caregiver for someone with a brain illness is hard on anyone, parents have an advantage over other kin relationships in that they already have an established caregiving role with their child. They experience somewhat less burden than spouses, for example (Kreutzer, Gervasio, & Camplair, 1994a, 1994b). Parents are frequently competent at advocating for and seeking out resources. Nevertheless, several problematic themes recur (Kay & Cavallo, 1994; Lezak, 1988). First are dashed hopes for the future of the child. Second is prolonging or returning to caregiving for parents who had looked forward to greater independence as their children reached maturity. This theme may be less dramatic in developing countries where multigenerational households are more common and parent-child relationships often remain close well into adulthood. For parents strongly identified with caregiving, the illness may present an excuse to continue the role longer than necessary, producing overprotection (see the following sections). Third, parents' marital relationship may be strained as they struggle over caregiving responsibilities and as they cope with emotions. Fourth, adolescent independence struggles may become intensified, prolonged, or relived, especially if the child has impaired judgment and has an impaired awareness of deficits.

### *Child and Siblings*

Children who have a parent or a sibling with a brain illness are often neglected in rehabilitation (Kay & Cavallo, 1994; Lezak, 1988). They are often confused about what is going on and why; and they may feel guilty, frightened, ashamed, and angry. Their social life may be disrupted because they cannot bring friends home. They may be thrust prematurely into caregiving. Many cope by learning to become numb (Spanbock, 1992). They are likely to resent the attention that the person with the illness takes away from them. Children may draw closer to the person with the illness, or they may withdraw, with different children in the same family sometimes taking opposite reactions. Adolescents may flee the family.

A parent with a brain illness who has lost some parenting capabilities may become abusive, or she may struggle to maintain an authority role or a position of competence of which she is not capable. Children may need to be protected from such a parent. In some cases, power struggles develop and children can take advantage of such a parent and can even ridicule her (Maitz & Sachs, 1995). Alternately the parent may become withdrawn and disinterested, leaving the child feeling unloved and perhaps guilty.

The major problems encountered in children of parents with a TBI are acting out, school problems, emotional difficulties, and relationship problems with the injured parent (Pessar, Coad, Linn, & Willer, 1993). Problems are more common in adolescents than in younger children and are more common when the injured parent is the father. Problems are related to the injured parent not fulfilling the parental role, showing negative behaviors (aggression, impatience), showing fewer positive behaviors, being depressed, and simply performing less as a parent.

Children need education about what is going on at a level they can understand. Their feelings need to be heard and to be addressed. Although this is often best done within the family, especially for younger children, clinicians can facilitate and guide family members who undertake this. The child's school should be notified so that teachers and school counselors can provide extra support and recognize and attend to problems that may arise. Adolescents may particularly benefit from having a knowledgeable confidant from outside the immediate family.

### *Adult Children*

Adult children of parents with brain illnesses are less studied than other relatives. Divided loyalties can occur between children, spouse, and parents. Moving the parent into the household may disrupt family dynamics, especially when there are significant parent-child or in-law conflicts. Intervening with the spouse of the adult child of the person with a brain illness may be the most effective way to stabilize a disrupted family (Kay & Cavallo, 1994). Caregiving conflicts may arise with the other parent. A reversal of childhood caregiving roles may be difficult for some. Adult children who were looking forward to independence as their own children matured may resent being tied down. On the other hand, many adult children derive satisfaction from being able to return caregiving to their own parents.

*Extended Family*

In rehabilitation settings of the developed world, the extended family is often on the outside looking in. They are not often directly involved in education or in rehabilitation and may be left to guess and to wonder at what is going on. Their criticisms and well-meaning suggestions become an added burden to the immediate family. When they do become actively involved, they can be a tremendous help and relief, offering respite care, a fresh perspective, energy, and different opportunities and resources. In the developing world, extended family is more often actively involved from the outset (see the Large Families section that follows).

Clinicians can facilitate extended family participation by asking the immediate family about their support network early in rehabilitation, by including the extended family in educational meetings, by giving literature to be passed on to others, by training the person with the brain illness and the family in what to say to others, and by encouraging support groups, family networking (Kay & Cavallo, 1994; Rogers & Kreutzer, 1984), and circles of support (Willer, Allen, Anthony, & Cowlan, 1993).

*Nontraditional Families*

Most research on the impact of brain illness on families appears to look at "traditional" nuclear families in a household of a heterosexual couple and their children or in one of an impaired elderly parent living with adult children. Other family constellations may require specific considerations.

*Gay Male Couples and Lesbian Couples.* Gay male couples and lesbian couples face a number of obstacles in addition to those of spouses, those of parents, and those of adult children (Mapou, 1990). If they are not fully "out of the closet" (public about the nature of their relationship), they may face choices of hiding or of abandoning the relationship to maintain secrecy or of not being able to play a fully supportive role in rehabilitation. If they are "out", they may face actual or feared prejudice from the rehabilitation system into which they have been sent (Case 13.1. Oscar). Whether out or not, they may face a loss of child custody or of access to their partner (depending on local laws and customs). Disapproving rela-

*Homophobia in Rehabilitation. Case 13.1. Oscar.* A professional, college-educated gay man in his 30s was admitted to a rehabilitation unit in the United States for a TBI. At the time of injury he had been living with his life partner, Jake, for several years in a stable, public, childless relationship in a large gay community. Jake had access to him denied during acute care because he was not regarded as immediate family. On rehabilitation Jake was identified as the primary caregiver for discharge to the home. Although Jake visited regularly and was an eager and competent student of caregiving techniques, some staff repeatedly questioned his commitment to caregiving. There was some difficulty making eye contact with him in family conference. He was not easily integrated into the unit's milieu of visiting families. One team member attempted to hold private prayer sessions with Oscar to convince him to change his sexual orientation. Sexually explicit get-well cards posted by Oscar's bed became the sensation of the staff. Visitors were scrutinized and were whispered about. The job of sexuality counseling was tossed about among team members like a hot potato. When Oscar and Jake showed doubts and inconsistencies common in families coping with severe and uncertain disability, these were often met with rolling eyes and implications of "What can you expect from *them*?" Fortunately, Oscar and Jake met all of this with humor and with appropriate assertiveness. Juggling of staff and reminders of professional ethics brought the situation under control. Discharge plans were successful.

tives, governments, or social service agencies may try to take advantage of the situation to destroy the relationship or to take over financial control. In working with such couples, clinicians need to be particularly sensitive to confidentiality and to the great damage that can be done by failing to guard it carefully, sensitive to their own values and the influence that these have on their work, and sensitive to avoiding stereotypes and unwarranted assumptions. Clinicians cannot assume that everyone with whom they work is heterosexual.

*Unmarried Heterosexual Couples.* Unmarried heterosexual couples face many of these same risks, but to a lesser degree, depending in large part on local values. Similar clinical cautions apply. Clinicians cannot assume that every couple with whom they work is formally married.

*Single Parents.* Single parents face all of the added strains of that often difficult role. Regardless of whether it is the parent or the child who is injured, the noncustodial parent may raise concerns of parental competence and/or responsibilities. If a single parent is injured, there is the problem of care for the children during recovery and the added risk of the loss of child custody (Case 13.2. Marilyn). Evaluating, mobilizing, and strengthening the support network of single parents is usually a clinical priority.

*Parenting. Case 13.2, Marilyn.* An attractive, struggling, single, working mother in her early 20s was hospitalized with a severe TBI. Her young daughter was left in the custody of her parents. Two different men came to the hospital to propose marriage to her within the same week in which she was barely emerging from posttraumatic amnesia. She rejected them both. Her judgment and her care of her daughter had apparently not been good prior to her injury, and she had continued struggles with her mother. Her injury further impaired her judgment, her attention and her memory, and she had very little awareness of her limitations. Marilyn's mother obtained legal custody of Marilyn's daughter. Marilyn was discharged to an apartment in her parents' basement where she sporadically cared for her daughter in between extended jaunts of socializing in the community. Her struggle with her mother continued. She periodically returned to the rehabilitation center to demand that she be proven competent to care for her daughter, getting abusive when the conclusion was not to her liking.

*Unrelated Roommates.* Brain illness tests the strength of virtually all relationships, including the one between unrelated friends sharing a home. Such roommates typically have more choices than do family members regarding how much responsibility they take. How long should parents of an adult child with a brain injury pay rent on a shared apartment with hopes that she will return there? How much can roommates be counted on to provide structure, limits, and help if needed? How long might that last? How long can a person with Alzheimer's disease continue to live with roommates (Case 13.3. Emma)? Such situations may need to be probed individually. Roommates may need to be educated carefully about the situation before they can make decisions, with particular care given regarding confidentiality.

*Large Families.* Although family size is not often addressed in the literature on this topic, in the author's experience large families often adapt relatively well to a brain illness in one member. There are more people to share the caregiving burden; it is less likely to fall as heavily on one or on a few people. They are often able to share the emotional burden and to get perceptions and feelings about the situation validated. The family often has diverse resources. One person may know how to build a wheelchair ramp, another may be good at paperwork, another may be patient and caring, another, may have a job available, and another may be good at talking with doctors. There is often a diversity of things that need doing that give the person a role and dignity. Someone with a mild dementia or a stroke who can no longer work for wages may still be able to care for children, cook for the household, feed chickens, teach someone to sew, or tell stories. The affinities

*An Unusual Housemate. Case 13.3. Emma.* During my student years I lived in a cooperative household with 11 adults between the ages of 20 and 43 and one 90 year old woman. Emma was a world traveler, an activist, and a local celebrity with no family. She would occasionally go off on speaking tours and on media interviews. Nevertheless, her repertoire of fascinating stories gradually became more restricted and repetitive. On her night to cook accidents and fires became increasingly frequent. She fiercely valued her independence and took pride in doing her share, and so we surreptitiously posted a guard when she cooked and filled in extra "work credits" for her on the chore chart. She was always present for house meetings, which made it difficult to talk about her. She became increasingly confused and incompetent. All of us had great affection for her, but none of us had the authority to do anything definitive. At length one household member sought help from a social worker friend who observed that the spirit of the house was gone, with Emma dominating the common space and everyone else feeling isolated, helpless, and worried. The social worker helped us contact Emma's friends who persuaded her to get a thorough medical evaluation and to move into assisted living from which she still ventured out to receive awards, give interviews, and attend ceremonies and demonstrations.

sometimes found among older people, young children, and people who are neurocognitively disabled are especially agreeable (Gronwall, Wrightson, & Waddell, 1990). They often have remarkable patience and tolerance and may get great satisfaction in helping each other. The challenge to the clinician may be to get to know all of these people, to make sure the right people get the right information, and to coordinate resources.

*Different Cultures.* Most research on brain illnesses and families comes from Europe, Israel, and North America. The findings suggest that effects vary considerably depending on characteristics of each family (Kay & Cavallo, 1994). Family structure and dynamics vary widely around the world, so considerable caution must be exercised in applying these results in other areas and cultures.

In working cross-culturally, neither the clinician nor the family may realize that they have different assumptions about family values. Even the alert clinician who asks about differences may not get the answers needed, because values and differences may be deeply ingrained and may not be accessible to introspection (Cavallo & Saucedo, 1995; Lynch & Hanson, 1992).

### *Overprotection*

An extremely common family problem in rehabilitation, especially in the developing world, is overprotection by families. In the rehabilitation unit of the

National Geriatric Hospital in Costa Rica, for example, the most common admission diagnosis is immobilization syndrome—the bedsores and contractures that typically result when a family does not allow a disabled member to leave the bed. A common related situation is a psychosocial immobilization syndrome—almost an atrophy of psychosocial skills resulting from confinement to the home.

Overprotection appears to have several sources, each best met with distinctive intervention strategies (Table 13.6):

1. An acute illness model, in which the person needs bedrest and assistance in most activities. Passive, medical-model rehabilitation reinforces this, so the person and the family all believe that this is what they should do.
2. The need of some family members (usually adult males) to exercise dominance and control over others (usually women and children, Galanti, 1991). When they are sick, they may order others to feed, bathe, and dress them, even when they are capable.
3. The need for family members to control the person they overprotect (Case 13.4. Tierno).

**TABLE 13.6. Sources of Overprotection and Clinical Strategies**

| General strategies |
|---|
| Evaluate carefully first and prioritize. |
| Educate all parties about recovery, prognosis, resources, and the active model of rehabilitation |
| Redirect fatalism; focus on small steps if necessary |
| Demonstrate the abilities of the person with the brain illness to the family (with videotape, one way mirror, etc. if their presence interferes with performance). |
| Model proper care for the family. |
| Train the family in proper care; observe them giving care and correct them. |
| Use a support group or the community to intervene and to facilitate the person doing more. |

| Overprotection source | Clinical strategy |
|---|---|
| Acute illness model | Present an active rehabilitation model (school metaphor) |
| Ill person exercising control | Give other ways of exercising control, explore relationship dynamics |
| Caregiver exercising control | Empower the person with the brain illness, explore relationship dynamics |
| Caregiver fulfilled by role | Look for other ways of fulfilling that role, present alternate model of caregiving as helping with recovery |
| Expressed love and caring | Look for other ways of expressing love and caring, present alternate model of caregiving as helping with recovery |
| Financial or other incentives | Make incentives for recovery more attractive, or eliminate disincentives for recovery |
| Embarrassment | Educate family and community, work on public presentation and reducing sources of embarrassment, work on attitude. |
| Following discharge orders | Update care plan, build in progression |

*Mommy Won't Let Me Come Out! Case 13.4. Tierno.* A 45-year-old, single, Costa Rican biologist was seen for evaluation 4 years after a stroke. He had a right hemiparesis and walked slowly but independently with a cane. He was independent in self-care. He had a moderately severe expressive aphasia. He was well aware of his deficits and had good attention, memory, and visual–spatial skills. He made professional-quality botanical drawings. He was depressed.

Following his stroke he had moved into his elderly mother's house. She hired a nurse to care for him (although he did not need it), but did not "allow" him to cross the street, even with the nurse, because she felt it would not be safe. Consequently, he spent almost all of his time with his mother, watching TV, trying to read, and sketching. When asked why he did not go ahead and do things outside of the house that he wanted to do, he shrugged and pointed at his mother.

4. The belief that overprotection shows love and caring.
5. Family members who find fulfillment in caregiving.
6. Financial incentives from disability payments.
7. Embarrassment about the person's disability or about their behavior in public.
8. Lack of follow-up. A family continues to carry out the level of care prescribed at discharge, not recognizing or allowing further recovery.

Overprotection needs to be carefully evaluated to distinguish it from appropriate care. Overprotection is often a voluntary relationship between the caregiver and the care receiver, so intervening to change it can be problematic from the perspective of customer service. In other words, if this is what they all want, what right does the clinician have to try to change it? The main answer to this is that, in fact, they may all want something else but do not know how to get there. The clinician can try to identify that something else and guide them there, which is likely to mean giving up overprotection.

In other cases, the person may not want to be overprotected, but she may be unable to change it due to her family role or her disabilities. The clinician's role is to find out about such situations, help her to assert herself, and advocate for her.

## *EVALUATION*

### *Screening*

Which families should be evaluated, and how thoroughly? Many medical and rehabilitation centers use the principle that the squeaky wheel gets the grease;

families that ask for help or show obvious problems get evaluated. This approach produces few false positives—almost every family evaluated needs help. The worry is the false negatives—how many families needing help are missed?

Some families of people with a TBI show a "command performance syndrome" (Sbordone, Kral, Gerard, & Katz, 1984). They mask their distress to the injured person and the rehabilitation staff. So do many careqivers of the elderly, who have high rates of depression and burden of care (Vitaliano, 1990). All caregivers should be screened for social support, for caregiver stresses, for depression (Gallo, 1990), for health, and for longstanding personality traits, particularly anger (Vitaliano; Table 13.7).

Screening should be directed toward the primary caregiver and possibly toward other family members. Often screening can be done incidentally, without making the family feel that they are under formal scrutiny. For example, a questionnaire might be experienced as intrusive and disempowering whereas many of the questions can be incorporated into the family interview for evaluating the person with the illness. When changes and problem areas are probed, for example, the family member can be asked, "How much of a problem is that for you?" or "How much does that bother you?" Care should be taken to avoid the "command performance syndrome" or cultural tendencies towards agreeableness (Galanti, 1991). For example, it is better to ask, "Who can you count on for help?" than "Do you have enough help?"

**TABLE 13.7. Areas for Screening Families of People with Brain Illnesses**

| | |
|---|---|
| Stressors | Characteristics of the person with the brain illness (especially behavioral)<br>Caregiving demands<br>Family conflict<br>Economic hardship<br>Subjective burden |
| Vulnerability | Physical health of caregivers<br>History of personality or psychiatric problems<br>Substance abuse problems<br>Personality characteristics (e.g., anger) |
| Psychological resources | Coping skills<br>Beliefs and values |
| Social resources | Number and quality of supporters<br>Perception of adequacy of that support<br>Community services |
| Distress | Depression |

### *Clinical Evaluation*

The needs and potential for intervention should be investigated in families identified for evaluation at three levels: individual members, family system, and family in the community (Table 13.8, Kay & Cavallo, 1994).

### *Empirical Evaluation*

The Family Assessment Device is the most consistently reliable and valid empirical family assessment technique from outside of the brain illness literature (Bishop & Miller, 1988). This is a 60-item questionnaire that assesses dimensions of problem solving, communication, role dimension, affective responsiveness, affective involvement, behavior control, and general functioning. However, Bishop and Miller recommended a combination of empirical and clinical assessment techniques, and a comparison of the results between the two.

Kay and Cavallo (1994) leveled a criticism at existing empirical family assessment techniques that are familiar from the discussion of personality assessment in brain illness (Chapter 5); namely, most of the developed instruments are not specific to the problems of brain illnesses. Kay and colleagues (1995) have developed the Head Injury Family Interview (Appendix B), which is so specified. It addresses the course of recovery and resource use and role changes for the person with the injury. It has sections specific for the spouse, for parents, for adult siblings, for younger siblings, for adult children, and for younger children

**TABLE 13.8. Evaluating the Family in Depth**[a]

| | |
|---|---|
| Individual family members | Personality structure<br>Knowledge, attitudes, relationship regarding the person with the brain illness<br>Role in the family<br>Skills and strengths |
| The family system | Structure and roles<br>Communication<br>Cohesion<br>Flexibility<br>Norms and values |
| The family in the community | Rehabilitation/medical community<br>Extended family<br>Friends<br>Other (work, school, recreation, religion, organizations) |

[a] From "The Family System: Impact, Assessment, and Intervention," by T. Kay and M. M. Cavallo, in *Neuropsychiatry of Traumatic Brain Injury* (pp. 533–567), edited by J. M. Silver, S. C. Yudofsky, & R. E. Hales, 1994, Washington, DC: American Psychiatric Press, Inc. Copyright 1994 by American Psychiatric Press, Inc. Adapted with permission.

of the person with the brain injury. The combination of multiple interviews and rating scales, when supplemented by behavioral observations, neuropsychological assessment, medical records, and so forth and informed by knowledge of family dynamics and of the effects of brain illness on the family, provides the combined clinical-empirical evaluation that Bishop and Miller (1988) recommended. It is adaptable to other forms of brain illness besides TBIs.

In assessing the burden of care in dementia, 8 of 10 measures were specifically designed for dementia, and 3 of those 8 are specific for Alzheimer's disease (Vitaliano, Young, & Russo, 1991). Only one, the *Screen for Caregiver Burden*, was specifically designed for one population of caregiver, namely spouses (Vitaliano, Russo, Young, Becker, & Maiuro, 1991).

The *Family Involvement Assessment Scale* (McNeill, Schuyler, & Ezrachi, 1997) is an experimental 37-item rating scale for evaluating families of persons receiving rehabilitation for a TBI. It produces subscales concerning involvement with staff, supportiveness, and involvement with the patient (Appendix B).

## *INTERVENTIONS*

A large variety of family interventions has been described, and flexibility in their application is usually advocated (DePompei & Zarski, 1989; Kay & Cavallo, 1994; Maitz & Sachs, 1995; Muir, Rosenthal, & Diehl, 1990; Rosenthal & Geckler, 1986; Sachs, 1991; Williams & Kay, 1991). All families affected by brain illness can benefit from education, support, problem solving, and cognitive restructuring; some families or individual members need formal therapy, usually because of issues outside of the brain illness (Figure 1.4, p. 5, Kay & Cavallo).

### *Education*

Prioritized and directed family education (see Chapters 3, 6, and 9-12) is fundamental to other interventions. This is not to say that a clinician should withhold support or empathetic listening until the family can draw an accurate representation of the limbic system, but any extended intervention for problem solving or for processing complex feelings must be based on accurate information. Education is not just giving information; it also involves training skills. If a mother complains that her son with a brain injury hits her, it is usually a higher priority to train her to keep him from hitting her than to ask her how she feels about being hit. Information about typical reactions, problems, and solutions of families dealing with similar problems often helps families normalize and make sense of a bewildering experience and helps them prepare for and anticipate later reactions.

### *Support and Problem Solving*

Emotional and practical support and problem solving are basic helping skills of most health care professionals and of many nonprofessionals. Often the only professional intervention needed is to allow family members to recognize and acknowledge their own stress levels and feelings and then direct them either to their own accustomed supports (family, friends, clergy, counselors) or to support groups. There they may grieve, sort through feelings, and tackle practical problems. Using natural supports instead of professionals, when effective, helps avoid the passivity and dependence on the rehabilitation industry that the medical service model suggests. It is likely that most people, given the choice, would rather cry out their grief in the arms of a loved one than in the office of a professional.

Beyond basic helping capacities, what is most important is knowledge of brain illnesses, of their consequences, and of possible solutions to problems they present. Problem-solving counseling regarding brain illness is much more likely to require the knowledge and skills of a professional than is supportive counseling. Perhaps the principal art in problem-solving counseling is finding the therapeutic window between being too directive and not providing enough structure. Often a family member, particularly when in crisis, looks for and wants someone to tell him what to do. He is not interested in a lengthy process to discover his own opinions on the matter. Provided that this is not a gambit for a relationship of dependency, of blame, or of litigation, it is best for the clinician to be quite directive. Other individuals resist all suggestions that they have not come up with themselves. Most people are somewhere in between. Additionally, the nature of the problem and of the family context dictate how directive one should be. Some problems have clear and standard solutions about which the family may not know. Others have solutions that depend on the circumstances. In these cases it is better either to help the family explore possible solutions or to present an array of solutions from which they can choose. Restructuring family beliefs and attitudes requires a bit more flexibility, sensitivity, and skill in helping families to see their situation in alternate ways.

### *Therapy*

Therapy for the family may take the form of individual therapy for family members, couples therapy, or family therapy (Sachs, 1991). If individual or family therapy is warranted, the therapist should carefully weigh the value of a referral to an outside, impartial therapist against the value of knowing the case and all of the actors. If a referral is made, the neuropsychotherapist may help prioritize issues and brief the other therapist on special issues related to the brain illness. What distinguishes therapy from counseling is that therapy goes beyond simply finding ways to cope with the person with the illness, with caregiving, and with the changes that illness has brought to the family (Rosenthal & Geckler, 1986). Therapy may be directed toward long-standing personality, psychiatric, couples, or family dynamics problems that have been stirred up or brought to attention by attempts to cope with the illness or toward malignant problems that have arisen primarily due to the illness. The focus may shift to individual personalities and behavior patterns or to dysfunctional interaction patterns. Although some of the content and timing of such interventions may be specific to brain illness as already described, the techniques can be essentially those of conventional individual, couples, and family therapy. For example, Maitz and Sachs (1995) have illustrated how a family systems perspective can be applied to family therapy in families affected by a brain illness. They describe a father of four children who lost his parental authority after he had a TBI. His children took advantage of him, teased him, and developed behavior problems at school, while his wife undermined his parental authority because he was too demanding on the children. The therapist convinced him to resume parental responsibilities while insisting that his wife support his authority. The therapist, wife, and husband worked together on the husband's parenting skills, on restoring his parenting role, and on resolving the children's school behavior problems. An individual, deficit-oriented approach focused only on parenting skills might not have had such an effect, because his attempts to parent would still be undermined by his wife and children.

Rosenthal and Geckler (1986) recommended the following techniques for family therapy when brain illness is involved:

1. Emphasize mutual responsibility for poor family communication and adaptation, shifting blame from individuals to the family system.
2. Reinforce healthy aspects of the family system.
3. Reenact family conflicts to explore dysfunctional patterns and problem-solving conflicts.
4. Use homework assignments to generalize behavioral change.

## *CONCLUSIONS*

Family members can range from being the most important member of the treatment team to the most important "patient," with many different roles in between, usually in combination. Often the family provides the most important long-term context of recovery and of life for the person with a brain illness. A great deal of rehabilitation and mental health effort may be expended on preparing that context. Further, family members themselves have losses, pain, and needs resulting from the brain illness that often can be addressed best by the neuropsychotherapist. Meeting those needs appropriately and efficiently takes flexibility and access to varied resources.

# 14

# The Community

## *THE MEDICAL/REHABILITATION COMMUNITY*

Imagine that one day, without warning, you are whisked away from your family and your daily routine by uniformed officials in a specialized official vehicle with sirens wailing. You arrive at a large institution, where you are guarded, for hours of waiting. You are stripped and examined down to your most private parts. Your possessions are taken away; you are issued institutional clothes. People of power and authority observe you closely and ask questions. They speak an unintelligible terminology. It is clear that your answers will help determine if and how long you are imprisoned, but it is not clear what answers will have what effect. Finally, you are shut in a room with strangers and are observed periodically by staff. You are fed an institutional diet. Eventually some of your family is permitted to visit. If your conduct is considered adequate, you may be permitted closely monitored outside communication. Periodic visits and meetings, usually unannounced, determine your fate. A string of authorities expect you to keep their slightly different roles straight.

The preceding narrative could as easily describe going to jail as having a brain injury or a stroke. This is the community and role into which people who develop brain illnesses are unwillingly thrust. For most, this is an unwelcome change, not only because of the illness, but also because the patient role, like imprisonment, involves loss of power, freedom, privacy, and dignity. The family does not fare much better. When these are the social realities, the consumer model is distorted by the double message: "You are the consumer, but you must do as we say."

To be sure, there are important differences between prisons and hospitals. However, some questioning of and resistance to the many losses of hospitalization is psychologically healthy. It is not surprising that most people want to flee such a system as soon as possible. The transition from medicine to rehabilitation is like a move from jail to prison and forced labor. Here roles are mixed again. You are a patient, but you are a student. Work will set you free. Relationships with staff and with therapists are within strict professional and economic roles. Relationships among patients are observed and regulated.

The professional rehabilitation community, no matter how caring and community-oriented, is an artificial community with respect to the patient. It may, in fact, be counterproductive for a rehabilitation community to be too caring; it may give the illusion that it can substitute for a real community, which it can do for only a few people for a limited time. Once the money runs out, these "bought" friends are on to the next patient. Unfortunately, the effect may be that the patient is kept away from his usual social network long enough for it to wither down to a few friends and family members while "fixing his problems," then he is sent out the door, "all dressed up with no place to go." Social skills (re)learned in rehabilitation are relevant only to the extent that the artificial community of rehabilitation resembles the community of return. There are limits to how much community reintegration can be achieved simply by "fixing" the person with the illness. Some people with TBIs experience successful job placement as a loss of psychosocial support from the rehabilitation program (Parenté et al., 1991). These individuals may need to transfer social support to a support group, because their experiences set them apart from their old communities. Some people with TBIs feel "that they are suspended in a *rehabilitation zone* [emphasis in original] and that their lives have become meaningless" (Slade & Burns, 1992, p. 10).

Professional rehabilitation has attempted to overcome these limitations by moving out into the community (Seaman, Roberts, Gilewski, & Nagai, 1993). The rehabilitation center may be in a store-front or in a similar location (Slade & Burns, 1992), making public excursions and vocational integration easier. Rehabilitation and team meetings may occur in the home (Kneipp, 1995). The financial and power structure of professional rehabilitation remains, however. A departure from this is the movement toward home health aides and adult foster care.

Willer and Corrigan (1994) advocate a "whatever it takes" model that collaborates with professional rehabilitation but goes much beyond it. They emphasized respect for the individual, predominant use of paraprofessionals and of natural supports, a preference for evaluating and changing environments rather than people, training in context, and lifetime resources. Freeman (1997) advocates supported home-based rehabilitation for severe brain injury. Malkmus (1989) favors a client-centered, flexible model of community reentry oriented toward wellness and normalcy. It involves home-like, open community residences with a naturalistic social learning environment. There may be a progress from group home to program apartment to independent apartment (a typical middle-class developmental sequence in developed countries, but perhaps less appropriate for other groups).

Limitations in professionally based rehabilitation are coming to be well-recognized in the developing world (Peat, 1991). Community-based rehabilitation, organized by the village or the neighborhood, trains local people as rehabilitation workers (Werner, 1990; World Health Organization, 1982). The World Health Organization has recommended that research and technology in rehabilitation training be redirected to emphasize teaching therapists to teach self-care to people with disabilities and their families rather than focusing exclusively on direct treatment (Peat, 1991). According to Peat,

> As in the developing countries, the role of rehabilitation specialists may shift towards teaching and coordination of programmes. Direct patient care in the traditional western model is proving inefficient, costly, and serving only a segment of the population in need [less than 2% in many countries, Johnston & Tjandrakusuma, 1982; World Health Organization, 1981]. . . . To the vast majority who may never get any help, professional concern over 'standards of care' might seem inconsequential. (p.234)

If it is unrealistic to think that the rehabilitation center can become a substitute community for the person with a brain illness, perhaps it is not unrealistic to think that the community can become a substitute rehabilitation center.

## *THE DISABILITY COMMUNITY*

Since the mid-1980s, many mutually reinforcing advances for people with brain illnesses have been seen, including the development of neuropsychological rehabilitation, increased legal rights and community acceptance, and the organization of the disability community through support groups, advocacy organizations, newsletters, computer networks, political advocacy, and direct action campaigns. Support groups are often initiated by rehabilitation centers, sometimes as group therapy or education. If they are to be true support groups they then pass into independence, setting their own agendas and inviting professionals as guest speakers and as advisors when needed.

Advocacy organizations are typically started in the middle class, often by families of people with disabilities, reaching into the upper classes for funding and for organizational know-how and into the lower classes by making resources available (and because some members become impoverished by their disabilities). Advocacy groups lobby for legislation, for policy change, and for increased resource allocation (Mann & Dittmar, 1992). They confront myths and discrimination, challenge attitudes, and provide role models and methods of self-advocacy. They help many people with disabilities develop an appropriate sense of entitlement as a necessary foundation for self-assertion. They have established the Independent Living Centers movement, providing support for and by people with disabilities for living in the community (Mathews, 1990). These centers typically offer accessible and affordable housing referral, skills training, advocacy, peer counseling, attendant services, transportation assistance, information, referral, recreation, and communication assistance. The independent living movement is moving into the developing world, just as community-based rehabilitation is moving into developed countries from developing countries (Lysack & Kaufert, 1994).

Advocacy groups also provide appropriate education for people with brain illnesses, for their families, and for other parts of the community (Aronson & Yatzkan, 1984). They provide emotional support, informal counseling, and problem solving from a knowledge base of experience. In these many ways they provide a valuable continuation of the work described in this book.

Able-brained rehabilitation professionals play important roles with these groups (Table 14.1; American Heart Association, n.d.; Miller, 1992, 1993). They help start groups where needed and withdraw when the group is established. They can consult to groups when asked and can refer appropriate people. One of the hardest things for a professional to do for a support/advocacy group is to not do too much, so as to allow it autonomy.

Another idea recently borrowed from the disabled community is circles of support (Willer et al., 1993). These are groups of volunteers organized in support of the dreams of a focus person with a disability, using whatever it takes (Willer & Corrigan, 1994) to get the job done. This may include professional rehabilitation, but much more often it involves overcoming community barriers. A facilitator, often someone from the organized disability community, helps the focus per-

**TABLE 14.1. Guidelines for Forming Brain Illness Support Groups[a]**

| |
|---|
| Focus on support, information, and advocacy |
| Assess the need |
| Put someone in charge |
| Enlist a facilitator |
| Invite guest speakers |
| Secure a location |
| Hook up to larger networks |
| Get the word out |
| Have time for: |
| Greetings and names |
| Information and news |
| Topic, speaker, or movie |
| Discussion |
| Separate support groups for the people with the brain illness and for family members |
| Reconvene for closing |

[a] From "When the Best Help is Self-Help, or Everything you Always Wanted to Know about Brain Injury Support Groups," by L. Miller, 1992, *The Journal of Cognitive Rehabilitation, 10*(6), 14–17. Copyright 1992 by Neuroscience Publishers; and from Miller (1993). Adapted with permission.

son organize the circle. The focus person chooses the members of the circle, although a facilitator may actually ask them to join. They may be friends, acquaintances, extended family members, people from the disability community, less often immediate family, and sometimes rehabilitation professionals participating voluntarily. Because these are private and voluntary organizations, not constrained by formal rules or regulations, their ways of functioning are very variable. Circles of support attempt to reconstruct the natural social support network that so often crumbles for people with brain illnesses (Finset, Dyrnes, Krogstad, & Berstad, 1995; Morton & Wehman, 1995).

## *THE WORK COMMUNITY*

An increasing number of vocational rehabilitation counselors are specializing in brain illnesses, because many assumptions and techniques of traditional vocational rehabilitation do not apply well to people with brain illnesses (Fraser, 1991; Kreutzer & Wehman, 1990; Wehman & Kreutzer, 1990; Ylvisaker & Gobble, 1987). When these specialized services are available, they should be used, because such expertise and community contacts typically go far beyond what other professionals or nonprofessionals can provide. In communities and countries where such services are not yet available, vocational rehabilitation falls to social workers, to psychologists, to counselors, to occupational therapists, or to the family. The following brief review of principles of vocational rehabilitation for people with brain illnesses (Table 14.2) is aimed at nonvocational rehabilitation counselors who find themselves in that role, and it should be supplemented by the literature. The discussion is directed primarily towards dealing with behavioral/emotional/personality problems.

**TABLE 14.2. Principles of Brain Illness Vocational Rehabilitation**

| |
|---|
| Be flexible |
| Build on pre-illness abilities |
| Assess learning style |
| Pay attention to motivation and to incentive |
| Pay attention to the social environment |
| Evaluate and train in context |
| Prepare the workplace |
| Use natural supports |
| Use cognitive compensations adapted to the job |
| Start part-time each day |
| Build in rest breaks |
| Take change slowly |

### *Be Flexible*

The variety of types of employment is enormous. So is the variety of types and combinations of problems resulting from brain illnesses (Table 14.3), making vocational rehabilitation for people with brain illnesses an extraordinarily complex job of matching variables. A fixed program offering a rigid set of workshop procedures may address itself to the "least common denominator" of participants and is not likely to meet the needs of very many of those people. Flexibility is required at all stages of vocational rehabilitation, from evaluation through repeat intervention for job advancement (Table 14.4). Even the decision of whether and how much to evaluate requires flexibility. In Chapter 5 the concepts of the no intervention/assess and assess/intervene thresholds were presented. These concepts also apply to vocational rehabilitation. Many individuals with enough recovery and a supportive workplace can attempt a return with no intervention. If the return fails they can go back to rehabilitation for interventions. Alternately, they may have a plan that requires little evaluation but does require intervention. For example, someone may return to work in his family's small business doing just a few tasks with a flexible schedule because the family is tolerant and supportive, with flexible productivity standards. However, he may require help adapting and facilitating tasks. Others show so little interest in work that evaluation is not needed.

Flexibility is also needed for finding solutions to work problems that fit the individual and the job. A written list of procedures for operating a machine that works for one person with memory impairment may not work for another with reading problems.

### *Build on Pre-Illness Abilities*

New learning difficulties and difficulty transferring and generalizing abilities are so common with brain illnesses that it is usually critically important to

**TABLE 14.3 Challenges to Employment in People with Traumatic Brain Injuries[a]**

| |
|---|
| Cognitive deficits |
| Communication impairments |
| Current emotional difficulties |
| Preexisting personality disorders |
| Financial disincentives |
| Motor and sensory deficits |
| Transportation difficulties |
| Vocational indecision/immaturity |
| Negative family influences |
| Medication concerns |

[a] From "Cross-Disciplinary Collaboration in the Removal of Work Barriers after Traumatic Brain Injury," by R. T. Fraser and R. Baarslag-Benson, 1994, *Topics in Language Disorders, 15*(1), 57. Copyright 1994 by Aspen Publishing. Adapted by permission

**TABLE 14.4. Vocational Rehabilitation Intervention Strategies**

| |
|---|
| None |
| Advocacy with employer |
| Education of co-workers |
| Supports in the workplace |
| Consultation regarding adaptations |
| Facilitating natural supports (co-worker or supervisor as job coach) |
| Outside job coach |
| Job simulation in the clinic |
| Job role-playing in the clinic |
| Job therapy experience |
| Training new job skills |
| Sheltered employment |

build on preexisting abilities. Old skills are often preserved or can be regained more easily than new skills can be acquired. The ideal is usually to return as close to previous employment as possible (Table 14.5).

### *Assess Learning Style*

For the person who will need to learn or to relearn skills it is important to know what types of instruction work best, whether it is verbal or visual, by principle or by example, by seeing or by doing, by written or oral orders, or by demonstration. Indications of learning style from the neuropsychological assessment need to be confirmed in the workplace.

**TABLE 14.5. Continuum of Vocational Placement Options**

| |
|---|
| Pre-illness job |
| Modified pre-illness job |
| Physically adapted |
| Cognitively adapted (compensations) |
| Reduced responsibilities |
| Reduced hours |
| Different profession, same employer |
| Pre-illness profession, new job |
| New profession, new job |
| Supported employment |
| Sheltered employment |
| Volunteer |
| Assisted volunteer |

### *Pay Attention to Motivation and to Incentive*

People have many and complex reasons for working. Pay is an obvious motivator for most, but feelings of contributing to a family or a society, taking pride in a job well done, pleasing customers, gaining status, helping others, having social relations at work, and getting fringe benefits all contribute. Reasons for working may be different after a brain illness than before, and they may not emerge until the person is working. Disability payments, attention from others, and more attractive alternatives to employment may be disincentives to work. Some people with brain illnesses may not recognize advantages to working and may be able to discover them through being educated or through trying it out.

Sale, West, Sherron, and Wehman (1991) studied 38 job separations in people placed in employment through a TBI vocational rehabilitation program. The main reasons for separation were a poor match between the person's job expectations and the actual job, a mismatch to the culture of the workplace, inflexibility, interpersonal difficulties, and mental health difficulties, whereas inability to do the job was almost never the reason. This suggests that motivation and social factors must be given high priority in job placements.

### *Pay Attention to the Social Environment*

The social environment in the workplace is tremendously important to successful placement (West, 1995). Flexibility, patience, tolerance, and support are important, but too much of these qualities can be problematic if there is not adequate structure and feedback. Such settings sometimes "carry" incompetent people to the detriment of all until resentments build. It is also important to match personality types and interests for camaraderie. Among 59 people completing a TBI rehabilitation program, the best predictors of employment were acceptance of the program, psychomotor dexterity, self-appraisal, verbal aptitude, and involvement with others (Ezrachi, Ben-Yishay, Kay, Diller, & Rattok, 1991). Attitudinal and social variables were at least as important as cognitive variables. Successful job placement depends on much more than the formal ability to meet the demands of the tasks.

### *Evaluate and Train in Context*

Because skills of people with brain illnesses frequently do not transfer or generalize easily, there has been much emphasis lately on placing people in work settings soon and evaluating and training them in context (Fraser, 1991; Willer & Corrigan, 1994). If training on site is not possible, the work situation should be simulated in the clinic (Parenté et al., 1991) or in a job training experience (Hurt & Raines, n.d.).

### *Prepare the Workplace*

Because many problems with a return to work for people with brain illnesses come from the workplace milieu, a priority should be set on preparing that milieu (Hurt and Raines, n. d.). This may be through advocacy with an employer, including reminding the employer of legal obligations not to discriminate against the disabled; education of employers, supervisors, and co-workers about the brain illness and about the requirements of the situation; and establishing feedback mechanisms to troubleshoot problems early. Flexibility is needed regarding who carries out this preparation: a rehabilitation professional, the person with the brain illness, or some other advocate. In many settings, personal contacts are more effective than professional authority. In hostile environments without enforced supportive legislation, intervention could do more harm than good. For this reason, confidentiality should be scrupulously protected, and how and what to say to whom should be carefully strategized.

*Job coaches* are individuals with appropriate personal characteristics and some training in brain illness, counseling, and rehabilitation (Parenté et al., Stapelton, and Wheatley, 1991). They supervise the person with the brain illness on the worksite, identify missing abilities, make and carry out training plans, restructure the work environment to facilitate success, and work with others in the workplace. Job coaches are especially useful when they know or quickly learn the job requirements and when the workplace is accepting of the placement.

### *Use Natural Supports*

Co-workers and supervisors can be natural supports to (re)train the person with the brain illness. This is more appropriate when likely candidates can be identified (often the case when a well-liked employee returns to an old job), when job coaches are not available, and when the job is complex so a job coach cannot learn it easily. This approach has the advantage that the workplace milieu takes on more responsibility for the success of the placement. Natural supports often know better how the job can be modified and how to work through dynamics of the milieu. Finally, natural supports are usually there long after a job coach leaves. Professional rehabilitation support is then directed toward educating the people who are providing natural support. Job coaches and natural supports can use cognitive rehabilitation and many of the techniques in this book.

### *Use Cognitive Compensations Adapted to the Job*

Cognitive compensations should be adapted to the specifics of the job and to the person's learning style (Parenté et al., 1991; Table 14.6, Case 14.1. G. P.). Cognitive compensations for emotional and for behavior problems, described in this book, can also be used (discretely).

**Table 14.6. Cognitive Compensations Adaptable to the Workplace**[a]

| |
|---|
| Organize workspace and access to tools |
| Place cue cards by equipment with which they are used |
| Place checklists in logical locations |
| Color code documents |
| Organize desktops with fixed locations for fixed materials |
| Color code keys with plastic jackets |
| Put commercial "key finder" beepers on keys or on other important objects |
| Telememo watches for recording and dialing telephone numbers |
| Appointment calendars with: |
| The day divided into half-hours |
| A blank, lined page for each day |
| A "Things to do" list each day |
| An appointment minder in the calendar that beeps for set appointments |
| Predial telephones, perhaps with voice recognition |
| Microcassette tape recorders for phone conversations, complex instructions, complex reading material |
| Word processors with grammar checker, spell checker, dictionary, and thesaurus |
| Expert system software |

[a] Adapted from Parenté et al. (1991).

### *Start Part-Time Each Day*

Fatigue is such a pervasive problem following brain illness that it is very frequently advisable to resume work part-time, a few hours each day (as contrasted with a few full days each week), gradually increasing hours as tolerated. When that is not possible, an alternative is to build in more rest time during the day and to make sure it is used to rest (see Case 12.1, p. 246, Lu Tan).

### *Take Change Slowly*

Many people with brain illnesses return to work at a level initially lower than their pre-illness work level. As they recover and master the job, they may be eager to advance. They may not realize that they are still slow to learn and to transfer skills. Advancements and other transitions should be handled gradually.

### *Cultural Considerations*

Most of the vocational rehabilitation programs for people with brain illnesses described in the literature are from the developed world. They tend to address reintegration into a formal, public economy with legal protections for disabled employees. These elaborate rehabilitation programs may reflect, in part, the interests of insurance companies that can avoid a lifetime of disability payments by returning someone to work. Such funding is sometimes available in the developing world, but few programs specific to brain illnesses have emerged as of yet.

*Quick! Which Key Locks up the Cobra? Case 14.1*[a]*. G. P.* G. P. worked in a pet store doing bookkeeping, billing, and sales, and was an expert on diagnosis and treatment of fish diseases. A TBI left him with a verbal/auditory memory impairment and difficulty with quick retrieval of facts, including facts concerning fish diseases. Other cognitive skills were adequate for his old job. With time, much of his old knowledge of fish diseases was retrieved and was entered into an expert system on a laptop computer. This allowed him to ask customers the questions on the screen, feed in the answers, and get treatment recommendations. With training he also used the computer for billing, for writing letters, and for inventory.

His 15 keys for the pet shop were color-coded and he was retrained in their functions. He learned to use a tape recorder to record phone conversations to avoid the embarrassment of asking people to repeat. He carried important work phone numbers on a telememo watch and used a daily calendar for appointments and for special duties. Cue cards on each cage gave feeding instructions, and a checklist by the back door gave him the "checkout sequence" for closing the shop.

[a]From "Practical Strategies for Vocational Reentry after Traumatic Brain Injury," by R. Parenté, M. C. Stapleton, and C. J. Wheatley, 1991, *Journal of Head Trauma Rehabilitation, 6*(3), 40. Copyright 1991 by Aspen Publishers. Adapted with permission.

Much of the developing world is characterized by a larger, informal economy—day labor, self-employment, street vendors, subsistence farming, family businesses, and so forth. Employment is often determined much more by family and by social contacts than by formal job criteria. There are more jobs with minimal cognitive requirements, but many require manual labor and/or are seasonal or unstable. Laws protecting the disabled are often weak and widely ignored. Disability myths are prevalent and often harmful. Viable transportation and modern communications are out of reach for many. Families are often large and close-knit; overprotection is common. Some of these characteristics and expectations come with these families when they emigrate to developed countries.

These conditions are an advantage for some, a disadvantage for many, and a potential opportunity for rehabilitation. The informal sector of the economy offers opportunities for graded return to meaningful work and for other contributions to the family. Supportive families offer potential natural supports who may be more disposed to be patient and invested in recovery than a professional. Community-based rehabilitation (Lysack & Kaufert, 1994; Peat, 1991), with emphasis on training family members and others in the community to promote recovery, may be a cost-effective way of improving the quality of life for many.

## *SCHOOL*

School for adults (for children and adolescents see Blosser & DePompei, 1989; Lehr, 1990; Rosen & Gerring, 1986; Savage & Wolcott, 1994; Ylvisaker et al., 1995) can be a transition between rehabilitation and work. Like rehabilitation, it is a service offered to clients, but it is less individualized, with standardized expectations. Its purpose is not fixing problems in a "sick" or a disabled individual but teaching skills and knowledge. It is for those who are between a dependent and a productive role. Unfortunately, being a student demands cognitive skills that are frequently impaired by brain illness, especially memory, attention, reasoning, planning, and initiation. Schooling after a brain illness is sometimes more for social reasons than for learning course content. In a young person with a progressive condition, school may be an end in itself, an intrinsically meaningful way to stay engaged with the world.

The transition from brain illness rehabilitation to full-time, career-path adult student can be eased by starting part-time with noncredit, noncareer path, personal growth courses. Initial goals may be to arrive at class on time consistently, to take notes, to interact with other students appropriately, and to attempt readings, assignments, and exams. Learning to resume the student role may be the priority, rather than grades or learning course content. When these goals are met, the course load can be gradually increased, and conventional priorities can be resumed.

Because the initial goals of a return to school may be more social, emotional, and behavioral than academic, support may be needed in these areas. This may be through old friends from school, organized into a circle of support if necessary, through a support group through disabled student services, or through natural supports from seeking out someone in particular in the class. A supportive family member or friend might take a first course with the person with the brain illness to act as a support and a coach.

Many community colleges in the United States have special programs and curricula for students with disabilities that include courses such as brain injury awareness, study skills, social skills, adapted physical education, and so forth. (Cook, 1990). Some of them sponsor support groups and have extensive teams of professionals, facilities, and programs that rival those of a rehabilitation center.

## *THE SOCIAL COMMUNITY*

Social isolation and loneliness are very common problems following brain illnesses (Finset et al., 1995; Morton & Wehman, 1995). Although it is possible to legislate against discrimination in employment, in housing, in transportation, in education, and in the social services, this will not work for friendships. Formal rehabilitation tends to approach this problem by trying to fix deficits in the social skills of the individual. However, when such deficits are of long duration, changes in the social environment must also be contemplated.

### *Changes in the Individual*

Many problems resulting from brain illness contribute to social isolation. Mobility problems may make it difficult to get together with family and with friends who do not live in the same home. Language impairments can make communication difficult. Attention and memory difficulties can make someone unrewarding to be with or unreliable. However, many of these types of difficulties can be compensated for, at least in part, with accessible transportation, telephones, computer networks, memory books, and so forth.

Those problems that seem to contribute more to social isolation are emotional reactions such as anxiety, depression, and embarrassment, and impaired social skills, particularly the executive functions such as communication pragmatics, social judgement, initiation, and impulse control (Levine, Van Horn, & Curtis, 1993; McGann & Werven, 1995; Santoro & Spiers, 1994).

Once some of the more socially disabling problems have been brought under control by individual work, social skills are often best treated through group therapy (Dikengil, King, & Monda, 1992; Dryovage & Seidman, 1992). The group can establish a specific goal or goals for the session for each participant and then monitor those behaviors through a group discussion, through role-play, through social problem-solving exercise, or through other activities. Specific skills and abilities can be practiced repeatedly. In a milieu rehabilitation setting, social skills goals may be monitored throughout the day and during community excursions. There can be social skills homework, such as initiating conversations, calling a friend, going to a public event, and so forth.

However, even in a community-oriented rehabilitation program, there may be limitations in how much such skills will then apply to the person's own more immediate community, friends, and family. McGann & Werven (1995) observed that the unwritten communication rules (communication pragmatics) of a rehabilitation center or a professional therapeutic relationship are quite restrictive compared to a family argument, to school friend chatter, to an off-color comedian, and to a politician's address. Rehabilitation center and therapy styles are only a very small proportion of possible communicative styles and are unlike what many people typically encounter outside of those contexts.

To overcome this intrinsic limitation of rehabilitation and therapy settings for social skills training, natural helper social skills coaches can be enlisted from the person's social circle. The coach is given permission and direction in giving feedback to the person with the brain illness, who then has someone to turn to for advice. The coach can also advocate for the person, intervene to straighten out misunderstandings, explain the person's condition to others, work out subtle cuing systems for social situations, and so forth. The role of the therapist may range from simply suggesting to the person with the brain illness that he seek out a coach through extended mentoring of the coach (see Tables 6.5, p. 99, and 6.6, p. 100, Blosser & DePompei, 1995), depending on how complicated the problems are, the abilities of the coach, and practicalities of the situation.

The advantages of such an approach are that the coach is likely to know the situation and the people better than the therapist, the coach is likely to be more available, the coach may be able to intervene in ways a therapist could not, and the coach's opinion may carry more weight with the person with the brain illness than that of the therapist. The coach should be someone whom the person with the brain illness trusts who is willing and mature enough to help. Different natural supports may serve for different contexts. For example, a young woman recovering from a brain injury and returning to work might use her husband to help her with parenting, a co-worker for the workplace, and her mother to help her deal with extended family members.

### *Changes in the Social Environment*

When the person has long-term impairments in social skills, changes in the person-environment fit may be needed. The least intrusive change may be to educate the people in the person's environment about what has happened and about what would be most helpful for them to do (see Table 6.4, p. 97). Beyond a few individuals in the immediate family who may receive their education from the medical/rehabilitation professionals, it is often best for the person with the brain illness, his family, or someone else from that social context to do this. For example, if a child is returning to school following a head injury it may be better if the teacher or the school counselor explains this to the class rather than an outside rehabilitation professional.

People who knew the person before the illness are more likely to have stayed friends and to help out from a sense of loyalty. Old friends who would like to continue with the friendship but who are not sure how to do so might be organized into a circle of support (described previously, p. 294) or a family network, an educational and problem-solving meeting of extended family and friends organized by professionals (Rogers & Kreutzer, 1984).

Making new friends is often much more difficult after brain illness than maintaining old friendships. Still, there may be no other option that to seek new friends. Support groups, the disability community, and friends made in rehabilitation may become part of this new circle because of shared experiences. People with brain illnesses may need help from social workers, from recreational therapists, or from others in finding new social opportunities. Support and encouragement may be needed to try out new opportunities. A confidant or other natural support person may be more appropriate for this than a professional.

### *Sexuality*

Sexuality assessment, levels of intervention for sexual dysfunction, and issues of sexuality in established couples are dealt with in Chapter 13 (p. 217). Only the secondary (psychosocial) aspects of sexuality in individuals without an established partner are addressed here, with the assumption that medical aspects will be addressed by a physician. Psychosocial problems with sexuality resulting from brain illness in a person without an established partner are of four major types: disinhibition, lack of interest, frustration, and vulnerability. Other rarer problems are discussed by Griffith and associates (1990).

### *Sexual Disinhibition*

This is the type of change that receives most of the attention in rehabilitation because it poses a risk to the community and/or to the person with the brain illness and is often offensive to rehabilitation staff. This can be a persistent problem that is not easy to treat. It can sometimes be controlled within an institution with a behavior management plan.

*Assessment.* Assessment of sexual disinhibition incidents can follow an AABCCC format (Table 14.7). How the person accounts for his behavior contributes to evaluating motivation, insight, potential for change, and possible strategies for change. Analysis of the antecedents should consider with whom the behavior takes place to predict the behavior. Does he appear to select people with whom he can "get away with it?" Have some individuals found ways to prevent the behavior? The behavior itself may give clues to its motivation. Someone with a progressive, subtle approach may think he is seductive, whereas someone who makes sudden, rude remarks or moves may be attempting to provoke anger or shock. Someone whose disinhibition is only verbal and gestural may present less risk to

**TABLE 14.7. AABCCC Analysis of Disinhibited Sexual Behavior**

| Step of analysis | Features to consider |
|---|---|
| Account | How does the person account for his behavior? Does he admit to it? Does he think it is acceptable? Does he recognize its impact? Does he want to change it? Why does he do it? |
| Antecedents | With what types of people (sex, physical characteristics, age, relationship to the person)? In what circumstances? (other people present? when physically close?) |
| Behavior | Verbal, gesture, touch? Does it appear intentional? Is it progressive or sudden? Is it crude or subtle? |
| Consequences 1 | Do people laugh, get angry, startle, ignore, move away, stop activity, distract, confront, talk about it, play along? |
| Consequences 2 (Reactions to the consequences) | How does he react to the reaction? Does he laugh, smile, show shock, apologize, stop, continue? |
| Change | Is this a change in his behavior compared to prior to his illness? |

the community and less legal liability than someone who touches. Someone who only touches may be stimulus-bound. Some behaviors seen as interpersonal sexual disinhibition may be more benign (Case 14.2. Mr. Bates). Some people, particularly those with dementia, may wander around nude while being unaware that others are present or that they are offensive to them.

Understanding the consequences the person receives is important in knowing if the behavior is being reinforced. Equally important, however, is knowing his reactions to those consequences. One person may be flirting and looking for a reciprocated response. If he is confronted or ignored he may stop. Another may be trying to provoke a reaction. Another may act in haste and regret at leisure as his pre-illness personality looks on in horror at what his post-illness disinhibition has done. Finally, is the behavior a change from pre-illness behavior (see Case 11.1, p. 215, Groucho)? Sexual mores vary widely and many people regularly violate those of others. The mores of the rehabilitation community may not match those of the person with the brain illness. Is there nonsexual disinhibition, and is it a change from pre-illness behavior?

Disinhibition is frequently a consequence of frontal orbital lesions that often leave people less responsive to social stimuli (Damasio et al., 1990). They may recognize and interpret social cues accurately; they simply do not change their behavior accordingly. Therefore, it is important to review the person's ability to respond to social stimuli.

*Intervention.* If the behavior is not interpersonally sexual by intention, then external structure, setting rules, and/or reinterpreting the behavior for those around the person may suffice.

If the person thinks he is flirting, social skills training may be in order, defining concretely with the person what is and what is not acceptable behavior, how to recognize that someone does not want to play along, and so forth. The best way to respond may be to firmly confront inappropriate behavior, kindly but firmly reject unwanted flirting, and play along with acceptable behavior if so desired.

> *If It Feels Good . . . Case 14.2. Mr. Bates.* A 40-year-old man had an anterior communicating artery aneurysm hemorrhage that left him with a profound amnesia and with disinhibition. One day he was sitting in the hospital corridor, completely absorbed in his open and vigorous masturbation. A female nurse approached him quietly and said, "That's not appropriate for here, Mr. B. Why don't you go to your room to do that." With neither embarrassment nor lechery he cheerfully answered, "OK!" and went to his room. He was not being exhibitionistic. He was simply oblivious to the possibility that others might come by or that his behavior was inappropriate.

This can be presented favorably to acknowledge when the intention is acceptable, but the execution is not, and to maintain motivation. For example, "flirting lessons" could be presented by someone to whom he has shown the behavior. "I'm going to teach you to flirt better. I'm going to tell you what I like and what turns me off and makes me go away."

If the person is attempting to shock others, it is best to ignore, to confront, and/or to redirect them, depending on the individual. For someone who is stimulus-bound it is most practical to avoid getting within grabbing distance or to provide something else of interest for him to hold. Firm but kind confrontation can be tried. If there is potential and motivation for self-control, this might be approached as follows: "I am going to come near you now. Please don't touch me. Say to yourself, `Don't touch. Don't touch.' Look for something to hold." If this is successful the cues can gradually be reduced (see Table 8.7, p. 149) and the strategy can be generalized to other people and locations.

If the person is aware of and embarrassed by his disinhibition, than the strategies in Chapter 8 can be applied.

If the behavior is the same as it was prior to the illness, it may not be organic disinhibition at all and can be dealt with as in someone with an intact brain (see Case 11.1, p. 215, Groucho).

Any of these approaches can be supplemented by a traditional behavioral approach. For instance, a concrete definition is given for inappropriate behavior. When the behavior occurs, the affected staff member gives a firm but calm message that the behavior is inappropriate. The person may then be redirected to some other activity. Counting inappropriate behaviors, setting goals, and giving feedback can then be used to try to reduce the offensive behavior. Generalization to the community must then be trained. Unless some insight and some motivation for maintaining the behavior change develops, however, the disinhibition may reemerge in other contexts or when the program is ended.

### *Lack of Sexual Interest*

A lack of sexual interest in people with brain illnesses without established partners has received little attention, perhaps because there is no partner to complain and caregivers may feel relieved not to have that to worry about. One legitimate perspective on the topic is that if no one complains about it, then it is not a problem and needs no intervention; it is not the business of rehabilitation to tell people that they ought to be interested in sex. However, a lack of interest may be an indicator of another problem deserving of intervention, such as depression, low self-esteem, unresolved sexual orientation, substance abuse, reduced emotional responsiveness, or impaired initiation. If intervention for a primary problem of a lack of sexual interest is decided upon, it might best begin by focusing on interest in social and potentially romantic relationships.

*Sexual Frustration*

Many people with brain illnesses without an established partner are frustrated because they are not seen as desirable and have difficulty encountering potential partners (Case 14.3. SWF). The feelings of frustration need to be acknowledged. Some individuals may seek solutions in sexual relationships that may not seem moral, healthy, or even safe. It is largely a personal decision for the therapist whether to facilitate, to discourage, or to stand aside from such efforts (within legal constraints). If frustration is felt as specifically sexual, then masturbation might be encouraged as a partial and temporary relief.

This frustration can be used as a motivator for therapy, especially for improving social skills and grooming. It can be particularly useful to arrange regular feedback from someone to whom the person might aspire as a potential partner. For instance, a teenager is much more likely to pay attention to the opinion of another teen, especially a friend, about what is cool and what is a turn-off than to the opinion of a middle-aged therapist (at least in most of North American culture).

The person may need to examine what he is interested in and why, and for what he is willing to settle. This can be difficult for someone with concrete thinking, with difficulty considering alternatives and with impaired awareness of deficits, and it may be facilitated by a neuropsychotherapist.

The person may also need a change in social environment to encounter potential partners. He may need help finding and following through on those opportunities. On occasion, support groups may be appropriate places to meet potential partners, but it is best not to encourage support groups to be used as singles clubs, because it can detract from their support function if people think they are going to be frequently approached by sexually disinhibited members. Some may consider disabled dating services or other dating services to be a viable option.

None of these ways of addressing sexual frustration need to be facilitated by a therapist. It is often better to have a friend provide most of the help with a therapist as guide or a mentor (see Tables 6.5, p. 99, and 6.6, p. 100, Blosser & DePompei, 1995) to the friend.

*Woman Seeking Man. Case 14.3. SWF.* The following Personals ad, taken from a local newspaper, reflects the dilemma in which many people with brain injuries may find themselves:

> Lost my brain a couple of years ago. Virtually homeless, really poor, little humor, not pretty, poor sense of smell, kinda fat, low self exteem (sic), walks into walls, holey clothes, desperately needs new shoes. No TV, no phone. Plays bingo and does ceramics, when not picking up horse poop or fixing car. Mid 30s, feel 80. hoping they have room for me at the funny farm when I decide to give up and check in. You: Normal, please. I'm weird enough for the both of us.

*Sexual Vulnerability*

Many people of both sexes are left sexually vulnerable by brain illness due to reduced physical mobility, poor social judgment, sexual frustration, and disinhibition. They may be gullible and susceptible to deceptive seduction, whereupon they could be left pregnant (or an expectant father), infected, impoverished, unwisely married, and/or emotionally devastated. Sexual assault is also a risk. These problems should be addressed early and frequently because they change considerably with changes in the person's abilities and social context. If sexual vulnerability appears possible, it should be assessed specifically, not simply inferred from other data. This includes assessing risks of the person's likely social contexts and the person's actual behavior. Direct observations from the different contexts and by different people are invaluable because behavior varies with circumstances (Case 14.4. Don). The person's behavior may also be quite different from what he says he would do.

There is no formulaic answer to problems of sexual vulnerability. In seeking solutions, various risks need to be weighed (pregnancy, disease, rape, psychological risks, Case 14.5. O.). Solutions need to respect the continuum of responsibility in combining external restrictions and self-control. In most circumstances, protection plans should be negotiated among the person, a caregiver, and someone who knows about brain illness and about the person's specific condition.

## *PRISONS*

The role of brain illnesses in violence is controversial. The prevalence of histories of TBIs in prison populations is high. What is not clear is how much this is true because violent, impulsive people are at risk for TBIs as well as for incarceration and to what extent brain injuries contribute to criminal behavior. Most experts agree that most violence is socially caused (Elliot, 1992) but also agree that some violence is caused primarily by brain illnesses, or that brain illness

*The Best Therapist in the World! Case 14.4. Don.* A 35-year-old married man was admitted to a rehabilitation unit with a severe TBI. Within 10 minutes of entering my office for evaluation he began praising my services and the help I had given him, concluding that I was one of the best therapists in the world. Much as I wanted to believe him, I suspected I was seeing an effect of his brain injury. Later at a team conference, the other therapists (all female) reported that he had been sexually inappropriate with them, ranging from excessive compliments to touching to frank sexual propositions. This behavior never happened in the presence of his wife.

*The Story of O. Case 14.5. O.* A 17-year-old woman with a moderate TBI had moderate impairments in attention, in memory, and in social judgment and was markedly impulsive. Prior to her injury she had done poorly in school and was marginally literate. She had a history of alcohol and drug abuse. She had been sexually abused by her stepfather, who was still living in the home where there were many fights. She had reportedly submitted herself to group sex as part of a gang initiation rite. She was not interested in rehabilitation. In negotiations with her and her mother it was concluded that the top priority, and the one to which O. would agree, was that she use a long-acting method of birth control.

symptoms make a contribution. Regardless of how much brain injuries contribute to criminal violence, it is worthwhile to consider what can be done about that proportion of criminal violence that is related to brain injury (Case 14.6. Nguyen).

Some people who experience impulsive anger feel that it is out of control and may want to change it, especially if it has gotten them into trouble, such as being put in prison. When it is out of character and is something they do not want to be doing, they may feel helpless about controlling it. Nevertheless, naming the problem, mobilizing hope for change, and giving simple, concrete techniques like a cue card for backing off can make a big difference (see Cases 7.2, p. 119, Douglass; 7.3, p. 119, Peleo). This is likely to be true of at least some members of the imprisoned community.

Likewise, there are probably many prisoners and guards who could benefit from rudimentary knowledge about the effects of brain injuries and how to manage them. The rehabilitation community and brain injury support group networks need to consider creative ways to apply what we know to this population which is not only often very disabled by their condition but is also a threat to society. It

*How Many Others? Case 14.6. Nguyen.* An 18-year-old southeast Asian refugee in the United States had a TBI resulting from a car accident. His family and his girlfriend reported a sudden change in his personality coincident with the accident in which he became withdrawn and impulsive. He had sudden outbursts of anger and violence regarding trivial matters for which he was immediately remorseful. He had no history of criminal activity, and his known substance abuse consisted of occasional use of small amounts of alcohol. One month after the accident he used a knife to brutally murder an elderly woman he had never previously met. He had no memory for the event. There was no clear motive. The court restricted the amount of medical evaluation he could receive. He was convicted and sentenced to a lengthy prison term.

seems unlikely that there will be comprehensive rehabilitation programs within prisons (even considering the high costs of imprisonment). Even adequate evaluations are the exception (Iverson, Demarest, & Franzen, 1994). Support group meetings and educational materials on topics such as anger, alcohol, recovery, mental fatigue, overstimulation, attention compensations, memory, concrete thinking, impulsivity, and self-regulation might be more realistic.

## *THE HOMELESS*

In all likelihood, the millions of homeless people who crowd the cities and the refugee camps of the world have an overrepresentation of people with brain dysfunction from a TBI, from malnutrition, from cerebral infections, from toxicities (both accidental and from substance abuse), and from developmental disorders. In many instances these dysfunctions probably contribute to their homelessness (Colman and Sandman, 1997). Clearly, the principal unmet needs of many of these people are much more basic than neuropsychotherapy and rehabilitation. Nevertheless, if programming for the homeless assumes that they have intact brains and can arrive for appointments, take advantage of employment opportunities unaided, conform to behavioral codes, or even maintain a simple household, then that programming runs the risk of failing some of those who are most in need. Rehabilitation and mental health professionals might help a few homeless people with brain illnesses by accepting them into their programs, recognizing that discharge planning will be a challenge. A more creative approach might be to consult with agencies already giving basic services concerning how they might identify, reach, and better serve those homeless people who have brain dysfunction (Case 14.7. Pega).

*Community Consultation. Case 14.7. Pega.* A 10-year-old boy who had been abandoned by his parents had lived in a small market in Managua, Nicaragua where he regularly sniffed cobbler's glue to get high on the toluene. He had a long history of prostitution, thievery, and glue abuse. He had a seizure disorder, apparently from the glue. He sometimes took anticonvulsants, prescribed by a community clinic and administered by a neighborhood rehabilitation program for glue-sniffing boys. In the program he had learned to read a few words. His was one of the most explosive of many high tempers among the participants. A typical episode occurred at a neighborhood religious celebration held in the courtyard of the program's center, a single room building with outdoor plumbing. While neighbors sang, many boys ran around, shouted, and threw firecrackers. Pega had already started several scuffles when a firecracker hit him in the back with no actual injury. He searched for the

*(continued)*

*Case 14.7. (Continued)*

offender with murder in his eyes. His friend pinioned his arms and took him off to the dorm. He curled up with a blanket on his sleeping place on the floor to cry.

This residential program is community organized and run. It costs about $3/day/child. It has served 67 children in 21 months, with about 75% success (off glue, off the streets, Roice, 1995).

A Nicaraguan neuropsychologist colleague and I visited the project to offer consultation, sitting on cinderblocks in a circle in the courtyard with the volunteers. Most of them had an elementary education or less; talking about white matter lesions of toluene toxicity would not be very helpful. However, we could listen to what their problems were. They had found that a few rules, a sense of community, and having adults around most of the time had taken care of most problems with fights, but a few boys, such as Pega, seemed different. We discussed what had worked, what might work, and what would not. We made suggestions for dealing with the limited attention spans of some of the boys that they found so disruptive to the center's activities. We talked about teaching anger management, behavior contracts, therapeutic communities, and time outs. We arrived at a plan to help the kids organize themselves to prevent fights and to teach each other to manage anger, as Pega's friend had tried. We suggested that a bucket of water might be handy for breaking up fights.

In the entire consultation we did not administer a single test or even mention the brain. Yet our profession is very relevant to such settings and has great potential to contribute to them.

The martyred Salvadoran Jesuit priest and psychologist, Ignacio Martín-Baró (1991), in his famous, "Towards a Liberation Psychology," emphasized the importance of spending time with poor people in their own settings to find out what they really need and shaping psychological research and interventions accordingly. These recommendations fit nicely with current directions in the North toward ecological neuropsychology and rehabilitation and with the emphasis on community reintegration following brain illness. In these ways it may be possible to follow Martín-Baró's direction in developing a liberation neuropsychology.

# 15

# Conclusions and Future Directions

What is neuropsychotherapy? Who is the neuropsychotherapist? How is neuropsychotherapy done? This book has tried to construct a vision of a professional role within a larger social context. That role will be recapitulated here.

The neuropsychotherapist is someone who can understand people in the full variety of their personalities, their social contexts, and the cultures from which they come. He understands well the physical, cognitive, executive, emotional, functional, and social changes that result from brain illnesses. He understands the many ways people react to those changes, both in themselves and in others. From these understandings, he can empathize with the person trying to cope with such a situation and with her family and others in her social network. He can communicate those understandings to people who differ widely in their personalities, emotional needs, cognitive abilities, education, and culture. He can help people reconstruct a self image and an image of their families from their experiences and from those insights.

He has a knowledge of and skills in techniques to help the person with the brain illness and those around her to cope with those changes. He knows how to find the right people to mobilize and/or train within that social network. He knows how to train those techniques and how to distribute them along a continuum of responsibility between the person with the brain illness and those around her. He can encounter the person's zone of recuperation in training such techniques. He knows how, where, and when to advocate for the person with the brain illness, to help develop a respectable place in society for that person.

He has the ability to turn all of those interventions and responsibilities over to the person and to her social network and to get out of the way when appropriate. He knows the limits of his role. He has the ability to turn over responsibility not only in the sense of individual cases, but also in the sense of the historical development of the neuropsychotherapist's role; that is, to turn over knowledge, techniques, and advocacy to other professions, to support groups, and to the general public, and to then turn his attention to tackling problems as yet unsolved.

That is quite a bit of expertise. However, it is notable that there are many things it does not include. The neuropsychotherapist need not be an expert in neuroanatomy, in neurophysiology, in neurology, in psychiatry, in cognitive testing, in cognitive rehabilitation, or in research (although it is helpful to be an informed consumer of research). Further, he can specialize by age range (children, adolescents, adults, the elderly), by disease type (developmental disorders, TBI, stroke, dementias), by culture (generally his own), and by personality type (refer out all cases of pre-illness major psychiatric disorder, substance abuse, or severe personality disorder). In this sense, someone with an elementary education with good interpersonal skills, working in his own community with a consistent population, could probably be trained and supervised in the necessary concepts and skills (Werner, 1990; Werner & Bower, 1982, see Case 14.7, p. 311, Pega). Alhough it may not be appropriate to call such a person a neuropsychotherapist, still, the essentials of the role would be fulfilled. Unless techniques are developed that can be so dissipated, and unless professionals teach these abilities, neuropsychotherapy will remain a service available to the elite few.

## *DIRECTIONS FOR FUTURE RESEARCH*

A drunk was searching the ground under a streetlamp one night. Someone walked up and asked "What are you looking for?" "My keys." "Where did you drop them?" "Way over there." "Why are you looking here?" "The light is better."

Neuropsychology has often looked where the light is better, where it is easiest to do research, especially in cognition. The effect has been to neglect (until recently) the important emotional, behavioral, family, and social impact of brain illnesses. Similarly, neuropsychology has often been blinded by the streetlamp in designing and in evaluating interventions. Some of the first attempts at cognitive rehabilitation consisted of little more than training the person to do the tests better, with the hope or assumption that this would improve the cognitive functions that the tests were designed to measure. This "teach to the test" strategy was not enormously successful.

There are places where the streetlamp shines clearly on the material in this book. Some directions for research are fairly clear, need little advocacy, and are discussed only briefly to emphasize areas that may be of more importance to public health but are perhaps less obvious or easy to research.

### *Efficacy*

Although there have been few efficacy studies of neuropsychotherapy techniques to date, they are in the economic interests of therapists and insurers and are likely to take place. Outcome measurement is not entirely straightforward (see Chapter 5, and Appendix B). Given the distortions of self-awareness that result from brain illnesses, self-report is insufficient as the only outcome measure. An intervention that improves self-awareness might produce a desirable temporary increase in reported distress.

Some techniques can be easily investigated, at least in part. Single subject designs should be adequate for demonstrating that cue cards are effective devices for teaching various routines and that therapy journals contribute to the efficiency of neuropsychotherapy. Some interventions are common sense or benign, and researching them does not appear to be a high priority; for example, speaking more slowly to someone with aphasia or with attention problems. However, some informal, small-scope research may help to define the best techniques for these problems; for instance, determining the optimal rate of speech for a given individual, which then permits imitating that rate, perhaps via a taped comprehension test at different speech rates.

The bigger questions of efficacy, however, concern the effects of various factors in the environment of recovery (including but not confined to professional interventions) on the recovery process. Table 5.12 (p. 59) lists variables in the environment of recovery that could be explored to determine their impact on recovery (or, in the case of a progressive illness, the rate of decline and quality of life). Such information could prove invaluable in planning interventions. Unfortunately, some of these variables are not easy to operationalize, particularly dimensions of the person-environment fit. This does not detract from their importance. The potential efficacy of techniques must not be confused with their suitability for research.

The effectiveness of cognitive rehabilitation was debated throughout the 1980s, but in the early 1990s it was accepted as at least sometimes effective. The questions were refined to ask which techniques are effective with whom and when. Research on neuropsychotherapy and on related interventions might do well to focus on global and specific efficacy simultaneously. Much of this book emphasizes the need to integrate cognitive and emotional rehabilitation and to look at functional outcomes. Global efficacy studies should look at flexible interventions that work with the whole person. Meanwhile, specific techniques for frustration, anosognosia, embarrassment, impulsive anger, reflex crying, disinhibition, and so forth can be studied through single subject designs. Some techniques suggested here need more development through clinical experience before they can be investigated, for example, interventions for overprotection, for diminished emotional responsiveness, and for personality changes sometimes accompanying temporal lobe epilepsy.

Results obtained in research centers need to be confirmed in other settings to have confidence of their applicability, especially for the developing world, for community-based rehabilitation programs, for support groups, and for homes, which vary quite significantly from university hospital settings in their personnel, their resources, and their populations. This book is biased toward techniques that it is hoped will prove to be appropriate, transferable technology.

### *Emotional Changes*

Research, much of it outside the confines of psychiatry's diagnostic categories, is needed to define more carefully the emotional changes accompanying brain illnesses. Structured interviews (Kay et al., 1995), combined with formal tests of emotional communication (Mountain & Spreen, 1993; Ross, 1981, 1993) and physiological measures (Damasio et al., 1990), may help determine the accuracy and clinical utility of the conceptualization of emotional changes presented here. Case study methodology (Shallice, 1979) has proven critical to the exploration of specific cognitive subsystems and may be useful here. If these conceptualizations are confirmed physiologically and phenomenologically, then well-identified exemplars could be studied with neuroimaging and with functional imaging, which may lead to better psychopharmacological interventions.

Current knowledge of emotional changes of brain illness needs to be extended to other populations, most notably children. Cultural variations also need to be considered. For example, Prigatano and Leathem (1993) found that anosognosia differed significantly between native Maoris and white New Zealanders.

### *Education*

Family education following a brain illness is widely espoused but little researched. Some public misconceptions about TBI result from misleading discussions with professionals (Gouvier, Prestholdt, & Warner, 1988), so research regarding the effectiveness of education is clearly needed. Investigations demonstrating that information is adequately conveyed and understood and that the recipient is satisfied are fairly straightforward. More important, but also more difficult, are investigations demonstrating that family behavior has changed, that skills were learned and applied, and that they were effective in dealing with the problems of the injured person.

Institutionally sponsored public education has a place in changing society's opinions and attitudes. However, such efforts can be dry and uninteresting and often do not reach people not already interested. What seems to reach public opinion much more broadly and effectively is the Lou Gehrig effect—the public takes notice when a celebrity has an illness. What is memorable and interesting are human interest stories, case studies, storytelling, and even talk shows. The stories of Lou Gehrig, Woody Guthrie, Betty Ford, Patricia Neal, James Brady, Annette Funicello, Ronald Reagan, Magic Johnson, and Muhammad Ali may have done more, for better or worse, to advance public awareness and knowledge regarding amyotrophic lateral sclerosis, Huntington's disease, alcohol and drug addiction, stroke, TBI, multiple sclerosis, Alzheimer's disease, AIDS, and Parkinson's disease, respectively, than government-sponsored public education programs on those conditions. Likewise, motion pictures such as *Rain Man, Regarding Henry, The Broken Cord, My Left Foot,* and *Awakenings* are often very far-reaching and compelling. Unfortunately, so are less accurate representations. Gouvier, Prestholdt, & Warner (1988) found that most public misconceptions about brain trauma—for example, that a second blow to the head restores memory—come from public media, especially television. Study of what the public knows regarding brain illnesses (Willer, Johnson, Rempel, & Linn, 1993), how they know it, and what their attitudes are (Devlieger et al., 1994) might allow public education efforts to be better focused.

Public knowledge, awareness, misconceptions, priorities for educational programs, and effective public education techniques are likely to vary widely by country and by culture (e.g., Devlieger et al., 1994). The work of rehabilitation professionals is likely to move from direct service toward educating and training others (World Health Organization, 1981). Research to support this change is needed to clarify what techniques consistently facilitate recovery and functioning in the community and how those techniques can be reliably and efficiently taught.

### *Social Context*

Research on the social context of the lives of people with brain illness is off to a good start (see Chapters 13 and 14). There is good reason to believe, however, that this context is likely to vary significantly from culture to culture (Cavallo & Saucedo, 1995; Dikengil et al., 1993; Galanti, 1991; Lynch & Hanson, 1992; Ramirez, 1991; D. Sue & W. Sue, 1990; Werner, 1990). For this reason, one priority in this field that carries considerable clinical significance is to study the generalizability of these findings to other cultures.

Although investigations reliably tell us that high percentages of people with brain illnesses and their families have major, enduring psychosocial problems, there has been little focus on individuals and families who do well and why this is the case (Ridley, 1989). Although the field of rehabilitation claims to be interested in successful coping with disability, it is but little studied when compared to unsuccessful coping (including this book).

## *DIRECTIONS FOR FUTURE ACTION*

The purpose of this book is not simply to teach professionals how to offer certain brain-illness mental health services, but rather to help make society more understanding, respectful, and accepting of people with brain illnesses. This book is directed primarily toward mental health and rehabilitation professionals because they can bring about some of that change. However, non-professionals, especially those personally affected by brain illnesses, are also critical in facilitating change (Chapter 14). This is not easily done. The behavior of many people with brain illnesses can be alienating and appears bizarre. Understanding comes both from scientific study and from personal openness. Understanding—both intellectual and emotional—may facilitate respect and acceptance, but it cannot guarantee them. These come from deeper values. At a minimum, professionals can facilitate respect and acceptance by modeling. The readers of this book are probably, for the most part, able-brained and economically comfortable. However that status could change for any of us at any time. Most of us will live to be old and are likely to experience at least some deterioration of mental functions. We have a personal stake in facilitating respect and acceptance.

Earlier parts of this book concern therapeutic empathy. However, this is often a shallow empathy for someone else's feelings of the moment or empathy as a clinical skill, not necessarily empathy as an existential experience. It is hoped that this book has stimulated its readers to go beyond this shallow sense of empathy, to think of people with brain illnesses as much more than patients, as collections of problems, as cases, or as clients, and instead, to think of them as neighbors, as friends, as family members, as community members, or as ourselves. Hopefully, such empathy will lead to interventions that we, ourselves, would be willing to receive; interventions that are respectful and not controlling, patronizing, condescending, or hateful. When as professionals we help make places in society for people with brain illnesses we can strive to make places that we would be glad to take in similar circumstances, because any of us may take those places tomorrow.

Public opinions and attitudes can change bit by bit through personal experience. As each person with a brain illness is helped back into the community with support and with education, family, friends, schoolmates, co-workers, and neighbors become informed and perhaps more supportive. However, the roles of professionals, professional organizations, and communities go beyond service one-by-one. One important form of community action is to facilitate support groups, their larger organizations, and the work they do in public education and policy and in legislative advocacy. However, professionals must not help such groups too much. Professionals and their institutions inevitably have interests distinct from those of people with brain illnesses and of their families. Professionals tend to seek professional solutions and to advocate for more professional services and research. People with brain illnesses may instead need more community acceptance, legal advocacy, accessible jobs and housing, opportunities, and protection from discrimination. At times, professionals can be more a part of the problem than a part of the solution, as is recognized by the independent living movement and the disabilities rights movement. The proper role of the professional often is to facilitate the founding of such organizations, to help out when asked, but otherwise to get out of the way and let them do what they need to do. That is true empowerment.

Most brain illnesses are preventable. Prevention is something all professionals working in the area can advocate for without ever worrying that it will drive us out of work. This is already well-entrenched in many U.S. rehabilitation programs for personal responsibility aspects of prevention, in keeping with mainstream U.S. values. Programs on seat belt and on helmet use, preventing drunk driving, drug abuse prevention, AIDS prevention, control of hypertension, stress reduction, and so forth are well established, if not yet universally effective. The social dimensions of prevention are less consistently attended to, but are also of tremendous importance. This is certainly true in the United States, but it is particularly true in those parts of the world where few can afford private vehicles, helmets, or even antihypertensive medication, and where a sense of personal responsibility is less highly regarded and less consistently rewarded. In this larger sense, brain injury and illness prevention also includes public health measures to reduce the spread of malaria, cysticercosis, meningitis, and so forth; to improve occupational health, including reducing industrial and agricultural toxic exposures; to assure universal primary health care; to improve perinatal nutrition; to assure economic justice; to prevent interpersonal violence; and, last but far from least, to prevent war.

# Appendix A

## Classification of Factors Affecting Personality following Brain Illness

(see Chapters 2 and 9–12 for detailed discussion.)
? = not yet well-accepted. * = described below but not in text.

I. Psychological Factors
- A. Pre-brain illness personality*
- B. Psychological reactions to illness
  1. Grief Reactions
     - a. Shock*
     - b. Denial
     - c. Anger
     - d. Depression
  2. Anxiety
  3. Perplexity
  4. Frustration
  5. Embarrassment
  6. Catastrophic reaction
  7. Post-traumatic stress disorder
  8. Paranoia*
  9. Obsessions/compulsions*
  10. Personal reformation

II. Neuropsychological (Organic) Factors
- A. Emotional changes
  1. Changes in emotional communication
     - a. Decreased emotional communication abilities
       - i. Impaired emotional expression
       - ii. Impaired emotional comprehension
       - iii. Alexithymia?*

        b. Increased involuntary emotional communication
            i. Reflex crying
            ii. Reflex laughing
            iii. Automatic cursing (aphasia, Tourette's)
    2. Changes in emotional reactivity
        a. Decreased emotional reactivity
        b. Increased emotional reactivity
            i. Labile emotions
            ii. Irritability, impulsive anger, agitation
            iii. Temporal lobe epilepsy personality?
        c. Changes in type of emotional reaction
B. Executive function impairments
    1. Lack of awareness of deficits (anosognosia)
    2. Disorders of activation
        a. Disorders of initiation
            i. Impaired initiation (abulia)
            ii. Excessive initiation (disinhibition)
        b. Disorders of termination
            i. Impaired termination (perseveration)
                1). Continuous (motor) perseveration
                2). Recurrent perseveration
                3). Stuck-in-set perseveration
                4). Memory perseveration
                5). Organic obsessions and compulsions?
            ii. Excessive termination (impersistence)*
    3. Concreteness (impaired abstraction/reasoning)
        a. Self-centeredness
        b. Lack of empathy
        c. Childishness
        d. Delusions
    4. Impaired monitoring and judgment
    5. Impaired planning and organization
    6. Impaired communication pragmatics
        a. Nonverbal behavior impairment
        b Turn-taking impairment
            i. Impaired awareness of listener
            ii. Impaired listening
        c. Topic maintenance impairment
        d. Social inappropriateness
        e. Impaired conversation repair
        f. Lack of cohesiveness of narrative

- C. Cognitively mediated changes of personality
  - 1. Attention impairments
    - a. Capacity impairment (speed, persistence)
    - b. Control impairment (distractibility, impaired selective, alternating, divided attention)
  - 2. Memory impairments
    - a. Anterograde amnesia
    - b. Retrograde amnesia
    - c. Procedural memory impairments
    - d. Semantic and episodic memory impairments
    - e. Material-specific amnesia
    - f. Prospective memory impairment
    - g. Confabulation
  - 3. Language impairments
    - a. Expression impairment
    - b. Comprehension impairment
    - c. Reading impairment
  - 4. Visual–spatial impairments*
  - 5. Apraxia*

III. Medical Factors
- A. Sensory impairments*
  - 1. Vision impairments
  - 2. Hearing impairments
  - 3. Somesthesis impairments
  - 4. Kinesthesis impairments
  - 5. Equilibrium impairments
- B. Motor impairments*
  - 1. Impaired strength
  - 2. Impaired coordination
  - 3. Movement disorders
- C. Pain*
- D. Orthopedic or other medical limitations
- E. Fatigue

## *Factors Not Elaborated in the Text*

### *Pre-Illness Personality Risk Factors*

Some types of brain illness have behavioral risk factors and are more likely to occur in some personality types than others:

1. TBI—angry, risk-taking, substance-abusing, young males.

2. Stroke—Type A personality, smokers, people prone to incomplete medical adherence.
3. AIDS—homosexual and bisexual males, multipartner heterosexuals, IV drug abusers, risk-takers.

Some behavioral patterns are predisposed to brain illness:

1. Substance abusers—at risk for toxicity, trauma, stroke, anoxia, dietary deficiencies.
2. Suicide attempters—at risk for trauma, toxicity, anoxia.

*Psychological Reactions*

*Shock.* Although awake and alert, the person in emotional shock has limited ability to respond to the environment beyond routine ways. He may show psychic numbing or extreme emotional reactions. This is usually a relatively short-lived experience, ranging from a few seconds to a few hours.

*Paranoia.* Loss of control over many aspects of one's life often results from brain illness. A paranoid interpretation of these losses and of other events can come from confusion, from amnesia, from denial, from a lack of awareness of deficits, from difficulty appreciating another person's perspective, and/or from misperceiving communication. Some pre-illness conditions may predispose one to paranoia, particularly dependency (Prigatano, O'Brien, & Klonoff, 1988).

*Obsessions/compulsions.* Some people adopt obsessions or compulsions as inefficient compensations for memory deficits.

*Alexithymia* (*emotional anomia? emotional agnosia?*).—This controversial concept is a selective verbal deficit in expressing emotions, particularly an inability to identify and label one's own emotions (Sifneos, 1994). Although it is clear that some people are poor at identifying and at labeling their own feelings (due to a lack of experience or to teaching?), it is not yet clear that alexithymia is a distinct, organic neuropsychological disorder.

*Excessive termination* (*impersistence*).—Some individuals have difficulty appropriately maintaining an activity they have started (Rosenbaum, Fischer, & Leavell, 1994), due, at least in part, to attention impairments or to fatigue.

*Impaired visual-spatial abilities.* Some subtypes of visual-spatial deficits can have a minor effect on personality. People with unilateral neglect (a tendency to ignore one side of personal space) may ignore people standing on their neglected side, and they may feel slighted. Impaired perception of emotion (see

Chapter 10) has a visual–spatial component in the interpretation of facial expression and of body language.

*Apraxia.* Impairments in skilled motor movements can be frustrating and disabling. It is possible that apraxia could affect sexual abilities, but this has not been well studied.

*Motor, sensory, and perceptual impairments.* People with notable motor impairments such as tremors, incoordination, or hemiplegia, or sensory impairments such as visual or auditory difficulties may have their independence, communication, and mobility compromised, limiting their social opportunities. How their visible disability is perceived by others can become a major issue (Eisenberg, Griggens, & Duvall, 1982; Wright, 1983).

*Chronic pain.* Chronic pain is fairly frequent in people with brain illnesses (and in the general population, as well). Chronic pain has a psychological dimension; moods, coping strategies, and attitudes impact the amount of disability, pain, and suffering experienced, regardless of organic injury. Many people with chronic pain benefit from behavioral (Fordyce, Roberts, & Sternbach, 1985), cognitive-behavioral (Hanson & Gerber, 1990), and/or psychodynamic (Coen & Sarno, 1989; Miller, 1993) psychological intervention (Benjamin, 1989).

*Rare conditions.* Many rare organic syndromes not included in this scheme have their own distinct peculiarities and personality effects. A few examples are Anton's syndrome (denial of blindness; Heilman, 1991; McGlynn & Schacter, 1989), prosopagnosia (inability to recognize people by their faces; A. R. Damasio, Damasio & Van Hoesen, 1982), reduplicative paramnesia (in which the person believes two or more, nearly identical locations exist; Stuss et al., 1992), and Capgras syndrome (in which the person believes that someone has been replaced by a duplicate; Stuss et al., 1992). Doubtless there are other conditions not yet discovered and described, which also produce unusual behavior and experiences.

# Appendix B

# Contemporary Neuropsychological Personality Assessment Tools

## *GENERAL*

*The Behavior Change Inventory* (BCI; Hartlage, 1991) is an adjective checklist that is completed both as a self-report and as a report by an informant, and refers to personality both before and after the brain injury, allowing for (cautious) interpretation of changes in personality and in self-awareness. Its ease of administration and of completion makes it useful for evaluating cognitively impaired subjects. Research data on the BCI are limited and there are intrinsic limits to the sophistication possible with an adjective checklist.

*The Head Injury Family Interview* (HI-FI; Kay et al., 1995) is a state-of-the-art, five-part structured interview, supplemented with a problem checklist. The interviews and checklist are for both the person with the injury and an informant; they allow for easy comparisons of perspectives. There are specific sections in the informant interviews for parents, for spouses, for siblings, and for children. The questions proceed from general and open-ended to specific. The interviews cover the pre-injury background, the history of the disability, community integration, and functional competencies. There is considerable detail concerning behavioral and affective changes, interpersonal skills, and actual functioning, as well as the impact of the injury on the family. Although it was designed for use with TBI, it can be easily and appropriately adapted to many other forms of brain insult.

The HI-FI requires 1 1/2 to 2 hours of clinician time to administer. However, when not used for research, a clinician can, with experience, use the HI-FI selectively, skipping parts of less relevance to the particular circumstances or where the information has been obtained from other sources, but using the interview as a model and a check on thoroughness. Some parts can be filled out as a questionnaire, but the interview format is preferred. Reliability is acceptable, and preliminary validity data are promising. Results of these studies have been factor analyzed, but the HI-FI has not been used to derive scales. The HI-FI was developed using public funds and is in the public domain. The authors encourage adaptations.

*The Behavioral Symptoms and Social Behavior scale (R1) of the Katz Adjustment Scale* (Katz & Lyerly, 1963) has been used in several studies of outcome from brain injuries (e.g., Fordyce, Roueche, & Prigatano, 1983; Goran & Fabiano, 1993; Hinkeldey & Corrigan, 1990; Klonoff, Snow, & Costa, 1986) and from multiple sclerosis (Rao et al., 1991). The person with a brain injury is assessed by a relative on 13 scales of general psychological functions, not unlike those of the MMPI, and comparisons are made to general and to psychiatric standardization norms (Hogarty & Katz, 1971). Data are accumulating to support validity in neurological groups along with findings that augment other sources of psychosocial data. The Katz has been modified and refactored for use with a brain-injured population (Jackson, Hopewell, Glass, & Warburg, 1992).

*The Coolidge Axis II Inventory* (CATI; Coolidge & Merwin, 1992) is a 200 item, 4-point true–false Likert scale self-report inventory of personality disorders that contains a Neuropsychological Dysfunction Scale (16 items) with Memory (6 items), Language (5 items), and Somatic (5 items) subscales. The Neuropsychological Dysfunction Scale items were theoretically derived and appear to discriminate mild TBI from normal adequately. However, the other scales are not specifically designed for neuropsychological use, and their usefulness in this context is unknown.

*The Memory Assessment Clinics–Psychiatric* (MAC–P; Crook, Feher, & Larrabee, 1993) is a clinician-rated instrument for dementia and for related disorders. It consists of 25 items based largely on in-clinic behavior. Its 8 empirically derived factors include 3 quasi-affective dimensions: general psychiatric, depression, and somatic complaints. Initial reliability and validity are satisfactory. This scale is specific to a neuropsychological population and is useful for some needs, but it is not sufficiently specific to give a great deal of direction to intervention for emotional and for behavioral problems.

*The Neurobehavioral Rating Scale* (Levin, et al., 1987) is a modification of the Brief Psychiatric Rating Scale with new scales reflecting functional issues of TBI, including diminished insight and disinhibition. These clinicians' ratings are based on observations of patients' behavior during interview, testing, and hospitalization. Levin and colleagues have presented excellent reliability data and early studies of validity. The scale is particularly useful for repeated measurements in an inpatient or in a similar setting where behavioral observations in a variety of conditions are possible. The scale does not require much time to complete, it covers a range of neurobehavioral problems well, and it is sufficiently sensitive to be used to measure change. It does not easily allow for comparisons of pre-injury with post-injury behavior or for a comparison of self-rating with informant rating.

*The Neuropsychology Behavior and Affect Profile* (Nelson et al. 1989, 1994) incorporates both "before" and "after" and self- and peer ratings. The lengthy development process has resulted in a scale of tolerable length with acceptable reliability and validity data. It has only five scales (Indifference, Inappropriateness, Pragnosia [impaired communication pragmatics], Depression, Mania), which are apparently based on *a priori* choices rather than on empirical criteria.

*The Rancho los Amigos Scale* (Hagen, 1982) is widely employed in rating the level of recovery from a TBI based on behavior, on cognition, and on emotional state. It is particularly popular in inpatient rehabilitation where rapid change often does not permit or require more detailed assessment. It is less adequate for outpatient and for chronic settings because of insufficient specificity. Reliability and validity data for its eight stages of recovery are not available.

## *SPECIFIC*

*The Neuropsychiatric Inventory* (Cummings, 1997) is a structured interview administered to caregivers of people with dementia concerning the person for whom they care. It has subscales of delusions, hallucinations, agitation, dysphoria, anxiety, apathy, irritability, euphoria, disinhibition, aberrant motor behavior, night-time behavior disturbances, appetite and eating abnormalities, and caregiver distress, all of which are rated for severity and frequency. Reliability, validity, and cross-cultural applicability are established.

*The Cornell Scale for Depression and Dementia* (Alexopoulos et al., 1988) and the *Dementia Mood Assessment Scale* (Sunderland et al., 1988) provide for either clinician's ratings of depression based on interview of the person with dementia and of professional caregivers or for direct observation of the affect and the behavior of the person with dementia during interview. These scales are specifically designed for the neurologically impaired, and they overcome many of the problems of overlapping symptoms in instruments not designed for these populations.

*The Structured Assessment of Depression in Brain-Damaged Individuals* (SADBD; Gordon et al., 1991) is a structured interview that has been modified both in content and in presentation to account for neurological dysfunction. It incorporates an assessment of the person's awareness of his own symptoms of neurological dysfunction, a modified *Hamilton Rating Scale for Depression* (Hamilton, 1960) and a modified *Beck Depression Inventory* (Beck et al., 1961). Visual cue cards are used to help overcome cognitive difficulties. Self-report and/or clinician ratings are used—depending on the accuracy of the self-report, cognitive impairment, and insight—to arrive at *DSM–III-R* diagnoses. Preliminary reliability and validity data from stroke populations are acceptable, and the SADBD holds promise for generalization to other neurological populations. The title says "Brain-Damaged Individuals," but the awareness questions are oriented toward stroke (although earlier versions were more generic). They would not be difficult to adapt to other populations.

*The Post-Stroke Depression Rating Scale* (Gainotti, et al., 1997) is a semistructured interview covering depressed mood, feelings of guilt, suicidal thoughts, vegetative disorders, apathy, anxiety, catastrophic reactions, hyperemotionalism, anhedonia, and diurnal variations. Preliminary studies in Italy found adequate reliability. The profile holds promise for differentiating aspects of depression and related phenomena in stroke.

The *Visual Analogue Mood Scales* are an elegant, if crude, approach to assessing the emotional state of people with severe aphasia (Nyenhuies et al., 1997). These scales use pictorial representations of moods, such as schematic faces (see Figure 9.1, p. 162). People with aphasia are asked by whatever means possible to indicate their mood by pointing to a place on a line between two moods. Such measures are often understood by people with aphasia who lack other means of reporting their moods.

*The Pathological Laughter and Crying Scale* (Robinson et al., 1993) is a quantified rating scale for reflex laughing and crying. It has very good interrater and test-retest reliability. The ratings dissociate from measures of depression.

*The Frontal Lobe Personality Scale* (Grace et al, 1996) consists of 42 items rated on a 5-point Likert scale completed by the person with the brain illness and by a family member describing the person's pre-illness and current behavior. Apathy, Disinhibition, and Executive Dysfunction subscales are derived. The Apathy subscale appears somewhat misnamed, in that the items mostly concern impaired initiation. The scale is reliable and distinguishes frontal lobe injury from unipolar depression and from bipolar disorder.

*The Emotional Perception Test* (Cognisyst, n.d.) consists of 45 nonsense and 45 meaningful sentences spoken by an actress on audio cassette in 5 different emotional tones—happy, angry, frightened, sad, and neutral—that the subject labels via multiple choice. Norms and reliability appear to be adequate.

*The Victoria Emotion Recognition Test* (Mountain & Spreen, 1993) asks subjects to judge the type and intensity of emotion displayed in photographs of faces and in taped voice clips. The instruments employed, although highly idiosyncratic, are shown to be reliable, and initial studies suggest the potential for considerable validity and utility in understanding the emotional behavior and communication of brain-injured individuals. This and similar tests are likely to become more important in the evaluation of disorders of emotional communication and for subsequent intervention planning.

*The Washington Psychosocial Seizure Inventory* (WPSI, Dodrill et al., 1980) and *The Adolescent Psychosocial Seizure Inventory* (Batzel et al., 1991) are well-researched instruments consisting of 132 and 139 (respectively) true–false items. Computer scoring produces 3 validity scales and 8 clinical scales, mostly oriented toward functional adjustment. These inventories are quite useful in screening epilepsy populations for individuals with significant psychosocial problems and for suggesting areas to probe. The WPSI has been translated into at least 13 languages. Limited data suggest that cross-cultural interpretation is not always straightforward (Dodrill et al., 1984; Tiberia & Froman, 1986).

*The Temporal Lobe Epilepsy Personality Inventory* (Bear & Fedio, 1977) makes explicit use of comparisons between self-report and family member report. It is more narrowly directed than the WPSI toward controversial interictal personality changes thought to be present in some individuals with temporal lobe epilepsy.

*The Structured Clinical Interview for Complex Partial Seizure-Like Symptoms* (Roberts et al., 1990) also has a narrow focus, looking for specific behaviors suggestive of one category of seizure. Its primary use is as a behavioral aid in the diagnosis of seizures, rather than as an aid to planning psychological intervention, although it could provide some help in reinterpreting some behaviors for selected individuals.

*The Overt Aggression Scale* (Yudofsky et al., 1986) is a quick, valid, and reliable rating scale that can be used by minimally trained individuals, and it is appropriate for use by family members of people with brain injuries. It rates four areas at four levels, covering verbal aggression and physical aggression against objects, self, and other people. It includes a checklist of interventions applied. It was designed for a brain-injured population, although it is not specific to that population or to differentiating organic from reactive, psychiatric, or characterological aggression.

*The Agitated Behavior Scale* (Corrigan, 1989; Corrigan & Mysiw, 1988) is a valid and reliable measure designed for use by minimally trained staff members in rating people with TBIs. Its 14 items are rated on a 4-point scale.

The *Family Involvement Assessment Scale* (McNeill et al., 1997) is an experimental 37-item rating scale for evaluating families of persons receiving rehabilitation for a TBI. It produces subscales concerning involvement with staff, supportiveness, and involvement with the patient. It has adequate construct validity, but reliability and criterion validity are not yet established. It holds promise for adapting rehabilitation strategies to different family styles.

# Glossary

Rehabilitation and mental health professionals often become so accustomed to their technical vocabulary that they do not realize that their language may confuse or alienate those with whom they work. Other terms may be unintentionally offensive or objectifying (American Psychological Association, 1994). The following is a "glossary" of common technical terms and suggested substitutes for communicating more clearly with the general public. Of course, some technical terms—such as the person's medical diagnosis—should be taught, because the person is likely to encounter them frequently and may need to know them in order to communicate clearly with others, especially other health care professionals. Likewise, people with higher education or with health care backgrounds will often be comfortable conversing in medical terms. However, vocabulary should usually be chosen to include the person with the least technical background who is participating in the discussion.

When it becomes necessary to refer to something repeatedly and the technical term, initials, or acronym is a convenient shorthand, then the term may be introduced and defined, with reminders of the definition on subsequent meetings as needed. Care still needs to be taken to avoid presenting too many new terms at once, especially when used in combination.

Some common words have technical meanings that should be specified the first few times they are used with nonprofessionals; for example, "transfer." Other common words have technical meanings very different from their variable common meanings that are that can produce miscommunication and are often best either avoided or carefully defined and used; for example, "memory," "amnesia," "intelligence," "verbal," and "trauma." For instance, a sentence such as "He has post-traumatic amnesia, but his verbal intelligence is intact," could plausibly—but quite inaccurately—be interpreted by a lay person to suggest, "He can't remember who he is because of his emotional shock, but he could organize and give a speech about yesterday's news."

Some alternatives offered here in italics come from people with brain illnesses and from their families. Such terms may be inaccurate in some regards or for some individuals, or may be insufficiently neutral or genteel for at least some professionals to offer, but may be accepted from certain families if it promotes understanding and rapport. This list is by no means exhaustive, but it may perhaps help to resensitize professionals to clearer communication. See Chapter 3, Family Education, Appropriate section (p. 31) for further discussion.

**Technical Term** **Substitute**

**Abulia** Initiation problems, trouble getting started, *apathy, no drive.*

**Acalculia** Arithmetic difficulties ("math problems" sounds like school exercises).

**Agraphia** Writing difficulty.

**Alexia** Reading difficulty.

**Afflicted With** (e.g. multiple sclerosis) Person with (e.g., multiple sclerosis).

**Agnosia** Trouble recognizing things.

**Ambulate** Walk ("use a wheelchair" for "wheelchair ambulation").

**Amnesia** Although many lay people know this word, it is often popularly associated with dissociative amnesia, with fugue states, or with other psychological causes. Where neurogenic amnesias are intended, it is often clearer to speak of the specific type of memory difficulty. See anterograde amnesia, retrograde amnesia, post-traumatic amnesia, procedural memory, prospective memory.

**Anomia** Difficulty finding words.

**Anosmia** Loss of the sense of smell.

**Anosognosia** Self-awareness problems, trouble recognizing his problems.

**Anterograde Amnesia** New learning difficulties, poor retention, forgets rapidly, *forgetfulness, C.R.S. (can't remember shit) syndrome.*

**Anoxia** Lack of oxygen (to the brain).

**Aphasia** Language difficulties.

**Apraxia** Problems with skilled movements.

**Auditory Impairment** Hearing problem.

**Aural Comprehension** Understanding what is said.

**Brain Damage** Brain injury, brain illness, or the specific condition, such as stroke, accident, meningitis, and so forth.

**Brain-injured** (used as a noun to refer to people) Person (or people) with (a) brain injury(ies).

**Brain Trauma** Brain injury, accident, assault (many people think of "trauma" as emotional trauma more readily than physical trauma, which may lead them to think of "effects of the trauma" as emotional reactions, compounding the miscommunication).

**Cerebral Vascular Accident** (CVA) Stroke.

**Challenged** (e.g.,"mobility challenged") (Considered euphemistic and offensive by some).

**Cognition** Thought.

**Cognitive** Thinking.

**Confabulation** Remembering things that didn't happen, false memories.

**Confined to a wheelchair** Uses a wheelchair.

**Constructional Disorder** Problem with drawing, putting things together, mechanical abilities, and so forth.

**Deficit** Difficulty, problem, weak area, loss.

**Diagnosis as Person** (as in, "the stroke in bed 6") Refer to people as people or by their names ("the person with a stroke in bed 6") When such shorthand must be used, it should be kept strictly among staff.

**Diplopia** Double vision.

**Dysarthria** Slurred speech, problems speaking clearly, difficulty articulating words clearly.

**Emotional Incontinence** Problems controlling emotional expression, reflex crying, reflex laughing.

**Executive Functions** Self-control abilities, the specific function or problem (planning, reasoning, organization, impulsiveness, initiation).

**Hematoma** Blood clot.

**Hemianopsia** Blind on his left (right) side (explaining that it is not the left [right] eye that is blind).

**Hemiplegia** Right (left) sided weakness.

**Hemispatial Neglect** Left (or right) neglect ("he doesn't pay attention to his left side").

**Hemorrhage** Bleeding.

**Hyperaesthesia** Noise (light, movement, touch, smell) intolerance, exaggerated startle.

**Iatrogenic** Caused by the treatment (medicine, etc.).

**Impairment** Difficulty, problem, weak area, loss.

**Impersistence** Trouble keeping going, *problems with stick-to-itiveness.*

**Infarct** Stroke.

**Initiation** Starting ability, *"my get-up-and-go got up and went".*

**Intelligence** Psychologists usually use this to mean "what IQ tests measure," whereas lay people have a variety of understandings of the term. ("If he still has his intelligence, why can't he figure out how to use the microwave oven?") Avoiding it can avoid misunderstandings. Describe more specific functions, instead.

**Lesion** Injury, bruise, wound, sore (on skin).

**Lower extremity** Leg.

**Memory** This word has many technical meanings and many lay meanings which can easily cause miscommunication. It is often better to be more specific. See anterograde amnesia, retrograde amnesia, posttraumatic amnesia, procedural memory, prospective memory.

**Mnemonic** Memory.

**Motor Impairment** Weakness, problem with movement, strength, coordination (as appropriate).

**Neologism** Nonsense word, word error that doesn't make sense.

**Neoplasm** Tumor.

**Neuroanatomy** Neuroanatomical terms beyond brain, spine, nerve, and nerve cell are rarely really necessary and should be avoided when possible.

**Neurogenic** Caused by the brain injury (illness).

**Nonverbal Functions** Nonlanguage functions, or name the specific function.

**Occlusion** Blockage, stroke.

**O.T.** Occupational Therapy (until the abbreviation is learned).

**Oral Expression** Talking, saying what he means.

**Organic** Resulting directly from the injury to the brain (nerves, body, etc.).

**Paraphasia** Speech error, word confusion, word substitution error.

**Patient** People with brain injuries, clients, Francois, and so forth.

**Perseveration** Abnormal repeating.

**Post-traumatic Amnesia** Memory loss resulting from the accident, loss of memory from around the time of the accident.

**Pragmatics** Conversation skills, or the specific function: facial expression, body language, eye contact, taking turns, listening, staying on topic, taking your audience into account, and so forth.

**Premorbid** Before the illness (injury).

**Procedural Memory** Skill memory, remembering how to do things.

**Prospective Memory** Remembering to do things at the right time.

**Pseudo-Bulbar Palsy** Problems controlling emotional expression, reflex crying, reflex laughing.

**P.T.** Physical Therapy (until the abbreviation is learned).

**Receptive Language** Listening (to speech), reading.

**Reduced Emotional Reactivity** Less intense feelings, *automaton, robot.*

**Retrograde Amnesia** Loss of old memories.

**Senility** Literally, this means old. When senile dementia is meant, "Alzheimer's disease" (or other specific disease, as appropriate) should be used instead.

**Somatosensory Deficit** Loss of sense of touch, reduced sensation.

**Stroke** Damage to the blood supply to the brain.

**"The Family," "The Wife," and so Forth** Your family, Joe's wife, Maria, his son, and so forth.

**Suffer (as in "He Suffered a Stroke")** Experience, have ("suffer" suggests pity).

**Survivor** This term is preferred by some support groups, but others feel it suggests false heroics.

**Transfer** Moving from bed to wheelchair and so forth.

**Trauma** Physical trauma can be confused with emotional trauma. The particular use should be specified.

**Upper Extremity** Arm.

**Verbal** This term is often used, even by professionals, to mean "oral" ("If he can't understand it verbally, write it down.") It is often better to avoid the term to avoid misunderstanding. Use "language."

**Verbal Comprehension** Understanding what is said (understanding what he reads).

**Verbal Expression** Talking, saying what he means (and writing).

**Victim (as in "Stroke Victim")** Person living with a stroke, person who had a brain injury, and so forth ("victim" suggests pity and puts the stroke rather than the person first, as if the person loses his identity and becomes the disease).

**Visual–Spatial Abilities** Artistic abilities, mechanical abilities, finding your way, and so on.

# References


Alexopoulos, G., Abrams, R., Young, R., & Shamoian, C. (1988). Cornell scale for depression in dementia. *Biological Psychiatry, 23,* 271–284.

Alfano, D., Finlayson, A., Stearns, G., & Neilson, P. (1990). The MMPI and neurologic dysfunction: Profile configuration and analysis. *The Clinical Neuropsychologist, 4,* 69–79.

Allen, S. N. (1994). Psychological assessment of post-traumatic stress disorder: Psychometrics, current trends, and future directions. *Psychiatric Clinics of North America.17,* 327–349.

American Heart Association (n.d.). *Guidelines for organizing stroke clubs.* (Available from author, Stroke Connection, 7272 Greenville Ave., Dallas, TX 75231–4596, U.S.A.)

American Heart Association of Wisconsin. (1988). *Sexuality After Stroke.* Milwaukee, WI: Author.

American Psychiatric Association. (1994). *Diagnostic and statistical manual of mental disorders* (4th ed.). Washington, DC: Author.

American Psychological Association. (1994). *Publication manual of the American Psychological Association* (4th Ed.). Washington, DC: Author.

Ames, D., Cummings, J. L., Wirshing, W. C., Quinn, B., & Mahler, M. (1994). Repetitive and compulsive behavior in frontal lobe degenerations. *Journal of Neuropsychiatry and Clinical Neurosciences. 6,* 100–113.

Antonak R. F., Livneh, H., & Antonak, C. (1993). A review of research on psychosocial adjustment to impairment in persons with traumatic brain injury. *Journal of Head Trauma Rehabilitation, 8*(4), 87–100.

Ardila, A., & Ostrosky–Solis, F. (1991). *Diagnóstico del Daño Cerebral: Enfoque Neuropsicológico.* [Diagnosis of Brain Damage: A Neuropsychological Focus]. Mexico City, Mexico: Trillas.

Ardila, A., & Rosselli, M., 1992. *Neuropsicología Clínica* [Clinical Neuropsychology]. Medellín, Colombia: Prensa Creativa.

Aronson, M. K., & Yatzkan, E. S. (1984). Coping with Alzheimer's disease through support groups. *Aging, 347,* 4–9.

Baddeley, A. D. (1992). Implicit memory and errorless learning: A link between cognitive theory and neuropsychological rehabilitation? In L. R. Squire & N. Butters (Eds.), *Neuropsychology of memory* (2nd ed., pp. 309–314). New York: Guilford.

Barkley, R. A. (1997). *ADHD and the nature of Self-Control.* New York: Guilford.

Barrett, K. (1991). Treating organic abulia with bromocriptine and lisuride: Four case studies. *Journal of Neurology, Neurosurgery and Psychiatry, 54,* 718–721.

Batzel, L. W., Dodrill, C. B., Dubinsky, B. L., Ziegler, R. G., Connolly, J. E., Freeman, R. D.,

Farwell, J. R., & Vening, E. P. G. (1991). An objective method for the assessment of psychosocial problems in adolescents with epilepsy. *Epilepsia, 32*, 202–211.

Bear, D. M. (1979). Temporal lobe epilepsy: A syndrome of sensory–limbic hyperconnection. *Cortex, 15*, 357–384.

Bear, D., & Fedio, P. (1977). Quantitative analysis of interictal behavior in temporal lobe epilepsy. *Archives of Neurology, 34*, 454–467.

Beck, A., Ward, C., Mendelson, M., Mock, J., & Erbaugh, J. (1961). An inventory for measuring depression. *Archives of General Psychiatry, 4*, 561–571.

Becker, M. E., & Vakil, E. (1993). Behavioural psychotherapy of the frontal-lobe-injured patient in an outpatient setting. *Brain Injury, 7*, 515–523.

Benjamin, S. (1989). Psychological treatment of chronic pain: A selective review. *Journal of Psychosomatic Research, 33*, 121–131.

Bennett, T. L. (Ed., 1992). *The Neuropsychology of epilepsy.* New York: Plenum.

Ben–Yishay, Y., & Lakin, P. (1989). Structured group treatment for brain-injury survivors. In D. W. Ellis & A. L. Christensen (Eds.), *Neuropsychological treatment after brain injury* (pp. 271–295). Boston: Kluwer.

Bergquist, T. F., & Jacket, M. P. (1993). Awareness and goal setting with the traumatically brain injured. *Brain Injury, 7*, 275–282.

Bhatia, K. P., & Marsden, C. D. (1994). The behavioural and motor consequences of focal lesions of the basal ganglia in man. *Brain, 117*, 859–876.

Binder, L. M. (1992). Deception and malingering. In A. E. Puente & R. J. McCaffrey (Eds.), *Handbook of neuropsychological assessment: A biopsychosocial perspective* (pp. 353–374). New York: Plenum.

Binder, L. M. (1993). An abbreviated form of the Portland Digit Recognition Test. *The Clinical Neuropsychologist, 7*, 104–107.

Bishop, D. S., & Miller, I. W. (1988). Traumatic brain injury: Empirical family assessment techniques. *The Journal of Head Trauma Rehabilitation, 3*(4), 16–30.

Bishop, G. D. (1994). *Health psychology: Integrating mind and body.* Boston: Allyn & Bacon.

Black, D. W. (1982). Pathological laughter: A review of the literature. *The Journal of Nervous and Mental Disease, 170*(2), 67–71.

Block, S. H. (1987). Psychotherapy of the individual with brain injury. *Brain Injury,1*, 203–220.

Blonder, L. X., Gur, R. E., & Gur, R. C. (1989). The effects of right and left hemiparkinsonism on prosody. *Brain and Language, 36*, 193–207.

Blosser, J. L., & DePompei, R. (1989). The head injured student returns to school: Recognizing and treating deficits. *Topics in Language Disorders, 9*(2), 67–77.

Blosser, J. L., & DePompei, R. (1995). Fostering effective family involvement through mentoring. *Journal of Head Trauma Rehabilitation, 10*(2), 46–56.

Blumer, D., & Benson, D. F., (1975). Personality changes with frontal and temporal lobe lesions. In D. F. Benson & D. Blumer (Eds.), *Psychiatric aspects of neurologic disease* (Vol. 1, pp. 151–170). New York: Grune & Stratton.

Bohnen, N., Twijnstra, A., Kroeze, J., & Jolles, J. (1991). A psychophysiological method for assessing visual and acoustic hyperaesthesia in patients with mild head injury. *British Journal of Psychiatry, 159*, 860–863.

Bornstein, R. A., & Kozora, E. (1990). Content bias of the MMPI scale Sc in neurological patients. *Neuropsychiatry, Neuropsychology, and Behavioral Neurology, 3*, 200–205.

Borod, J. C. (1992). Interhemispheric and intrahemispheric control of emotion: A focus on unilateral brain damage. *Journal of Consulting and Clinical Psychology, 60*, 339–348.

Boudewyns, P. A., Hyer, L., Woods, M. G., Harrison, W., & McCranie, E. (1990). PTSD among Vietnam veterans: An early look at treatment outcome using direct therapeutic exposure. *Journal of Traumatic Stress, 3*(3), 359–368.

Brannon, L., & Feist, J. (1992). *Health psychology : An introduction to behavior and health.* Belmont, CA: Wadsworth.
Brodal, A. (1973). Self-observations and neuroanatomical considerations after a stroke. *Brain, 96,* 675–694.
Brumback, R. A. (1993). *Neurology and clinical neuroscience.* New York: Springer–Verlag.
Brooks, N. (1991). The head-injured family. *Journal of Clinical and Experimental Neuropsychology, 13,* 155–188.
Bullis, R. K., & Cherry, A. D. (1994). Pastoral care for the head-injured: A biopsychosocial/spiritual perspective. *Pastoral Psychology, 42,* 321–333.
Burgess, P. W., & Alderman, N. (1990). Rehabilitation of dyscontrol syndromes following frontal lobe damage: A cognitive neuropsychological approach. In R. L. Wood & I. Fussey (Eds.), *Cognitive rehabilitation in perspective* (pp. 183–203). London: Taylor & Francis.
Burke, J. M., Danick, J. A., Bemis, B., & Durgin, C. J. (1994). A process approach to memory book training for neurological patients. *Brain Injury, 8,* 71–81.
Burke, W. H., & Wesolowski, M. D. (1988). *Applied behavior analysis in brain injury rehabilitation.* Houston, TX: HDI.
Burns, D. (1981). *Feeling good: The new mood therapy.* New York: Signet.
Busch, C. R., & Alpern, H. P. (1998). Depression after mild traumatic brain injury: A review of current research. *Neuropsychology Review, 8,* 95–108.
Butcher, J. N., Dahlstrom, W. G., Graham, J. R., Tellegen, A., & Kaemmer, B. (1989). *Minnesota Multiphasic Personality Inventory–2: Manual for administration and scoring.* Minneapolis, MN: University of Minnesota Press.
Campbell, J. J., Duffy, J. D., & Salloway, S. P. (1994). Treatment strategies for patients with dysexecutive syndromes. *Journal of Neuropsychiatry and Clinical Neurosciences, 6,* 411–418.
Carberry, H. (1991). Psychotherapy in an adult rehabilitation setting. *Cognitive Rehabilitation,* 9(2), 16–18.
Carroll, D. (1992). *Health psychology : Stress, behaviour and disease.* Washington, DC: Falmer Press.
Cavallo, M. M., & Saucedo, C. (1995). Traumatic brain injury in families from culturally diverse populations. *Journal of Head Trauma Rehabilitation, 10*(2), 66–77.
Chittum, W. R., Johnson, K., Chittum, J. M., Guercio, J. M., & McMorrow, M. J. (1996). Road to awareness: An individualized training package for increasing knowledge and comprehension of personal deficits in persons with acquired brain injury. *Brain Injury, 10,* 763–776.
Christensen, A. L. (1989). The neuropsychological investigation as a therapeutic and rehabilitative technique. In D.W. Ellis & A. L. Christensen (Eds.), *Neuropsychological treatment after brain injury* (pp. 127–153). Boston: Kluwer.
Christensen, A. L. & Rosenberg, N. K. (1991). A critique of the role of psychotherapy in brain injury rehabilitation. *Journal of Head Trauma Rehabilitation, 6*(4), 56–61.
Cicerone, K. D. (1991). Psychotherapy after mild traumatic brain injury: Relation to the nature and severity of subjective complaints. *Journal of Head Trauma Rehabilitation, 6*(4), 30–43.
Cicerone, K. D. (1992). Psychological management of post–concussion disorders. In L. J. Horn & N. D. Zasler, (Eds.), *Rehabilitation of post-concussive disorders* (pp. 129–142). Philadelphia: Hanley & Belfus.
Cicerone, K. D., & Giacino, J. T. (1992). Remediation of executive function deficits after traumatic brain injury. *NeuroRehabilitation, 2,* 12–22.
Cicerone, K. D., & Tupper, D. E. (1990). Neuropsychological rehabilitation: Treatment of errors in everyday functioning. In D. E. Tupper & K. D. Cicerone (Eds.), *The neuropsychology of everyday life: Issues in development and rehabilitation.* Boston: Kluwer.
Coen, S. J., & Sarno, J. E. (1989). Psychosomatic avoidance of conflict in back pain. *Journal of the American Academy of Psychoanalysis, 17.* 359–376.

CogniSyst (n.d.). *Emotional Perception Test.* Durham, NC: CogniSyst.

Cohen, H. (Ed., 1993). *Neuroscience for rehabilitation.* Philadelphia, PA: Lippincott.

Cohen, N. J., & Squire, L. R. (1980). Preserved learning and retention of pattern-analyzing skills in amnesia: Dissociation of knowing how and knowing that. *Science, 210,* 207–210.

Coolidge, F. L., & Merwin, M. M. (1992). Reliability and validity of the Coolidge Axis II Inventory: A new inventory for the assessment of personality disorders. *Journal of Personality Assessment, 59,* 223–238.

Comfort, A. (Ed., 1998). *Sexual consequences of disability.* Philadelphia, PA: George F. Stickley.

Cook, J. V. (1990). Returning to work after traumatic head injury. In M. Rosenthal, E. R. Griffity, J. R. Bond, & J. D. Miller (Eds.), *Rehabilitation of the adult and child with traumatic brain injury* (2nd ed., pp. 493–505). Philadelphia, PA: F. A. Davis.

Corman, A., & Sandman, C. (1997). Cognitive deficits and their remediation in the homeless. *Journal of Cognitive Rehabilitation, 15*(1), 16–23.

Corrigan, J. D. (1989). Development of a scale for assessment of agitation following traumatic brain injury. *Journal of Clinical and Experimental Neuropsychology, 11,* 261–277.

Corrigan, J. D. (1995). Substance abuse as a mediating factor in outcome from traumatic brain injury. *Archives of Physical Medicine and Rehabilitation, 76,* 302–309.

Corrigan, J. D., Lamb–Hart, G. L. & Rust, E. (1995). A programme of intervention for substance abuse following traumatic brain injury. *Brain Injury, 9,* 221–232.

Corrigan, J. D., & Mysiw, J. (1988). Agitation following traumatic head injury: Equivocal evidence for a discrete stage of cognitive recovery. *Archives of Physical Medicine and Rehabilitation, 69,* 487–492.

Corsini, R. J., & Wedding, D. (Eds., 1995). *Current psychotherapies.* Itasca, IL: F. E. Peacock.

Cowell, L. C., & Cohen, R. F. (1995). Amantadine: A potential adjuvant therapy following traumatic brain injury. *Journal of Head Trauma Rehabilitation, 10*(2), 91–94.

Crook, T. H., Feher, E. P., & Larrabee, G. J. (1993). Initial validation of the MAC–P: A new clinician-rated scale for cognitive and affective changes in dementia. *Clinical Neuropsychologist, 7,* 420–429.

Crosson, B., Barco, P. P., Velozo, C. A., Bolesta, M. M., Cooper, P. V., Werts, D., & Brobeck, T. C. (1989). Awareness and compensation in postacute head injury rehabilitation. *Journal of Head Trauma Rehabilitation, 4*(3), 46–54.

Cummings, J. L. (1985). Organic delusions. *British Journal of Psychiatry, 146,* 184–197.

Cummings, J. L. (1997). The Neuropsychiatric Inventory: Assessing psychopathology in dementia patients. *Neurology, 48*(5 Suppl. 6), 910–918.

Damasio, A. R., Damasio, H., & Van Hoesen, G. W. (1982). Prosopagnosia: Anatomic basis and behavioral mechanisms. *Neurology, 32,* 331–341.

Damasio, A. R., Tranel, D., & Damasio, H. (1990). Individuals with sociopathic behavior caused by frontal damage fail to respond autonomically to social stimuli. *Behavioural Brain Research, 41,* 81–94.

DeBoskey, D. S., Hecht, J. S. & Calub, C. J. (1991). *Educating families of the head injured: A guide to medical, cognitive, and social issues.* Gaithersburg, MD: Aspen.

DeJong, R. N. (1979). *The neurologic examination.* Hagerstown, MD: Harper.

DePompei, R., & Zarski, J. J. (1989). Families, head injury, and cognitive–communicative impairments: Issues for family counseling. *Topics in Language Disorders, 9*(2), 78–89.

Devinsky, O., & Bear, D. (1984). Varieties of aggressive behavior in temporal lobe epilepsy. *American Journal of Psychiatry, 141,* 651–656.

Devinsky, O., Bear, D., Moya, K., & Benowitz, L. (1993). Perception of emotion in patients with Tourette's syndrome. *Neuropsychiatry, Neuropsychology, and Behavioral Neurology, 6,* 166–169.

Devlieger, P., Piachaud, J., Leung, P., & George, N. (1994). Coping with epilepsy in Zimbabwe and the Midwest, USA. *International Journal of Rehabilitation Research, 17,* 251–264.

Dikengil, A., Jones, G., & Byrne, M. (1993). Orientation of foreign language interpreters working with brain-injured patients. *The Journal of Cognitive Rehabilitation, 11*(4), 10–13.

Dikengil, A., King, C., & Monda, D. (1992). Communication functional skills group: An integrated group therapy approach to head injury rehabilitation. *The Journal of Cognitive Rehabilitation, 10*(4), 28–31.

Dikmen, S., McLean, A., & Temkin, N. (1986). Neuropsychological and psychosocial consequences of minor head injury. *Journal of Neurology, Neurosurgery and Psychiatry, 49*, 1227–1232.

Direnfeld, G. (1991). Traumatic brain injury: Getting to the underbelly and getting through it. *Cognitive Rehabilitation, 9*(2), 20–22.

Dodrill, C., Batzel, L. W., Queisser, H. R., & Temkin, N. (1980). An objective method for the assessment of psychological and social problems among epileptics. *Epilepsia, 21*, 123–135.

Dodrill, C., Beier, R., Kasparich, M., Tacke, I., Tacke, U., & Tan, S. Y. (1984). Psychosocial problems in adults with epilepsy: Comparison of findings from four countries. *Epilepsia, 25*, 176–183.

Dowling, J. R. (1995). *Keeping busy: A handbook of activities for persons with dementia.* Baltimore, MD: Johns Hopkins University Press.

Dryovage, J., & Seidman, K. (1992). Interdisciplinary approach to community reintegration. *The Journal of Cognitive Rehabilitation, 10*(4), 12–21.

Eames, P., Haffey, W. J., & Cope, D. N. (1990). Treatment of behavioral disorders. In M. Rosenthal, E. R. Griffity, J. R. Bond, & J. D. Miller (Eds.), *Rehabilitation of the adult and child with traumatic brain injury* (2nd ed., pp. 410–432). Philadelphia, PA: F. A. Davis.

Eisenberg, M. G., Griggens, C., & Duvall, R. J. (Eds., 1982). *Disabled people as second class citizens.* New York: Springer.

Elliott, F. A. (1992). The neurologic contribution: An overview. *Archives of Neurology, 49*, 595–603.

Ellis, D. W. (1989). Neuropsychotherapy. In D. W. Ellis & A. L. Christensen (Eds.), *Neuropsychological treatment after brain injury* (pp. 241–269). Boston: Kluwer.

Eslinger, P. J. (1998). Neurological and neuropsychological bases of empathy. *European Neurology, 39*, 193–199.

Evans, J. J., Emslie, H., & Wilson, B. A. (1998). External cueing systems in the rehabilitation of executive impairments of action. *Journal of the International Neuropsychological Society, 4*, 399–408.

Ezrachi, O., Ben–Yishay, Y., Kay, T., Diller, L., & Rattok, J. (1991). Predicting employment in traumatic brain injury following neuropsychological rehabilitation. *Journal of Head Trauma Rehabilitation, 6*(3), 71–84.

Feil, N. (1986). Validation therapy for the time-confused. *Geriatric Care, 18*(5), 1–2.

Feil, N. (1993). *The validation breakthrough: Simple techniques for communicating with people with Alzheimer's-type dementia.* Baltimore, MD: Health Professions Press.

Finset, A., Dyrnes, S., Krogstad, J. M., & Berstad, J. (1995). Self-reported social networks and interpersonal support 2 years after severe traumatic brain injury. *Brain Injury, 9*, 141–150.

Fisher, A., Murray, E., & Bundy, A. (1991). *Sensory integration: Theory and practice.* Philadelphia, PA: F. A. Davis.

Fishman, S. (1988). *A bomb in the brain: A heroic tale of science, surgery, and survival.* New York: Scribner.

Fordyce, D. J., Roueche, J. R., & Prigatano, G. P. (1983). Enhanced emotional reactions in chronic head trauma patients. *Journal of Neurology, Neurosurgery, and Psychiatry. 46*, 620–624.

Fordyce, W. E., Roberts, A. H., & Sternbach, R. A. (1985). The behavioral management of chronic pain: A response to critics. *Pain, 22*, 113–125.

Fox, D. D., Lees-Haley, P. R., Earnest, K., & Dolezal-Wood, S. (1995). Base rates of postconcussive symptoms in health maintenance organization patients and controls. *Neuropsychology, 9*, 606–611.

Frankl, V. (1962). *Man's search for meaning: An introduction to logotherapy.* Boston: Beacon Press.

Fraser, R. T. (1991). Vocational evaluation. *Journal of Head Trauma Rehabilitation, 6*(3), 46–58.

Fraser, R. T., & Baarslag-Benson, R. (1994). Cross-disciplinary collaboration in the removal of work barriers after traumatic brain injury. *Topics in Language Disorders, 15*(1), 55–67.

Freeman, E. A. (1997). Community-based rehabilitation of the person with a severe brain injury. *Brain Injury, 11,* 143–153.

Gacono, C. B., & Hutton, H. E., (1994). Suggestions for the clinical and forensic use of the Hare Psychopathy Checklist–Revised (PCL–R). *International Journal of Law and Psychiatry, 17,* 303–317.

Gainotti, G., Azzoni, A., Razzano, C., Lanzillota, C., Marra, C., & Gasparini, F. (1997). The post–stroke depression rating scale: A test specifically devised to investigate affective disorders of stroke patients. *Journal of Clinical and Experimental Neuropsychology, 19,* 340–356.

Galanti, G. A. (1991) *Caring for patients from different cultures: Case studies from American hospitals.* Philadelphia, PA: University of Pennsylvania Press.

Gallo, J. J. (1990). The effect of social support on depression in caregivers of the elderly. *Journal of Family Practice, 30,* 430–436.

Gans, J. S. (1983). Hate in the rehabilitation setting. *Archives of Physical Medicine and Rehabilitation, 64,* 176–179.

Garyfallos, G., Manos, N., & Adamopoulou, A. (1988). Psychopathology and personality characteristics of epileptic patients: Epilepsy, psychopathology and personality. *Acta Psychiatrica Scandinavica, 78,* 87–95.

Gass, C. S., & Brown, M. C. (1992). Neuropsychological test feedback to patients with brain dysfunction. *Psychological Assessment, 4,* 272–277.

Gass, C. S., & Russell, E. W. (1986). Differential impact of brain damage and depression on memory test performance. *Journal of Consulting and Clinical Psychology, 54,* 261–263.

Gerber, D. J., & Schraa, J. C. (1995). Mild traumatic brain injury: Searching for the syndrome. *Journal of Head Trauma Rehabilitation, 10*(4), 28–40.

Gil, T., Calev, A., Greenberg, D., & Kugelmass, S., (1990). Cognitive functioning in Post-Traumatic Stress Disorder. *Journal of Traumatic Stress, 3*(1), 29–45.

Gilley, D. W. (1993). Behavioral and affective disturbances in Alzheimer's disease. In R. W. Parks, R. F. Zec, & R. S. Wilson (Eds.), *Neuropsychology of Alzheimer's disease and other dementias* (pp. 112–137). New York: Oxford University Press.

Gilley, D. W., & Wilson, R. S. (1997). Criterion–related validity of the Geriatric Depression Scale in Alzheimer's disease. *Journal of Clinical and Experimental Neuropsychology, 19,* 489–499.

Glenn, M. B. (1987). Update on pharmacology: A pharmacologic approach to aggressive and disruptive behaviors after traumatic brain injury (Part 1). *Journal of Head Trauma Rehabilitation, 2*(1), 71–73.

Goldstein, K. (1952). The effects of brain damage on the personality. *Psychiatry, 15,* 245–260.

Goran, D .A., & Fabiano, R. J. (1993). The scaling of the Katz Adjustment Scale in a traumatic brain injury rehabilitation sample. *Brain Injury, 7,* 219–229.

Gordon, W. A., Hibbard, M. R., Egelko, S., Riley, E., Simon, D., Diller, L., Ross, E. D., & Lieberman, A. (1991). Issues in the diagnosis of post–stroke depression. *Rehabilitation Psychology, 36*(2), 71–87.

Gouvier, W. D., Presthold, P. H., & Warner, M. S. (1988). A survey of common misconceptions about head injury and recovery. *Archives of Clinical Neuropsychology, 3,* 331–343.

Grace, J., Malloy, P. F., & Stout, J. C. (1996, October). Assessing frontal behavioral syndromes: Reliability and validity of the Frontal Lobe Personality Scale. Paper presented at the National Academy of Neuropsychology, New Orleans, LA.

Griffith, E. R., Cole, S., & Cole, T. M. (1990). Sexuality and sexual dysfunction. In M. Rosenthal,

E. R. Griffity, J. R. Bond, & J. D. Miller (Eds.), *Rehabilitation of the adult and child with traumatic brain injury* (2nd ed., pp. 206–224). Philadelphia, PA: F. A. Davis.

Griffith, E. R., & Lemberg, S. (1993). *Sexuality and the person with traumatic brain injury: A guide for families*. Philadelphia, PA: F. A. Davis.

Gronwall, D., Wrightson, P., & Waddell, P. (1990). *Head injury: The facts: A guide for families and care-givers*. Oxford, England: Oxford University Press.

Gualtieri, C. T. (1991). *Neuropsychiatry and behavioral pharmacology*. New York: Springer-Verlag.

Hagen, C. (1982). Language–cognitive disorganization following closed head injury: A conceptualization. In L. E. Trexler (Ed.), *Cognitive rehabilitation: Conceptualization and intervention*. New York: Plenum.

Hallett, J. D., Zasler, N. D., Maurer, P., & Cash, S. (1994). Role change after traumatic brain injury in adults. *The American Journal of Occupational Therapy, 48*, 241–246.

Hamilton, M. (1960). A rating scale for depression. *Journal of Neurology, Neurosurgery, and Psychiatry, 23*, 56–62.

Hanson R. W., & Gerber, K. E. (1990). *Coping with chronic pain: A guide to patient self–management*. New York: Guilford.

Hanson, S., & Tucker, D., (Eds., 1992). Neuropsychological assessment. *Physical Medicine and Rehabilitation: State of the Art Reviews, 6*(3). Philadelphia, PA: Hanley & Belfus.

Hartlage, L. (1991). Assessment of behavioral sequelae of traumatic and chemical CNS insult. *Archives of Clinical Neuropsychology, 6*, 279–286.

Hartman, D. E. (1995). *Neuropsychological toxicology: Identification and assessment of human neurotoxic syndromes* (2nd ed.). New York: Plenum.

Haynes, S. D. (1994), The experience of grief in the head-injured adult. *Archives of Clinical Neuropsychology, 9*, 323–336.

Hecaen, H., & Albert, M. L. (1978). *Human neuropsychology*. New York: Wiley.

Heilman, K. M. (1991). Anosognosia: Possible neuropsychological mechanisms. In G. P. Prigatano & D. L. Schacter (Eds.), *Awareness of deficit after brain injury: Clinical and theoretical issues* (pp.53–62). New York: Oxford University Press.

Heilman, K. M., & Valenstein, E. (Eds., 1985). *Clinical neuropsychology* (2nd ed.). New York: Oxford University Press.

Herman, J. (1992). *Trauma and recovery*. New York: Basic Books.

Hibbard, M. R., Gordon, W. A., Egelko, S., & Langer, K. (1987). Issues in the diagnosis and cognitive therapy of depression in brain–damaged individuals. In A. Freeman & V. Greenwood (Eds.), *Cognitive therapy: Applications in psychiatric and medical settings* (pp. 183–198). New York: Human Sciences.

Hibbard, M. R., Grober, S. E., Gordon, W. A., Aletta, E. G., & Freeman, A. (1990). Cognitive therapy and the treatment of poststroke depression. *Topics in Geriatric Rehabilitation, 5*(3), 43–55.

Hickling, E. J., Gillen, R., Blanchard, E. B., Buckley, T., & Taylor, A. (1998). Traumatic brain injury and posttraumatic stress disorder: A preliminary investigation of neuropsychological test results in PTSD secondary to motor vehicle accidents. *Brain Injury, 12*, 265–274.

Hinkeldey, N., & Corrigan, J. (1990). The structure of head-injured patients' neurobehavioral complaints: A preliminary study. *Brain Injury, 4*, 111–114.

Hogarty, G., & Katz, M. (1971). Norms of adjustment and social behavior. *Archives of General Psychiatry, 25*, 470–480.

Hopewell, C. A., Burke, W. H., Weslowski, M. & Zawlocki, T. (1990). Behavioral learning therapies for the traumatically brain–injured patient. In R. L. Wood & I. Fussey (Eds.), *Cognitive rehabilitation in perspective* (pp. 229–245). London: Taylor & Francis.

Horton, A. M., Jr. (1994). *Behavioral interventions with brain injured children*. New York: Plenum.

Hotz, G., & Helm-Estabrooks, N. (1995a). Perseveration. Part I: A review. *Brain Injury, 9*, 151–159.

Hotz, G., & Helm–Estabrooks, N. (1995b). Perseveration. Part II: A study of perseveration in closed-head injury. *Brain Injury, 9*, 161–172.

Howard, M. E. (1988). Behavior management in the acute care rehabilitation setting. *Journal of Head Trauma Rehabilitation, 3*(3), 14–22.

Howard, R., & Ford, R. (1992). From the jumping Frenchmen of Maine to post-traumatic stress disorder: The startle response in neuropsychiatry. *Psychological Medicine, 22*, 695–707.

Hurt, G. D., & Raines, J. (n.d.). *Job Therapy experience: Developing and implementing JTE programs.* (Available from Good Samaritan Community Healthcare Rehabilitation Center, 407–14th Ave. SE, Puyallup, WA 98371–0192)

Iverson, G. L., Demarest, D. S., & Franzen, M. D. (1994). Case studies of neuropsychological assessment in a correctional setting. *International Journal of Offender Therapy and Comparative Criminology, 38*, 231–240.

Jackson, H. F., Hopewell, C. A., Glass, C. A., & Warburg, R., (1992). The Katz Adjustment Scale: Modification for use with victims of traumatic brain and spinal injury. *Brain Injury, 6*, 109–127.

Jacobs, H. E. (1993). *Behavior analysis guidelines and brain injury rehabilitation.* Gaithersberg, MD: Aspen.

Johnston, M., & Tjandrakusuma, H. (1982). Reaching the disabled. *World Health Forum, 3*, 307–310.

Jones, M. (1996). *GENTLECARE—Changing the experience of Alzheimer's disease in a positive way.* British Columbia, Canada: Chelsea Printers.

Jones, T. (1993). *The pugilist at rest: Stories.* Boston: Little, Brown & Co.

Jochims, S. (1995). Emotional processes of coping with disease in the early stages of acquired brain lesions. *Arts in Psychotherapy, 22*, 21–30.

Joraski, M. (1986). The role of creative arts in cognitive rehabilitation. *Cognitive Rehabilitation, 4*(2), 18–21.

*Journal of Head Trauma Rehabilitation, 5*(2) (1990). Special issue: Sexuality and head injury.

Judd, T. (n.d.) Reflex crying. In *Emotional aspects of stroke.* (Available from American Heart Association Stroke Connection, 7272 Greenville Ave., Dallas, TX 75231–4596, U.S.A.)

Judd, T. (1988). The varieties of musical talent. In L. K. Obler & D. Fein (Eds), *The exceptional brain: Neuropsychology of talent and special abilities* (pp. 127–155). New York: Guilford.

Judd, T. (1996). Natural recovery: An ecological approach to neuropsychological recuperation. Unpublished manuscript.

Judd, T., & Fordyce, D. (1996). Personality tests. In R. Sbordone & D. Long (Eds.), *Ecological validity of neuropsychological tests.* Winter Park, FL: GP Press.

Judd, T., & Stoffel, C. (1989, December). *Reflex crying.* Paper presented at the annual meeting of the Pacific Northwest Neuropsychology Society, Seattle, WA.

Jutagir, R. (1992). Prospects for rehabilitation of cognitive functions in the elderly. *NeuroRehabilitation, 2*(3), 55–61.

Kapur, N. (Ed., 1997). *Injured brains of medical minds: Views from within.* New York: Oxford University Press.

Kasowski, J. C. (1994). Family recovery: An insider's view. *The American Journal of Occupational Therapy, 48*, 257–258.

Kassirer, J. P., & Kopelman, R. I. (1991). *Learning clinical reasoning.* Baltimore, MD: Williams & Wilkins.

Katz, M., & Lyerely, S. (1963). Methods of measuring adjustment and behavior in the community: I. Rationale, description, discriminative validity, and scale development. *Psychological Reports. 13*, 503–535.

Kay, T. (1992). Neuropsychological diagnosis: Disentangling the multiple determinants of functional disability after mild traumatic brain injury. In L. J. Horn & N. D. Zasler (Eds.), *Physical medicine and rehabilitation: State of the art reviews, 6*(1), 109–127. Philadelphia, PA: Hanley & Belfus.

Kay, T. (1995). Question and answer. *Journal of Head Trauma Rehabilitation, 10*(6), 78–79.

Kay, T., & Cavallo, M. M. (1994). The family system: Impact, assessment, and intervention. In J. M., Silver, S. C. Yudofsky, & R. E. Hales (Eds.), *Neuropsychiatry of traumatic brain injury* (pp.533–567). Washington, DC: American Psychiatric Press.

Kay, T., Cavallo, M. M., Ezrachi, O., & Vavagiakis, P. (1995). The head injury family interview: A clinical and research tool. *Journal of Head Trauma Rehabilitation, 10*(2), 12–31.

Kennedy, M., & DeRuyter, F. (1991). Cognitive and language bases for communication disorders. In D. Beukleman & K. Yorkston (Eds.), *Communication disorders following brain injury* (pp. 123–190). Austin, TX: Pro-Ed.

King, D. A., Cox, C., Lyness, J. M., & Caine, E. D. (1995). Neuropsychological effects of depression and age in an elderly sample: A confirmatory study. *Neuropsychology, 9*, 399–408.

Klonoff, P. S., & Lage, G. A. (1991). Narcissistic injury in patients with traumatic brain injury. *Journal of Head Trauma Rehabilitation, 6*(4), 11–21.

Klonoff, P., Snow, W., & Costa, L. (1986). Quality of life in patients 2 to 4 years after closed head injury. *Neurosurgery, 19*, 735–743.

Kneipp, S. (1995). A model for team meetings in nonresidential community integrated programs. *Journal of Head Trauma Rehabilitation, 10*(2), 50–59.

Kokkinidis, L., & McCarter, B. D. (1990). Behavioral evidence implicating dopamine in sensorimotor arousal and norepinephrine in the sedative effects of antidepressant drugs. *Psychopharmacology, 100*, 542–547.

Kolb, B., & Whishaw, I. Q. (1985). *Fundamentals of human neuropsychology* (2nd ed.). New York: Freeman.

Kreutzer, J. S., Gervasio, A. H., & Camplair, P. S. (1994a). Patient correlates of caregivers' distress and family functioning after traumatic brain injury. *Brain Injury, 8*, 211–230.

Kreutzer, J. S., Gervasio, A. H., & Camplair, P. S. (1994b). Primary caregivers' psychological status and family functioning after traumatic brain injury. *Brain Injury, 8*, 197–210.

Kreutzer, J. S., Gordon, W. A., & Wehman, P. (1989). Cognitive remediation following traumatic brain injury. *Rehabilitation Psychology, 34*, 117–130.

Kreutzer, J., & Wehman, P. (Eds., 1990). *Community integration following traumatic brain injury.* Baltimore, MD: Paul H. Brookes.

Kubler-Ross, E. (1969). *On death and dying.* New York: McMillan.

Kushner, H. S. (1981). *When bad things happen to good people.* New York: Schocken.

LaChapelle, D. L., & Finlayson, M. A. J. (1998). An evaluation of subjective and objective measures of fatigue in patients with brain injury and healthy controls. *Brain Injury, 12*, 649–659.

Lamberty, G. A., & Bieliauskas, L. A. (1993). Distinguishing between depression and dementia in the elderly: A review of neuropsychological findings. *Archives of Clinical Neuropsychology, 8*, 149–170.

Langer, S. (1992). Psychotherapy with the neuropsychologically impaired adult. *American Journal of Psychotherapy, 46*, 620–639.

Langley, M. J., Lindsay, W. P., Lam, C. S., & Priddy, D. A. (1990). A comprehensive alcohol abuse treatment programme for persons with traumatic brain injury. *Brain Injury, 4*, 77–86.

LaPlante, E. (1993). *Seized: Temporal lobe epilepsy as a medical, historical, and artistic phenomenon.* New York: HarperCollins.

Layton, B. S., & Wardi-Zonna, K. (February 1994). *Post-traumatic stress disorder with neurogenic amnesia for the traumatic event.* Paper presented at the meeting of the International Neuropsychological Society, Cincinnati, OH.

Lazes, P. M., Kaplan, L. H., & Gordon, K. A. (Eds., 1987). *The handbook of health education.* Gaithersburg, MD: Aspen.

Leaf, L. E. (1991). Relationship therapy: A psychotherapeutic approach with persons sustaining brain injury. *Cognitive Rehabilitation, 9*(6), 14–16.

Leaf, L. E. (1993). Traumatic brain injury: Affecting family recovery. *Brain Injury, 7*, 543–546.

Lefebvre, K. A. (1988). Sexual assessment planning. *Sexuality Update, 1*(1), 6–8.

Lefebvre, K. A. (1990). Sexual assessment planning. *Journal of Head Trauma Rehabilitation, 5*(2), 25–30.

Lehr, E. (1990). *Psychological management of traumatic brain injuries in children and adolescents*. Rockville, MD: Aspen.

Lennox, D. B., & Brune, P. (1993). Incidental teaching for training communication in individuals with traumatic brain injury. *Brain Injury, 7*, 449–454.

Levin, H. S., Eisenberg, H. M., & Benton, A. L. (Eds., 1989). *Mild head injury.* New York: Oxford University Press.

Levin, H. S., High, W. M., Goethe, K. E., Sisson, R. A., Overall, J. E., Rhoades, H. M., Eisenberg, H. M., Kalisky, Z., & Gary, H. E. (1987). The neurobehavioral rating scale: Assessment of the behavioral sequelae of head injury by the clinician. *Journal of Neurology, Neurosurgery and Psychiatry, 50*, 183–193.

Levine, M. J., Van Horn, R., & Curtis, A. B. (1993). Developmental models of social cognition in assessing psychosocial adjustments in head injury. *Brain Injury, 7*, 153–167.

Lewis, L. (1991). A framework for developing a psychotherapy treatment plan with brain–injured patients. *Journal of Head Trauma Rehabilitation, 6*(4), 22–29.

Lewis, L. & Rosenberg, S. J. (1990). Psychoanalytic psychotherapy with brain–injured adult psychiatric patients. *Journal of Nervous and Mental Disease, 178*, 69–77.

Lezak, M. D. (1978). Subtle sequelae of brain damage: Perplexity, distractibility, and fatigue. *American Journal of Physical Medicine, 67*, 9–15.

Lezak, M. D. (1986). Psychological implications of traumatic brain damage for the patient's family. *Rehabilitation Psychology, 31*, 241–250.

Lezak, M. D. (1988). Brain damage is a family affair. *Journal of Clinical and Experimental Neuropsychology, 10*, 111–123.

Lezak, M. D. (1995). *Neuropsychological Assessment* (3rd ed.). New York: Oxford University Press.

Lieberman, A., & Benson, D. F. (1977). Control of emotional expression in pseudobulbar palsy: A personal experience. *Archives of Neurology, 34*, 717–719.

Linge, F. R. (1980). *What does it feel like to be brain damaged?* Framingham, MA: National Head Injury Foundation.

Linge, F. R. (1990). Faith, hope, and love: Non–traditional therapy in recovery from serious head injury: A personal account. *Canadian Journal of Psychology, 44*, 116–129.

Livingston, M. G., & Brooks, D. N. (1988). The burden on families of the brain injured: A review. *Journal of Head Trauma Rehabilitation, 4*, 6–15.

Lloyd, L. G., & Cuvo, A. J. (1994). Maintenance and generalization of behaviours after treatment of persons with traumatic brain injury. *Brain Injury, 8*, 529–540.

Love, R. J. (1992). *Neurology for the speech–language pathologist* (2nd ed.). Boston: Butterworth–Heinemann.

Luria, A. R. (1973). *The working brain: An introduction to neuropsychology.* New York: Basic Books.

Lynch, E. W., & Hanson, M. J. (Eds., 1992). *Developing cross–cultural competence: A guide for working with young children and their families*. Baltimore, MD: Paul H. Brookes.

Lysack, C., & Kaufert, J. (1994). Comparing the origins and ideologies of the independent living movement and community-based rehabilitation. *International Journal of Rehabilitation Research, 17*, 231–240.

Mace, N. L., & Rabins, P. V. (1991). *The 36-hour day.* Baltimore, MD: Johns Hopkins University Press.

Maitz, E. A., & Sachs, P. P. (1995). Treating families of individuals with traumatic brain injury from a family systems perspective. *Journal of Head Trauma Rehabilitation, 10*(2), 1–11.

Malec, J. F. (1993). Ethics in brain injury rehabilitation: Existential choices among Western cultural beliefs. *Brain Injury, 7*, 383–400.

Malkmus, D. D. (1989). Community reentry: Cognitive-communicative intervention within a social skill context. *Topics in Language Disorders, 9*(2), 50–66.

Malloy, P., Bihrle, A., Duffy, J., & Cimino, C. (1993). The orbitomedial frontal syndrome. *Archives of Clinical Neuropsychology, 8*, 185–201.

Mann, W. C., & Dittmar, S. S. (1992). Consumer advocacy and professional education: Traumatic brain injury. *The Journal of Cognitive Rehabilitation, 10*(6), 8–11.

Mapou, R. (1990). Traumatic brain injury rehabilitation with gay and lesbian individuals. *Journal of Head Trauma Rehabilitation, 5*(2), 67–72.

Marshall, L. F., & Ruff, R. M. (1989). Neurosurgeon as victim. In H. S. Levin, H. M. Eisenberg, & A. L. Benton (Eds.), *Mild head injury* (pp. 276–280). New York: Oxford University Press.

Martin, J. ("Miss Manners", 1984, April 23). Memory slips: Show respect when elderly forget. *Seattle Times*, p. A–23.

Martín-Baró, I. (1991). Towards a liberation psychology. In J. Hassett & H. Lacey (Eds.), *Towards a society that serves its people: The intellectual contributions of El Salvador's murdered Jesuits* (pp. 319–332). Washington, DC:Georgetown University Press.

Masters, W. H., & Johnson, V. E. (1970). *Human sexual inadequacy.* Boston: Little, Brown, & Co.

Mateer, C., & Judd, T. (1993). Language. In H. Cohen (Ed.), *Neuroscience for rehabilitation* (pp. 282–299). Philadelphia, PA: J. B. Lippencott.

Mateer, C. A., Sohlberg, M. M., & Crinean, J. (1987). Focus on clinical research: Perceptions of memory function in individuals with closed-head injury. *Journal of Head Trauma Rehabilitation, 2*(3), 74–84.

Mathews, R. M. (1990). Independent living as a lifelong community service. *The Journal of Head Trauma Rehabilitation, 5*, 23–30.

Max, J. E., Smith, W. L., Jr., Lindgren, S. D., Robin, D. A., Mattheis, P., Stierwalt, J., & Morrisey, M. (1995). Case study: obsessive–compulsive disorder after severe traumatic brain injury in an adolescent. *Journal of the American Academy of Child and Adolescent Psychiatry 34*, 45–49.

McDonald, S. (1992). Communication disorders following closed head injury: New approaches to assessment and rehabilitation. *Brain Injury, 6*, 283–292.

McGann, W., & Werven, G. (1995). Social competence and head injury: A new emphasis. *Brain Injury, 9*, 93–102.

McGlynn, S. M. ,& Schacter, D. L. (1989). Unawareness of deficits in neuropsychological syndromes. *Journal of Clinical and Experimental Neuropsychology, 11*, 143–205.

McGuire, P. K., Bench, C. J., Frith, C. D., Marks, I. M., Frackowiak, R. S., & Dolan, R. J. (1994). Functional anatomy of obsessive–compulsive phenomena. *British Journal of Psychiatry 164*, 459–468.

McMillan, T. M. (1991). Post-traumatic stress disorder and severe head injury. *British Journal of Psychiatry, 159*, 431–433.

McNeill, D. E., Schuyler, B. A., & Ezrachi, O. (1997). Assessing family involvement in traumatic brain injury rehabilitation: The development of a new instrument. *Archives of Clinical Neuropsychology, 12*, 645–660.

Meichenbaum, D. (1977). *Cognitive behavior modification: An integrative approach.* New York: Plenum.

Meichenbaum, D. (1985). *Stress inoculation training.* Elmsford, NY: Pergamon.

Meichenbaum, D. (1992). Stress inoculation training: A twenty year update. In R. L. Woolfold & P. M. Lehrer (Eds.), *Principles and practices of stress management.* New York: Guilford.

Meichenbaum, D. (1993). The "potential" contributions of cognitive behavior modification to the rehabilitation of individuals with traumatic brain injury. *Seminars in Speech and Language, 14*, 18–31.

Meltzer, M. L. (1983). Poor memory: A case report. *Journal of Clinical Psychology, 39*, 3–10.

Miller, L. (1992). When the best help is self–help, or, everything you always wanted to know about brain injury support groups. *The Journal of Cognitive Rehabilitation, 10*(6), 14–17.

Miller, L. (1993). *Psychotherapy of the brain-injured patient: Reclaiming the shattered self*. New York: Norton.

Milner, B. (1962). Les troubles de la memoire accompagnant des lesions hippocampiques bilaterales [Memory difficulties accompanying bilateral hippocampal lesions]. In *Physiologie de l'hippocampe* (pp. 257–272). Paris: Centre National de la Recherche Scientifique.

Mintz, M. C., Van Horn, K. R., & Levine, M. J. (1995). Developmental models of social cognition in assessing the role of family stress in relatives' predictions following traumatic brain injury. *Brain Injury, 9*, 173–186.

Mirsky, A. F., Anthony, B. J., Duncan, C. C., Ahearn, M. B., & Kellam, S. G. (1991). Analysis of the elements of attention: A neuropsychological approach. *Neuropsychology Review, 2*(2), 109–145.

Mittenberg, W., Zielinski, R. & Fichera, S. (1993). Recovery from mild head injury: A treatment manual for patients. *Psychotherapy in Private Practice, 12*(2), 37–52.

Moore, A., & Stambrook, M. (1995). Cognitive moderators of outcome following traumatic brain injury: A conceptual model and implications for rehabilitation. *Brain Injury, 9*, 109–130.

Moore, A., Stambrook, M., & Peters, L. (1993). Centripetal and centrifugal family life cycle factors in long-term outcome following traumatic brain injury. *Brain Injury, 7*, 247–255.

Morton, M. V., & Wehman, P. (1995). Psychosocial and emotional sequelae of individuals with traumatic brain injury: A literature review and recommendations. *Brain Injury, 9*, 81–92.

Mountain, M., & Spreen, O. (June 1993). *Implications of impaired ability in brain damaged patients to recognize emotion*. Paper presented to the International Neuropsychological Society, Funchal, Madiera, Portugal.

Muir, C. A., Rosenthal M., & Diehl, L. N. (1990). Methods of family intervention. In M. Rosenthal, E. R. Griffity, J. R. Bond, & J. D. Miller, J. D. (Eds.) *Rehabilitation of the adult and child with traumatic brain injury* (2nd ed., pp. 433–448). Philadelphia, PA: F. A. Davis.

Nelson, L., Satz, P., & D'Elia, L. (1994). *Neuropsychology Behavior and Affect Profile*. Palo Alto, CA: Mind Garden.

Nelson, L., Satz, P., Mitrushina, D., Van Gorp, W., Cicchetti, D., Lewis, R., & Van Lancker, D. (1989). Development and validation of the neuropsychology behavior and affect profile. *Psychological Assessment, 1*, 266–272.

Nigro, M. A., & Lim, H. C. (1992). Hyperekplexia and sudden neonatal death. *Pediatric Neurology, 8*, 221–225.

Novaco, R. (1975). *Anger control: The development and evaluation of an experimental treatment*. Lexington, MA: Lexington Books.

Nyenhuis, D. L., Stern, R. A., Yamamoto, C., Luchetta, T., & Arruda, J. E. (1997). Standardization and validation of the Visual Analog Mood Scales. *The Clinical Neuropsychologist, 11*, 407–415.

O'Hara, C. C., & Harrell, M. (1991). *Rehabilitation with brain injury survivors: An empowerment approach*. Gaithersburg, MD: Aspen.

Olsen, R. V., Ehrenkrantz, E., & Hutchings, B. (1993). *Homes that help: Advice from caregivers for creating a supportive home*. Newark, NJ: New Jersey Institute of Technology Press.

Olshansky, S. (1966). Parent responses to a mentally defective child. *Mental Retardation, 4*(4), 21–23.

Parenté, R., Stapleton, M. C., & Wheatley, C. J. (1991). Practical strategies for vocational reentry after traumatic brain injury. *Journal of Head Trauma Rehabilitation, 6*(3), 35–45.

Parks, R. W., Zec, R. F., & Wilson, R. S. (1993). *Neuropsychology of Alzheimer's disease and other dementias.* New York: Oxford University Press.

Peat, M. (1991). Community based rehabilitation: Development and structure (Part I). *Clinical Rehabilitation, 5,* 231–239.

Peppard, N. R. (1991). *Special needs dementia units: Design, development, and operations.* New York: Springer.

Pepping, M., & Roueche, D. (1991). Psychosocial consequences of significant brain injury. In D. E. Tupper & K. D. Cicerone (Eds.), *The neuropsychology of everyday life: Issues in development and rehabilitation.* Boston: Kluwer.

Perani, D., Colombo, C., Bressi, S., Bonfanti, A., Grassi, F., Scarone, S., Bellodi, L., Smeraldi, E., & Fazio, F. (1995). [18F]FDG PET study in obsessive–compulsive disorder. A clinical/metabolic correlation study after treatment. *British Journal of Psychiatry, 166,* 244–250.

Pessar, L. F., Coad, M. L., Linn, R. T., & Willer, B. S. (1993). The effects of parental traumatic brain injury on the behaviour of parents and children. *Brain Injury, 7,* 231–240.

Prigatano, G. P. (1991). Disorder mind, wounded soul: The emerging role of psychotherapy in rehabilitation after brain injury. *Journal of Head Trauma Rehabilitation, 6,*1–10.

Prigatano, G. P. (1992). Personality disturbances associated with traumatic brain injury. *Journal of Consulting and Clinical Psychology, 60,* 360–368.

Prigatano, G. P., & Leathem, J. M. (1993). Awareness of behavioral limitations after traumatic brain injury: A cross-cultural study of New Zealand Maoris and non-Maoris. *The Clinical Neuropsychologist, 7,* 123–135.

Prigatano, G. P., O'Brien, K. P., & Klonoff, P. S. (1988). The clinical management of paranoid delusions in postacute traumatic brain-injured patients. *Journal of Head Trauma Rehabilitation, 3,* 23–32.

Prigatano, G. P., & Schacter, D. L. (Eds., 1991). *Awareness of deficit after brain injury: Clinical and theoretical issues.* New York: Oxford University Press.

Puente, A. E., & McCaffrey, R. J. (Eds., 1992). *Handbook of neuropsychological assessment: A biopsychosocial perspective.* New York: Plenum Press.

Ramirez, M., III (1991). *Psychotherapy and counseling with minorities: A cognitive approach to individual and cultural differences.* Elmsford, NY: Pergamon.

Ranseen, J. (1990). Positive personality change following traumatic head injury: Four case studies. *Cognitive Rehabilitation, 8*(2), 8–12.

Rao, S., Huber, S. J., & Bornstein, R. A. (1992). Emotional changes with multiple sclerosis and Parkinson's disease. *Journal of Consulting and Clinical Psychology, 60,* 369–378.

Rao, S., Leo, G., Ellington, L., Nauertz, T., Bernardin, L., & Unverzagt, F. (1991). Cognitive dysfunction in multiple sclerosis: 2. Impact on social functioning. *Neurology, 41,* 692–696.

Rape, R. N., Busch, J. P., & Slavin, L. A. (1992). Toward a conceptualization of the family's adaptation to a member's head injury: A critique of developmental stage models. *Rehabilitation Psychology, 37,* 3–22.

Raskin, S. A. (1997). The relationship between sexual abuse and mild traumatic brain injury. *Brain Injury, 11,* 587–603.

Raskin, S. A., & Gordon, W. A. (1992). The impact of different approaches to cognitive remediation on generalization. *NeuroRehabilitation, 2*(3), 38–45.

Rawling, P., & Brooks, N., (1990). Simulation Index: A method for detecting factitious errors on the WAIS—R and WMS. *Special Section: Forensic–legal medical issues of neuropsychology. Neuropsychology, 4,* 223–238.

Rees, R. J., & Storry, C. J. (1996). Static and dynamic assessment practices after head injury. *Brain Injury, 10,* 247–257.

Reisberg, B. (1983). *A guide to Alzheimer's disease: For families, spouses and friends.* New York: Free Press.

Renshaw, D. C. (1978). Stroke and sex. In A. Comfort (Ed.), *Sexual consequences of disability* (pp. 121–131). Philadelphia, PA: George F. Stickley.

Riddoch, M. J., & Humphreys, G. W. (Eds., 1994). *Cognitive neuropsychology and cognitive rehabilitation.* Hove, U.K.:Lawrence Erlbaum Associates.

Ridley, B. (1989). Family response in head injury: Denial . . . or hope for the future. *Social Science and Medicine, 29,* 555–561.

Roberts, R. J., Varney, N. R., Hulbert, J. R., Paulsen, J. S., Richardson, E. D., Springer, J. A., Shepherd, J. S., Swan, C. M., Legrand, J. A., Harvey, J. H., & Struchen, M. A. (1990). The neuropathology of everyday life: The frequency of partial seizure symptoms among normals. *Neuropsychology, 4,* 65–85.

Robinson, A., Spencer, B., & White, L. (1989). *Understanding difficult behaviors: Some practical suggestions for coping with Alzheimer's disease and related illnesses.* Ypsilanti, MI: Geriatric Education Center of Michigan, Eastern Michigan University.

Robinson, R. G. (1987). Depression and stroke. *Psychiatric Annals, 17,* 731–740.

Robinson, R. G., Parikh, R. M, Lipsey, J. R., Starkstein, S. E., & Price, T. R. (1993). Pathological laughing and crying following stroke: Validation of a measurement scale and a double-bind treatment study. American Journal of Psychiatry, 150, 286–293.

Rogers, C. (1980). *A way of being.* Boston: Houghton Mifflin.

Rogers, P. M., & Kreutzer, J. (1984). Family crises following head injury: A network intervention strategy. *Journal of Neurosurgical Nursing, 16,* 343–346.

Roice, J. (1995). Overview. *Sí a la vida!* [Yes to life!] (3)1–2,5. (Newsletter available from UFM Committee on Peace and Social Concerns, 2046 Westlake Ave. N, #101, Seattle, WA 98109, USA)

Rolls, E. T., Hornad, J., Wade, D., & McGrath, J. (1994). Emotion–related learning in patients with social and emotional changes associated with frontal lobe damage. *Journal of Neurology, Neurosurgery, and Psychiatry, 57,* 1518–1524.

Rosen, C. D., & Gerring, J. P. (1986). *Head trauma: Educational reintegration.* San Diego, CA, College-Hill Press.

Rosenbaum, J., Fischer, R. S., & Leavell, C. A. (February 1994). *Motor impersistence and relationship to rehabilitation outcome.* Paper presented at the meeting of the International Neuropsychological Society, Cincinnati, OH.

Rosenthal, M., & Geckler, C. (1986). Family therapy issues in neuropsychology. In D. Wedding, A. M. Horton, & J. Webster (Eds.), *The neuropsychology handbook* (pp. 325–344). New York: Springer.

Rosenthal, M., & Muir, C. (1983). Methods of family intervention. In M. Rosenthal, E. Griffith, M. Bond, & J. D. Miller (Eds.), *Rehabilitation of the head injured adult* (pp. 407–419). Philadelphia, PA: R. A. Davis.

Ross, E. D. (1981). The aprosodias: Functional–anatomic organization of the affective components of language in the right hemisphere. *Archives of Neurology, 38,* 561–569.

Ross, E. D. (1993). Nonverbal aspects of language. *Behavioral Neurology, 11,* 9–23.

Ross, E. D., & Stewart, R. S. (1987). Pathological display of affect in patients with depression and right frontal brain damage: An alternative mechanism. *Journal of Nervous and Mental Disease, 175,* 165–172.

Rubens, A. B. & Garrett, M. F. (1991). Anosognosia of linguistic deficits in patients with neurological deficits. In G. P. Prigatano & D. L. Schacter (Eds.), *Awareness of deficit after brain injury: Clinical and theoretical issues* (pp. 40–52). New York: Oxford University Press.

Ruckdeschel-Hibbard, M., Gordon, W. A., & Diller, L. (1986). Affective disturbances associated with brain damage. In S. Filskov & T. Boll (Eds.), *Handbook of clinical neuropsychology* (pp.305–337). New York: Wiley.

Ruff, R. M., Camenzuli, L., & Mueller, J. (1996). Miserable minority: Emotional risk factors that influence the outcome of a mild traumatic brain injury. *Brain Injury, 10,* 551–565.

Sachs, P. R. (1985). Beyond support: Traumatic head injury as a growth experience for families. *Rehabilitation Nursing, 10*(1), 21–23.

Sachs, P. R. (1991). *Treating families of brain-injury survivors* (Vol. 9, Springer series on rehabilitation), New York: Springer.

Sale, P., West, M., Sherron, P., & Wehman, P. H. (1991). Exploratory analysis of job separations from supported employment for persons with traumatic brain injury. *Journal of Head Trauma Rehabilitation, 6*(3), 1–11.

Sandson, J., & Albert, M. L. (1984). The varieties of perseveration. *Neuropsychologia, 22,* 715–732.

Santoro, J., & Spiers, M. (1994). Social cognitive factors in brain injury-associated personality change. *Brain Injury, 8,* 265–276.

Savage, R. G., & Wolcott, G. F. (Eds., 1994). *Educational dimensions of acquired brain injury.* Austin, TX: Pro-Ed.

Sbordone, R. J. (1991). Psychotherapeutic treatment of the client with traumatic brain injury: A conceptual model. In J. S. Kreutzer & P. H. Wehman (Eds.), *Cognitive rehabilitation for persons with traumatic brain injury: A functional approach.* Baltimore, MD: Paul H. Brookes.

Sbordone, R. J., Kral, M., Gerard, M., & Katz, J. (1984). Evidence of a "Command Performance Syndrome" in the significant others of the victims of severe traumatic head injury. *International Journal of Clinical Neuropsychology, 6,* 183–185.

Sbordone, R. J., & Liter, J. C. (1995). Mild traumatic brain injury does not produce post–traumatic stress disorder. *Brain Injury, 9,* 405–412.

Schiffer, R. B., Cash, J., & Herndon, R. M. (1983). Treatment of emotional lability with low–dosage tricyclic antidepressants. *Psychosomatics, 24,* 1094–1096.

Schover, L. R. (1986). Sexual problems. In L. Tem & P. M. Lewinsohn (Eds.), *Geropsychological assessment and treatment* (pp. 145–187). New York: Springer.

Seaman, B., Roberts, P., Gilewski, M., & Nagai, J. (1993). Clinic to the real world: Community reintegration of head injured patients. *The Journal of Cognitive Rehabilitation, 11*(2), 6–17.

Serio, C. D., Kreutzer, J. S., & Witol, A. D. (1997). Family needs after traumatic brain injury: A factor analytic study of the Family Needs Questionnaire. *Brain Injury, 11,* 1–9.

Shaibani, A. T., Sabbagh, M. N., & Doody, R. (1994). Laughter and crying in neurologic disorders. *Neuropsychiatry, Neuropsychology, and Behavioral Neurology, 7,* 243–250.

Shallice, T. (1979). Case study approach in neuropsychological research. *Journal of Clinical Neuropsychology, 1,* 183–211.

Shallice, T. (1988). *From neuropsychology to mental structure.* New York: Cambridge University Press.

Shapiro, F. (1989). Efficacy of the eye movement desensitization procedure in the treatment of traumatic memories. *Journal of Traumatic Stress, 2*(2), 199–223.

Sherer, M., Boake, C., Levin, E., Silver, B. V., Ringholz, G., & High, W. M. (1998). Characteristics of impaired awareness after traumatic brain injury. *Journal of the International Neuropsychological Society, 4,* 380–387.

Sheridan, C. (1987). *Failure–free activities for the Alzheimer patient.* New York: Bell.

Sifneos, P. E. (1994). Affect deficit and alexithymia. *New Trends in Experimental and Clinical Psychiatry, 10*(4), 193–195.

Silver, J. M., & Yudofsky, S. C. (1994). Aggressive disorders. In J. M. Silver, S. C. Yudofsky, & R. E. Hales (Eds.), *Neuropsychiatry of traumatic brain injury* (pp. 533–567). Washington, DC: American Psychiatric Press.

Silver, J. M., Yudofsky, S. C., & Hales, R. E. (Eds., 1994). *Neuropsychiatry of traumatic brain injury.* Washington, DC: American Psychiatric Press.

Slade, C., & Burns, R. (1992). Cognitive rehabilitation at a retail work site. *The Journal of Cognitive Rehabilitation, 10*(3), 10–13.

Slater, E., & Beard, A. W. (1963). The schizophrenia-like psychoses of epilepsy: Psychiatric aspects. *British Journal of Psychiatry, 109*, 90–150.

Small, L. (1980). *Neuropsychodiagnosis in psychotherapy* (rev. ed.). New York: Brunner/Mazel.

Sohlberg, M. M., & Mateer, C. A. (1989). *Introduction to cognitive rehabilitation: Theory and practice*. New York: Guilford.

Sonkin, D. J., & Durphy, M. (1989). *Learning to live without violence : A handbook for men.* Volcano, CA: Volcano Press.

Spanbock, P. (1992). Children and siblings of head injury survivors: A need to be understood. *The Journal of Cognitive Rehabilitation, 10*(4), 8–9.

Squire, L. R. (1987). *Memory and brain.* New York: Oxford University Press.

Starch, S., & Falltrick, E. (1990). The importance of a home evaluation for brain injured clients: A team approach. *Cognitive Rehabilitation, 8*(6), 28–32.

Starr, A., & Phillips, L. (1970). Verbal and motor memory in the amnestic syndrome. *Neuropsychologia, 8,* 75–88.

Stuss, D. T. (1991). Disturbance of self–awareness after frontal system damage. In G. P. Prigatano & D. L. Schacter (Eds.), *Awareness of deficit after brain injury: Clinical and theoretical issues* (pp.63–83). New York: Oxford University Press.

Stuss, D. T., & Benson, D. F. (1986). *The frontal lobes.* New York: Raven.

Stuss, D. T., Gow, C. A., & Hetherington, C. R. (1992). "No longer Gage": Frontal lobe dysfunction and emotional changes. *Journal of Consulting and Clinical Psychology, 60,* 349–359.

Sue, D. W., & Sue, D. (1990). *Counseling the culturally different: Theory and practice* (2nd ed.). New York: Wiley.

Sunderland, T., Alterman, I., Yount, D., Hill, J., Tariot, P., Newhouse, P., Mueller, E., Mellow, A., & Cohen, R. (1988). A new scale for the assessment of depressed mood in demented patients. *American Journal of Psychiatry, 145*, 955–959.

Teri, L., & Wagner, A. (1992). Alzheimer's disease and depression. *Journal of Consulting and Clinical Psychology, 60*, 379–391.

Tiberia, V. A., & Froman, T. (1986). The development and standardization of a Spanish version of the Washington Psychosocial Seizure Inventory. *Epilepsia, 27,* 51–54.

The tough case: Life care plan for a behaviorally challenging patient. (1993, March/April). *Headlines, 4*(2), 18–19.

Treiman, D. M. (1991). Psychobiology of ictal aggression. In D. Smith, D. Treiman, & M. Trimble (Eds.), *Advances in neurology* (Vol. 55, pp.341–356). New York: Raven.

Udaka, F., Yamao, S., Nagata, H., Nakamura, S., & Kameyama, M. (1984). Pathologic laughing and crying treated with levodopa. *Archives of Neurology, 41*, 1095–1096.

Van Allen, M. W., & Rodnitzky, R. L. (1981). *Pictorial manual of neurologic tests.* Chicago: Year Book.

Vidailhet, M., Rothwell, J. C., Thompson, P. D., Lees, A. J., & Marsden, C. D. (1992). The auditory startle response in the Steele–Richardson–Olszewski syndrome and Parkinson's disease. *Brain, 115,* 1181–1192.

Vitaliano, P. P. (1990). Commentary. *Journal of Family Practice, 30*, 437–440.

Vitaliano, P. P., Maiuro, R. D., Ochs, H., & Russo, J. (1989). A model of burden in caregivers of DAT patients. In E. Light & B. Lebowitz (Eds.), *Alzheimer's disease treatment and family stress: Future directions of research* (pp. 267–291). Washington, DC: Government Printing Office.

Vitaliano, P. P., Russo, J., Young, H. M., Becker, J., & Maiuro, R. D. (1991). The Screen for Caregiver Burden. *The Gerontologist, 31,* 76–83.

Vitaliano, P. P., Young, H. M., & Russo, J. (1991). Burden: A review of measures used among caregivers of individuals with dementia. *The Gerontologist, 31*, 68–75.

Vygotsky, L. S. (1978). *Mind in society: The development of higher psychological processes.* Cambridge, MA: Harvard University Press.

Waaland, P. K., & Kreutzer, J. S. (1988). Family response to childhood traumatic brain injury. *Journal of Head Trauma Rehabilitation, 3*(4), 51–63.

Walsh, K. W. (1978). *Neuropsychology: A clinical approach.* London: Churchill Livingston.

Webb, D. (1991). Increasing carryover and independent use of compensatory strategies in brain injured patients. *Cognitive Rehabilitation, 9*(3), 28–35.

Weber, A. M. (1990). A practical clinical approach to understanding and treating attentional problems. *Journal of Head Trauma Rehabilitation, 5,* 73–85.

Wehman, P., & Kreutzer, J. (Eds., 1990). *Vocational rehabilitation of persons with traumatic brain injury.* Rockville, MD: Aspen.

Weiger, W. A., & Bear, D. M. (1988). An approach to the neurology of aggression. *Journal of Psychiatric Research, 22,* 85–98.

Werner, D. (1990). *Disabled village children.* Palo Alto, CA: Hesperian Foundation, 1919 Addison St. #304, Berkeley, CA 94704.

Werner, D., & Bower, B. (1982). *Helping health workers learn.* Palo Alto, CA: Hesperian Foundation.

West, M. D. (1995). Aspects of the workplace and return to work for persons with brain injury in supported employment. *Brain Injury, 9,* 301–313.

Wiederholt, W. G. (Ed., 1988). *Neurology for non-neurologists.* Philadelphia, PA: W. B. Saunders.

Willer, B. S., Allen, K., Anthony, J., & Cowlan, G. (1993). *Circles of support for individuals with acquired brain injury.* Buffalo, NY: Rehabilitation Research and Training Center on Community Integration of Persons with Traumatic Brain Injury.

Willer, B., & Corrigan, J. D. (1994). Whatever it takes: A model for community-based services. *Brain Injury, 8,* 647–659.

Willer, B., Johnson, W. E., Rempel, R. G., & Linn, R. (1993). A note concerning misconceptions of the general public about brain injury. *Archives of Clinical Neuropsychology, 8,* 461–465.

Williams, J. M., & Kay, T. (1991). *Head injury: A family matter.* Baltimore, MD: Paul H. Brookes.

Williams, J. M., & Long, C. J. (Eds., 1987) *The rehabilitation of cognitive disabilities.* New York: Plenum.

Wilson, B. A. (1987). *Rehabilitation of memory.* New York: Guilford.

Wilson, B. A. (1992). Rehabilitation and memory disorders. In L. R. Squire & N. Butters (Eds.). *Neuropsychology of memory* (2nd ed., pp. 315–321). New York: Guilford.

Wilson, B. A. (1997). Cognitive rehabilitation: How it is and how it might be. *Journal of the International Neuropsychological Society, 3,* 487–496.

Woessner, R., & Kaplan, B. (1995). Affective disorders following mild to moderate brain injury: Interpretive hazards of the SCL–90–R. *Journal of Head Trauma Rehabilitation, 10*(2), 78–89.

Wood, F., Ebert, V., & Kinsbourne, M. (1982). The episodic–semantic memory distinction in memory and amnesia: Clinical and experimental observations. In L. Cermak (Ed.), *Memory and amnesia.* Hillsdale, NJ: Lawrence Erlbaum Associates.

Woodward, J. R. (1993). A secret in the family. *Mouth, the voice of disability rights, 3*(5), 22–23. (Available from Mouth, 61 Brighton St., Rochester, NY 14607, USA)

World Health Organization. (1981). *Disability prevention and rehabilitation: Report of the WHO expert committee on disability prevention and rehabilitation.* Geneva, Switzerland: World Health Organization.

World Health Organization. (1982). *Community based rehabilitation.* (Report of a WHO interregional consultation Columbo, Sri Lanka, June 28–July 3). Geneva, Switzerland: World Health Organization.

Wright, B. A. (1983). *Physical disability: A psychosocial approach.* New York: Harper & Row.

Yehuda, R., Keefe, R. S., Harvey, P. D., Levengood, R. A., Gerber, D. K., Geni, J., & Siever, L. J. (1995). Learning and memory in combat veterans with posttraumatic stress disorder. *American Journal of Psychiatry, 152,* 137–139.

Ylvisaker, M., Feeney, T., & Mullins, K. (1995). School reentry following mild traumatic brain injury: A proposed hospital-to-school protocol. *Journal of Head Injury Rehabilitation, 10*(6), 42–49.

Ylvisaker, M., & Gobble, E. M. R. (Eds., 1987) *Community reentry for head injured adults.* Boston: Little, Brown & Co.

Youngjohn, J. R., Davis, D., & Wolf, I. (1997). Head injury and the MMPI–2: Paradoxical severity effects and the influence of litigation. *Psychological Assessment, 9,* 177–184.

Yudofsky, S. C., Silver, J. M., & Hales, R. E. (1990). Pharmacologic management of aggression in the elderly. *Journal of Clinical Psychiatry, 51 (supplement 10),* 22–28.

Yudofsky, S. C., Silver, J. M., Jackson, M., Endicott, J., & Williams, D. (1986). The Overt Aggression Scale: An operationalized rating scale for verbal and physical aggression. *American Journal of Psychiatry, 143,* 35–39.

Yudofsky, S. C., Silver, J., & Yudofsky, B. (1989). Organic personality disorder, explosive type. In *Treatment of psychiatric disorders: A task force report of the American Psychiatric Association* (pp. 839–852). Washington, DC: American Psychiatric Association.

Zalewski, C., Thompson, W., & Gottesman, I., (1994). Comparison of neuropsychological test performance in PTSD, generalized anxiety disorder, and control Vietnam veterans. *Assessment, 1*(2), 133–142.

Zasler, N. D. (1988). Sexuality issues after traumatic brain injury. *Sexuality Update, 1*(1), 1–3.

Zeigler, E. A. (1987). Spouses of persons who are brain injured: Overlooked victims. *Journal of Rehabilitation, 10,* 50–53.

Zeilig, G., Drubach, D. A., Katz–Zeilig, M., & Karatinos, J. 1996). Pathological laughter and crying in patients with closed traumatic head injury. *Brain Injury, 10,* 591–597.

Zgola, J. M. (1987). *Doing things: A guide to programming activities for persons with Alzheimer's disease and related disorders.* Baltimore, MD: Johns Hopkins University Press.

Zung, W. (1965). A self–rating depression scale. *Archives of General Psychiatry, 12,* 63–70.

# Index

A. L. S. (Case), 184
AABCCC (technique for assessment of sexual problems), 305
ABC (technique of behavioral analysis), 91–93
Abuela (Case), 76
Abulia, 28, 216–221, 322, 334
Acquired brain injury: *see* Traumatic Brain Injury
Activation, disturbances of, 28, 322
Active listening, 41, 109, 111, 115, 120–121, 208, 233
Acute illness onset: *see* Illness onset, sudden
Adolescent, 90, 277–278, 301, 314, 340, 348, 349
Adolescent Psychosocial Seizure Inventory, 210, 331
Advocacy, viii, 2–3, 11–13, 53–54, 60, 105, 133, 211, 261,277, 284, 287, 293–294,297, 299, 303, 313–314, 318–319, 349
Affect
  flat: *see* Abulia; Communication Pragmatics; Emotional expressiveness
  labile: *see* Emotions, labile; Reflex crying; Reflex laughing
Africa, 270–271
Agenda
  for family education, 96
  for therapy session, 67, 87, 90, 110, 112
Agitated Behavior Scale, 331
Agitation, 20, 55, 94, 159, 166, 194–202, 322, 329, 331, 342; *see also* Anger
Aggression, 9, 55, 82, 119, 126, 137, 159, 173, 194, 197, 198, 206, 214, 219, 223, 278, 331, 342, 344, 353, 354, 355, 356; *see also* Anger
Agraphia, 57, 334
AIDS, 7, 17, 317, 319, 324
Alcohol, viii, 7, 24, 25, 55, 59, 70, 75, 79, 88, 91, 96, 109, 128, 148, 178–179, 195–199, 206, 222, 223, 234, 258; *see also* Substance abuse
Alexia, 47, 57, 334
Alexithymia, 321, 324, 353
Alexopoulos, G., 163, 329, 339
Alfano, D., 72, 339
Alzheimer's disease, 7, 10, 18, 22, 24, 56, 58, 61, 70, 118, 120–121, 140, 159–160, 190, 229, 258, 268–270, 281, 287, 317, 336; *see also* Dementia
Amantadine: *see* Medication, amantadine
American Heart Association, 277, 294, 339, 346
American Psychiatric Association: *see* DSM IV
Ames, D., 227, 339
Amnesia, vii, 4, 11, 37, 56, 66, 70, 88–91, 94, 145, 155–161, 166–168, 174–176, 194, 211, 227, 248–253, 306, 324, 333, 334, 342, 347, 355; *see also* Memory, impairments in

Amnesia (*cont.*)
anterograde, 42, 174, 249–250, 323, 334, 336
posttraumatic, 68, 70, 107, 128, 140, 160, 202, 249, 252–253, 281, 334, 336
psychogenic, 174, 249, 323, 334, 336,
retrograde, 68, 334, 336
Amphetamine: *see* Medication, stimulant
Amygdala, 197, 210
Anger
characteristics of, 167, 171, 196–197, 209, 221
cue cards for, 111, 114, 117, 119, 203–205
of family, 54, 85, 193, 264, 266–267, 270, 285
impulsive, 7, 28, 32, 48, 55–56, 69, 119, 123, 135, 137–138, 159, 170, 175–176, 193–197, 209, 310, 311, 315, 322
interventions for, 21, 48, 86, 95, 104, 109, 141–143, 149, 198, 203–209, 247, 311–312, 350
irritability, 55, 59, 68, 94, 109–111, 117, 119, 159, 170, 175–177, 194–195, 197, 209, 214, 222, 256, 258, 305, 322, 329
sources of, 55, 155–156, 167, 171, 176, 194–195, 222, 237, 247, 273, 321
Anhedonia, 159, 330
Anosognosia, 28, 48, 66, 78, 86, 105, 120, 124–129, 155–164, 170, 172, 217, 234–236, 315–316, 322, 334, 345, 352
Anoxia, 7, 18–19, 324, 334
Anticholinergic effects: *see* Medication, anticholinergic effects of
Anticonvulsant: *see* Medication, anticonvulsant
Antidepressant: *see* Medication, antidepressant
Antipsychotic: *see* Medication, antipsychotic
Antonak, R. F., 27, 339
Anxiety, 23, 24, 48, 53–55, 58, 66, 68, 91–94, 114, 126, 137–138, 143, 155, 159, 164–169, 173, 174, 189, 199, 200, 211, 219, 227, 229, 232, 247, 258, 263–264, 267, 273, 276–277, 303, 321, 329–330, 356
Anxiolytic: *see* Medication, anxiolytic
Aphasia, *see also* Communication; Language; Speech
activities for people with, 47, 255
defined, 334, 336
emotional dimensions, 253–257, 276, 284, 322
family interaction, 33, 52–53, 66, 98
intervention for, 120, 140, 145, 161, 164, 188, 257, 315
managing, 88, 117, 189
as symptom, 56–57, 104, 161, 170, 187–188, 195, 226–227, 234, 240–241, 250–251, 273
testing for, 52–53, 188, 330
Apraxia
defined, 334
emotional dimensions, 272–273
family interaction, 33
as symptom, 56–57, 227, 323, 325
Aprosodia: *see* Emotional communication; Monotone voice
Aronson, M. K., 294, 339, 209, 255, 346
Art, 68, 87, 89, 100
Assault, 20, 70, 119, 165, 172, 309, 334
Assessment
adjusting the conclusions of, 82–83
as a cognitive problem-solving process, 51–65
of environment of recovery, 72, 74–77
of families: *see* Family, assessment
feedback, 32, 81–82
hypotheses in, 52–58
incident log in: *see* Incident log
neuropsychological, 8–9, 14, 20, 32, 51–83, 329
neurobehavioral, 63–77, 191, 328–329, 345, 348
role of cognitive testing in, 39–40, 59–63
role of personality testing in, 59–63, 73
of sexuality problems: *see* Sexuality, assessment planning
use of informants, 59, 66, 71, 77, 197, 235, 327
Attention
concentration, 68, 73, 109, 123, 159–160, 166, 168, 174–176, 184, 247–248, 262
deficit disorder, 7, 214, 237, 245–248

Automatic cursing, 28, 172, 187–189, 192, 195, 196, 221–222, 322
Awareness, *see also* Anosognosia
lack of, 7, 28, 48, 56, 67–68, 72–75, 156, 161
self–awareness training, 53, 82, 95–96, 108, 109–111, 118, 122–134, 138, 151

B. B. (Case), 12
Backing off, 93, 98, 109, 111, 116, 119, 137, 141–152, 202–205, 224, 229, 310, 312
Barkley, R. A., 214, 247, 339,
Barbiturates: *see* Medication, barbiturates
Basal ganglia, 57, 182, 190, 217, 227, 340
Batzel, L. W., 73, 210, 331, 339, 343
Bear, D. M., 10, 187, 197, 208–210, 235, 331, 340, 342, 354, 355
Beck, A., 73, 162, 329, 340
Becker, M. E., 5, 287, 340, 354
Behavior
analysis, 91–93, 341, 346; *see also* Incident log; Record-keeping
Change Inventory, 191, 198, 235, 327
cognitive-behavioral: *see* Cognitive-behavioral
control, 7, 18–22, 45–46, 72, 91–96, 138–146, 184, 187–189, 197, 206–208, 213–214, 223–224, 270, 286–287, 303, 310, 318
flash cards, 113–117, 243
modification, 34–37, 94–95, 349, 350
problem: *see* Problem behavior
reinterpreting, 64, 94, 306, 331
Ben-Yishay, Y., 37, 298
Benzodiazapine: *see* Medication, anxiolytic
Bergquist, T. F., 120, 340
Binder, L. M., 250, 340
Bipolar disorder: *see* Depression; Manic-depressive disorder
Bishop, D. S., 24, 286–287, 340
Black, D. W., 184, 340
Blame, 25–26, 32, 85, 91, 195, 207, 251–253, 266, 270, 289
Block, S. H., 5, 35, 85, 87–88, 340
Blonder, L. X., 182, 340
Blosser, J. L., viii, 98, 99–100, 301, 303, 308, 340
Blumer, D., 5, 190, 340
Bohnen, N., 258, 340
Borod, J. C., 26, 181, 182, 340
Brain
growth, 44
injury: *see* Traumatic brain injury
Brain illness
in children: *see* Children
depression in: *see* Depression
education concerning: *see* Education
emotions and: *see* Emotional; Emotions
grief in: *see* Grief
infection: *see* Infection, brain
onset of: *see* Illness onset
personality in: *see* Personality
psychotherapy in: *see* Psychotherapy in brain illness
responsibility for behavior in: *see* Responsibility
toxicity: *see* Toxicity, brain
Brainstem, 37, 179
Brodal, A., 87, 341
Bromocriptine: *see* Medications, bromocriptine
Brooks, N., 250, 263–264, 341, 348, 351
Brother: *see* Family, sibling
Bullis, R. K., 85, 341
Burden, of caregiving: *see* Caregiving, burden of
Burgess, P. W., 341
Burke, W. H., 35, 43, 91, 116, 139, 341, 345
Burns, D., 124, 145, 292, 341, 353
Busch, C. R., 158, 264, 341, 351

Calm down, 20, 102, 138, 141–145, 149, 168, 171, 202, 205–206
Campbell, J. J., 215, 341
Caregivers: *see* Caregiving
Caregiving
burdens of, 23–24, 122–123, 263–268, 270, 277–281, 284–285, 287, 348, 354
depression: *see* Depression, in caregivers
Caretakers: *see* Caregiving
Catastrophic reaction, 7, 28, 48, 56, 61, 122–123, 173–174, 247, 253, 321, 330
Caudate nucleus, 217

Causality
  and blame, 85
  of symptoms, 6–7, 51, 55, 88, 101, 122–123, 134, 160, 162, 198, 210, 273
Cavallo, M. M., viii, 11, 65, 263, 264, 271, 277–279, 282, 286–287, 317, 341, 347
Cerebra (Case), 126–127
Cerebral vascular accident (CVA): *see* Stroke
Chemical dependency: *see* Substance abuse
Child
  and brain illness, viii, 52, 117, 187, 214, 277, 304, 312, 316, 342, 343, 345, 348, 350, 355
  custody, 152, 157, 179, 203–204, 279–281, 289
  of persons with brain illnesses, 61, 102, 246, 248, 270, 271–272, 278–282, 286, 289, 327, 351, 354
Chittum, W. R., 131, 341
Christensen, A.-L., 8–9, 32, 72, 81, 340, 341, 343
Chronic pain: *see* Pain, chronic
Chronic sorrow: *see* Grief
Cicerone, K. D., 18–19, 45, 122, 124, 213–214, 224, 230, 239, 341, 351
Cingulum, 197
Circles of support: *see* Support, circles of
Coaches
  job: *see* Vocational job coaches
  social skills, 97–98, 183, 225, 232, 243, 302–304
Cognisyst, 183, 330
Cognitive
  analysis of assessment process: *see* Assessment, as a cognitive problem-solving process
  -behavioral: *see* Psychotherapy, cognitive-behavioral
  compensation, 4–5, 14, 37, 107, 113, 118, 251, 259, 295, 299–300
  errors in diagnostic reasoning, 51, 62, 65, 351
  impairment, 8, 28–29, 37, 39, 41, 48, 55–57, 86, 122, 166, 181, 195, 211, 245
  orthotics, 102, 219, 221
  prosthetics, 102, 219
Cognitive (*cont.*)
  psychotherapy: *see* Psychotherapy, cognitive
  rehabilitation: *see* Rehabilitation, cognitive
  remediation: *see* Rehabilitation, cognitive
  rigidity: *see* Concreteness; Perseveration
  strategies, 45, 144
  task analysis, 15, 34
  testing, 71–72, 215, 314
Coolidge Axis II Inventory, 328, 342
Coolidge, F. L., 328, 342
Comfort, A., 277, 342
Command performance syndrome, 285, 353
Communication, *see also* Language; Aphasia
  emotional: *see* Emotional communication
  pragmatics, 4, 21, 28, 68, 72, 87, 90, 240–243, 303, 322, 329, 336
  style in neuropsychotherapy, *see* Neuropsychotherapy, communication style in
  word-finding, 41, 45, 68, 161, 250, 254, 266
Community
  -based rehabilitation, 293–294, 301, 315, 344, 348, 351, 355
  disability, 293–295
  homeless, 311–312
  integration, 11, 80, 130, 135, 261, 292, 300, 312, 327, 343, 347, 353
  medical/rehabilitation, 48, 291, 304
  prison, 309–311
  school, 301–302
  social, 302–309
  workplace, 295–301
Compensation, 5–6, 19, 21, 41–43, 46, 79–80, 88, 110, 117, 126–127, 131–134, 168, 179, 183, 189–190, 216–239, 243, 311, 324, 342, 355; *see also* Cognitive, compensation
Concentration: *see* Attention
Concreteness, 34, 56, 175, 189, 211, 214, 217, 228, 230–233, 275, 308, 311, 322
Confrontation, 58, 61, 66, 82, 121, 127, 133, 141, 156–158, 164, 173, 196, 199, 305–307
Conjoint interview: *see* Informant

Continuum of responsibility: *see* Responsibility, continuum of
Cook, J. V., 302. 342
Cornell Scale for Depression and Dementia, 162–163, 329, 339
Corpus striatum. 247
Corrections: *see* Community, prison
Corrigan, J. D, viii, 76, 195, 198, 292, 294, 298, 328. 331, 342, 345, 355
Cost
of assessment, 51–53, 58, 60–61
benefit analysis, 48, 61, 83
of care and rehabilitation, 11–12, 60, 64, 252, 293
of intervention, 59, 82
Costa Rica, viii, ix, 47, 52–53, 76, 119, 283, 284
Counseling, *see also* Neuropsychotherapy
for problem-solving, 2, 11–12, 99, 100, 101, 103. 151–152, 173, 186, 191, 211, 224-225, 287–288, 294, 303–304
for sexuality, 272–277, 306–309
Cowell, L. C., 221, 342
Crook, T. H., 328, 342
Crosson, B., 126, 234, 342
Crying, reflex: *see* Reflex crying
Cue cards
for anger, 119, 142–144, 202–206, 310
for anxiety, 114
for depression, 114, 179, 329
for emotional control, 45–46, 109, 111, 116–117. 134–135, 151, 173, 186, 188, 228-229
examples of, 111, 113–115, 117–118
flash cards: *see* Behavior flash cards
forms of, 113. 225
for procedures and routines, 41, 102, 114, 145. 224, 243, 300–301, 315
for stressful events, 21, 115, 223
uses in neuropsychotherapy, 113–118, 254
writing, 113–118
Cuing, 41, 81, 98, 132, 143, 148–149, 194, 218–219. 221, 228, 303
Cultural considerations, viii, 10, 35, 66, 70, 90, 112, 118, 135, 150, 172, 189, 195. 196, 207–208, 215, 222, 238, 240. 242, 262, 270, 282, 285, 300, 308. 313–314, 316–317, 329, 331, 341. 344, 348, 349, 351, 354
Cummings, J. L., 70, 73, 191, 227, 329, 339, 342
Cursing, automatic: *see* Automatic cursing

Damasio, A. R., 92, 306, 316, 325, 342
Death, 30, 70, 155, 163, 178, 264, 268, 347, 350
DeBoskey, D. S., 133, 342
Delusions, 24, 68, 69, 105, 121, 140, 195, 201, 322, 329, 342, 351
Dementia, 13, 17, 24, 56, 64, 120–121, 140, 162–163, 198–199, 266, 272, 287, 306, 314, 328, 329, 339, 342, 344, 347, 351, 354; *see also* Alzheimer's disease; Huntington's disease; Illness onset, progressive; Jacob-Creutzfeldt disease; Multi-infarct dementia; Parkinson's disease
activities for people with, 281, 343
and depression: *see* Depression and dementia
Dementia Mood Assessment Scale, 163, 329
Denial, 33, 54, 67, 125–127, 155–158, 196, 234–235, 264, 266, 321, 324, 325, 352; *see also* Anosognosia; Awareness
Dependency
chemical: *see* Substance abuse
emotional: *see* Emotional, dependency
DePompei, R., viii, 98–100, 287, 301, 303, 308, 340, 342
Depression, *see also* Beck Depression Inventory; Cornell Scale for Depression and Dementia; Dementia Mood Assessment Scale; Geriatric Depression Scale; Hamilton Depression Rating Scale; Manic-depressive disorder; Post-Stroke Depression Rating Scale; Zung Depression Scale
in caregivers, 24, 263–264, 273, 285, 344
and confusable neurological symptoms, 1, 5, 58, 119–120, 185, 189, 217, 238, 242, 247, 252
and dementia, 328, 339, 347, 354
evaluation, 55–58, 68, 321, 328–330, 340, 345, 356

Depression (*cont.*)
in persons with brain illness, 12, 24, 48, 53–54, 76, 95–96, 101, 114, 122–124, 127, 130, 137–138, 143, 155, 158–165, 172, 176, 177, 179, 182, 209, 218, 252, 253, 275, 284, 303, 307, 341, 344, 347, 352
post-stroke rating scale, 330, 344, 352
psychotherapy for: *see* Psychotherapy, depression
sudden, 114, 138, 143, 179
Devinsky, O., 187, 208, 209, 342
Devlieger, P., 271, 317, 342
Diagnostic and Statistical Manual, 4th Edition, American Psychiatric Association: *see* DSM IV
Dikengil, A., viii, 303, 317, 343
Dikmen, S., 67, 343
Direnfeld, G., 85, 343
Disability
awareness of: *see* Awareness
community: *see* Community, disability
overestimation of, 122–124, 170
rights, viii, 87, 105, 221, 261, 293, 318–319, 355
underestimation of, 122, 124–134
Disorientation: *see* Orientation, disorientation
Distraction
as an attention problem, 40, 68, 74, 109–110, 120, 160, 175–177, 214, 245–248, 258, 323, 348
as a behavior management strategy, 20, 114, 128, 139, 141, 143, 152, 186, 193–194, 199, 202, 228, 253, 275
Dodrill, C., 73, 210, 211, 330–331, 339, 343
Don (Case), 309
Doris (Case), 254
Douglass (Case), 118–119, 310
Drug use/abuse, viii, 7, 24, 59, 91, 114, 148, 179, 199, 223, 258, 310, 317, 319, 324
DSM IV, 81, 159–160, 174, 198
Dumi (Case), 218, 220–221, 243
Dysarthria, 12, 117, 182, 254, 335
Dysthymia: *see* Depression

Eames, P., 35, 91, 92, 343
Education, *see also interventions for specific problems*
contents of, 86, 89, 96–97, 130, 133, 272–276, 347
Education (*cont.*)
in neuropsychotherapy, 3, 18, 24, 349
of family and community, 2–3, 12, 20, 25, 31–37, 52, 64–65, 76, 81, 86, 89, 96–103, 151, 164, 186, 219, 272–289, 293–312, 316–318, 342
of persons with brain illness, 2–3, 12, 21, 31–37, 52, 61–65, 81, 89, 164, 169, 171, 218, 293, 352, 353
techniques of, 82, 97–103, 124
Efficacy, 314–316
El Salvador, 78, 349
Elizabeth (Case), 45–46
Elliott, F. A., 343
Ellis, D. W., 8, 35, 107, 128, 340, 341, 343
Elvis (Case), 129–130
Embarrassment, 1–2, 45–46, 91, 113, 117, 123, 141–143, 172–173, 184–188, 193, 222, 254, 266, 283–284, 307, 321
Emma (Case), 281–282
Emotional
changes, organic, 181–211
changes, reactive, 54, 127, 156, 169–170, 196, 207, 211, 331
communication, 27–28, 68, 73, 104, 161, 163, 181–183, 241, 266, 316, 321–322; *see also* Automatic cursing; Reflex crying; Reflex laughing
comprehension, 57, 182–183, 211, 266, 321
dependency, 56–58, 70–71, 82, 122–123, 131, 209, 219, 288, 292–294, 324–325
expressiveness, 28, 52–53, 56, 79–80, 120, 161, 170, 175, 181, 189, 240, 253
incontinence: *see* Reflex crying; Reflex laughing
obsessiveness, 155, 197, 205, 208–211, 247, 321
Perception Test, 183, 330, 342
reactivity, 27–28, 57, 68, 79, 159, 170, 189–191, 195, 266, 322, 336
rehabilitation: *see* Rehabilitation, emotional
Emotions, *see also* Mood
labile, 159, 192–194, 322

Empathy
and concrete thinking, 175, 189, 231
deficits in, 120
false, vii
therapeutic, 318
Employment, 40, 295–300, 343, 353, 355
Encephalitis: *see* Infection, brain
Epilepsy
as intermittent disorder, 24–25
temporal lobe, 10, 192, 195, 208–211, 247, 315, 322, 331, 340, 342, 343, 344, 347, 354
Eslinger, P .J., 231, 343
Ethics, 13, 81, 104–105, 209, 280, 349
Evaluation: *see* Assessment
Evans, J. J., 239, 343
Executive functions, 213–243; *see also* Abulia; Anosognosia; Awareness; Communication pragmatics; Concreteness; Disinhibition; Impersistence; Impulsiveness; Initiation; Judgment; Monitoring; Organization; Perseveration; Planning
impairments, 12, 28, 32, 55–56, 86, 119, 195, 322
personality, 68, 86, 122, 205, 218, 232, 303
treatment of, general scheme, 213–244, 341
Existential aspects, 85, 262, 318, 349

Faith, vii, 27, 109, 145, 178, 263, 348; *see also* Religion; Spirituality
Family
adult child of the person with brain illness, 270, 278–279, 286
assessment, 59–60, 65–66, 70–71, 340
Assessment Device, 286–287
child, 203–204, 246, 248, 271–272, 278, 282, 289, 301, 327, 351, 354
extended, 76, 98, 103, 135, 264, 271, 279, 286, 304
gay male and lesbian, 271, 279–280, 349
Head Injury Family Interview, 198, 235, 286, 327–328, 347
Involvement Assessment Scale, 287, 331
large, 279, 281–282
nontraditional, 279
Family (*cont.*)
parent, 53, 128, 220, 264, 277–281, 286, 289, 311, 350, 351
roles, 264–265, 271, 284
siblings, 53–54, 278, 286, 327, 354
spouse, 24, 48, 190, 264, 267, 271–277, 279, 286–287, 327, 351, 356
Fatigue, 21, 55, 57, 69, 87, 91–92, 117, 139, 147, 159–160, 163–164, 166, 192, 199, 206, 227, 245–246, 255–257, 300, 323, 347, 348
Feedback, 32, 56, 79–83, 88, 99, 110, 119, 128–132, 183, 205, 214, 234, 236–237, 242–243, 298–299, 303, 308, 344
Feil, N., 8, 24, 120–121, 140, 343
Finset, A., 295, 302, 343
Fishman, S., 87, 343
Fordyce, D. J., 9, 63, 73, 325, 328, 343, 346
Fox, D. D., 67, 343
Frank (Case), 255, 276
Frankl, V., 261, 344
Fraser, R. T., 295–296, 298, 344
Freeman, E. A., 5, 292, 339, 344, 345
Frontal lobes
dorsolateral, 56, 78, 190, 217, 227
and executive functions, 213, 217, 222, 231, 234, 238, 242, 341, 354
orbital, 56, 92, 192, 197, 222, 224, 306
Personality Scale, 191, 235, 330, 344
posterior, 56, 182, 213, 227
Frustration, 41, 45–46, 53–54, 56, 61, 72, 75, 92, 111, 122, 138, 146–147, 150, 170–173, 195, 199, 200, 207, 257, 275, 308, 321
Fyodor (Case), 9, 10, 209

G. P. (Case), 301
Gabby (Case), 116–117, 243
Gainotti, G., 162, 330, 344
Gallo, J. J., 272, 285, 344
Gans, J. S., 85, 344
Gass, C. S., 81–83, 161, 344
Gay male: *see* Family, gay male and lesbian
Gehrig, Lou, 316
Generalization, 21, 32, 35, 40–44, 56, 88, 118, 125–126, 151, 216–243, 296, 348, 351, 356
Georgia (Case), 9, 10
Geriatric Depression Scale, 72, 344

Gigi (Case), 178–179
Gil, T., 176, 344
Gilles de la Tourette's syndrome: *see* Tourette's syndrome
Gilley, D. W., 70, 72, 159, 344
Glenn, M. B., 201, 344
Goldstein, K., 173, 230, 344
Gordon, W. A., 5, 13, 18, 40, 103, 158, 161, 162, 173, 329, 344, 345, 347, 351, 352
Grace, J., 191, 215, 218, 235, 330, 344
Gramps (Case), 245–246
Grief, *see also* Depression
  in acute illness, 283
  in family members, 251–252, 264, 271, 275, 288
  in intermittent illness, 270
  mobile mourning, 264
  in people with brain illnesses, 22–23, 56–58, 82–83, 155–156, 158, 163–164, 195, 206–207, 321, 345
  in progressive illness, 266–267
Griffith, E. R., 273–274, 277, 305, 344, 345, 352
Groucho (Case), 215, 306, 307
Guilt, 25, 55–58, 85, 91, 159, 177, 199, 209, 222, 264, 271, 278

Hagen, C., 21, 198, 329, 345
Hallucinations, 68–69, 174, 250, 329
Hamilton, M., 73, 162, 329, 345
Hare Psychopathy Checklist, 198, 344
Hartlage, L., 191, 198, 235, 327, 345
Haynes, S. D., 155, 345
Head injury: *see* Traumatic Brain Injury
Headache: *see* Pain, headache
Heilman, K. M., 28, 325, 345
Hibbard, M. R.: *see* Ruckdeschel-Hibbard, M.
Hickling, E. J., 176, 345
Hippocampus, 210, 250
Homework, 43, 90, 108, 110–113, 130, 133, 134, 289, 303
Homophobia, 280
Hotz, G., 225–228, 345, 346
Howard, M. E., 35, 91, 93, 139, 258, 346
Huntington's disease, 7, 8, 22, 268, 317
Hyperaesthesia, 56–57, 106, 139, 246–247, 257–259, 335, 340
Hypergraphia, 10, 209, 211
Hypersensitivity: *see* Hyperaesthesia
Hypersexuality: *see* Sexuality, hypersexuality
Hypervigilance, 167, 174–178
Hypoglycemia, 7, 24–26, 199, 206
Hyposexuality: *see* Sexuality, hyposexuality
Hypothalamus, 197
Hypotheses
  in assessment: *see* Assessment, hypotheses in
  testing of, 47

Illness onset,
  intermittent, 19, 25–26, 58, 270–271
  progressive, 17–19, 22–26, 58, 123, 125, 139, 142, 221, 266–270, 302, 315
  sudden, 17–22, 58, 64, 122–125, 137–138, 152, 264–267, 283
Impersistence, 28, 190, 214, 216, 322, 324, 335, 352
Impulsiveness, 7, 28, 32, 48, 55–56, 68, 78, 135, 137–138, 159, 194–208, 221–225, 310–311
Incident log, 131, 144–149, 205–206; *see also* Behavior analysis; Record-keeping
Independent living, 292–294, 302, 318, 325, 348, 349, 355
Indifference, 28, 56, 182, 189–190, 214, 252, 269, 329; *see also* Abulia; Emotional communication
Infection, brain, 7, 13, 123, 319
Informants, 34, 66, 71, 77, 197, 251, 327, 329
Ingrid (Case), 128–129
Insomnia: *see* Sleep
Intermittent illness onset: *see* Illness onset, intermittent
Initiation, *see also* Abulia
  impaired, 34, 78, 102, 159, 175, 216–221, 275, 307, 330
  rehabilitation of, 218–221
Irritability, 55, 59, 68, 94, 109–111, 117, 119, 159, 170, 175–177, 194–195, 197, 209, 214, 222, 256, 258, 305, 322, 329
Iverson, G. L., 311, 346

J. D. (Case), 86, 129
Jacob-Creutzfeldt disease, 268
Janaki's mother (Case), 100–101
Jones, M., 24, 121, 142, 201, 268, 346

Jochims, S., 255, 346
Journal, therapy
  cultural considerations, 112
  feelings journal, 93, 116, 131, 204–205
  responsibility for, 107–108, 151
  sections, 93, 108–112, 204
  uses of, 107–113
Juan (Case), 128, 133
Judd, T., 9, 39, 43, 63, 73, 184, 185, 186, 190, 235, 252, 346, 349
Judgment, impaired, 126, 195, 205, 234, 236–237, 277

Kassirer, J. P., 52, 58–60, 65, 346
Katz Adjustment Scale, 328, 344, 346
Katz, M., 184, 285, 328, 345, 346, 353
Kay, T., 11, 61, 65, 71, 87, 124, 191, 198, 235, 263, 264, 271, 277, 278, 279, 282, 286–287, 298, 316, 327, 343, 346, 347, 355
Klonoff, P. S., 35, 36, 324, 328, 347, 351
Kreutzer, J. S., viii, 13, 265, 277, 279, 295, 296, 304, 347, 352, 353, 355
Kubler-Ross, E., 340
Kushner, H. S., 85, 347

Lability: *see* Emotions, labile; Reflex crying; Reflex laughing
LaChapelle, D. L., 347
Lamberty, G. A., 160, 161, 347
Language, *see also* Communication; Dysarthria; Word–finding
  impairment, 89, 172, 254–255, 303, 323; *see also* Aphasia
  reading, 47, 53–54, 68, 74, 108, 111–112, 119, 129, 220, 300, 323
  writing, 10, 34, 53, 68, 90, 104, 107–108, 112, 128, 143, 173, 190, 226, 229, 243, 301
Laughing
  inappropriate
  reflex: *see* Reflex laughing
Layton, B. S., 166, 176, 249, 347
Laziness
Learning, procedural: *see* Memory, procedural learning
Lefebvre, K. A.
Left
  hemisphere, 52, 161, 188
  neglect: *see* Neglect, unilateral

Lesbian: *see* Family, gay male and lesbian
Levin, H. S., 17, 191, 198, 328, 348, 349, 353
Lezak, M. D., 7, 9, 40, 51, 59, 71, 168, 213, 215, 218, 264, 271, 272, 277, 278, 348
Liberation psychology and neuropsychology, 312, 349
Libido: *see* Sexuality, libido
Lieberman, A., 184, 344, 348
Limbic
  epilepsy: *see* Epilepsy, temporal lobe
  system, 190, 192, 210, 213, 250–251, 287
Listening, active: *see* Active listening
Livingston, M. G., 263, 264, 348, 355
Lobe: *see* Frontal lobes; Occipital lobes; Parietal lobes; Temporal lobes
Love, 145, 255, 262, 271–275, 278, 283, 348
Lu Tan (Case), 245–247, 300
Ludwig (Case), 189, 190, 234–235
Lysack, C., 294, 301, 348

Maitz, E. A., 278, 287, 289, 349
Malec, J. F., 11, 349
Malloy, P., 191, 215, 344, 349
Malingering, 26, 247, 340
Manic-depressive disorder, 6, 195, 208, 214, 222, 234, 242, 329; *see also* Depression
Maori, 316, 351
Mapou, R., 279, 349
Marcel (Case), 32–33
Marilyn (Case), 280–281
Martín-Baró, I., 312, 349
Masters, W. H., 276, 349
Mateer, C., ix, 26, 39–43, 107, 218, 248, 250–252, 349, 354
McGann, W., 303, 349
McNeill, D. E.
Meaning
  of life, 58, 86, 262
  of words, 121, 230, 241
Medication
  amantadine, 201, 221, 342
  amphetamine: *see* Medication, stimulant
  anticholinergic effects of, 206
  anxiolytic, 142, 194, 201
  anticonvulsant, 142, 194, 201, 211, 311

Medication (*cont.*)
antidepressant, 1, 142, 161, 164–168, 178, 187, 194, 201, 206, 259, 347, 454
antipsychotic, 168, 194, 201, 206
barbiturates, 206
bromocriptine, 221, 339
dopamine agonists, 201, 221, 339, 342 347
opiates, 206
tranquilizer, major: *see* Medication, anti-psychotic
tranquilizer, minor: *see* Medication, anxiolytic
stimulant, 195, 202, 206, 259, 275
Meichenbaum, D., 18–19, 35, 41, 44, 100, 145, 149, 168, 349, 350
Memory
Assessment Clinics–Psychiatric (instrument), 328
compensations, 41, 168, 179, 251–252
confabulation, 56, 79–80, 88, 223, 250–251, 256, 323, 335
impairments, 43, 56–57, 170, 217, 227, 237, 241, 269, 296, 301, 323; *see also* Amnesia
procedural learning, 42–43, 145, 168, 229, 249, 252
prospective, 90, 217, 249–250, 323, 336
Meningitis: *see* Infection, brain
Mentoring, 97–100, 303, 340
Metaphor, use in education, 31, 89–90, 97, 102, 219, 230, 233
Migraine, 7, 24, 92, 270
Miller, L., viii, 8, 9, 35, 195–196, 245, 286, 287, 294, 375, 340, 342, 343, 345, 350, 352
Minnesota Multiphasic Personality Inventory: *see* MMPI
Mr. Bates (Case), 306
Mittenberg, W., 124, 350
MMPI, 72, 157, 177, 328, 339, 340, 356
Modeling, as form of education, 97–99, 186, 205, 254, 233–237, 303, 322
Monitoring, 20–21, 44, 53, 131, 171, 214
Monotone voice, 28, 181; *see also* Abulia; Communication pragmatics; Emotional expressiveness
Mood, 12, 43–44, 67, 76, 159–161, 165, 185, 190, 198, 325, 329, 330, 341, 350, 354;*see also* Emotional; Emotions
visual mood scale, 161–162, 330, 359
Morton, M. V., 8, 158, 166, 295, 302, 350
Motivation, 54, 60, 95, 109, 171, 216, 218–219, 257, 295, 298, 307–308
Mourning: *see* Grief
Mountain, M., 183, 316, 330, 359
Muir, C. A., 264, 287, 350, 352
Multi-infarct dementia, 17, 268
Multiple sclerosis, 7, 8, 17, 19, 268, 270, 328, 351
Music, 43, 56, 57, 121, 129–130, 143, 177, 190, 229, 235, 255, 269, 346

Naricio (Case), 52–54
Natural helper, support: *see* Support, natural
Neglect, unilateral, 47, 56–57, 104, 120, 127, 129, 234, 256
Nelson, L., 191, 235, 329, 350
Neuroanatomy, 8, 58, 336; *see also characteristics of specific problems*, 155–257
Neurobehavioral Rating Scale, 191, 198, 328, 348
Neuropsychiatric Inventory, 73, 191, 329, 342
Neuropsychologist, 2–3, 8–9, 104, 127, 312
Neuropsychological
report, 32, 108, 130
test: *see* Assessment, role of cognitive tests in; Assessment, role of personality tests in; Test
Neuropsychology Behavior and Affect Profile, 191, 235, 329, 350
Neuropsychotherapist, qualifications and training, 8–9, 28–29
Neuropsychotherapy
appropriate patients, 6
balance with psychotherapy, 33, 36–37
cognitive compensations in, 4–5, 37, 107, 113, 252, 295, 299–300
and cognitive rehabilitation, 3–5, 8, 39–48
communication style in, 87–90
defined, 3–6
need for, 8
roadmap to this book, 14
role of the neuropsychotherapist, 8–9, 20–21, 24–25, 27, 28, 47, 63, 104, 105, 127, 142, 208, 211, 253, 288, 289, 308, 313–314
theoretical foundations
treatable problems, 6–8

Neuropsychotherapy (*cont.*)
validation therapy, 120–121, 140–141, 343
when needed, 9–14
Neurotoxicity: *see* Toxicity, brain
New person, 85--87, 265
New Zealand, 316, 351
Nguyen (Case), 310
Nicaragua, viii–ix, 311–312
Nightmares, 156, 174, 177
Novaco, R., 203, 350

O. (Case), 310
Obsession, 34, 159, 177, 205, 208–211, 226–227, 321–322, 324, 349, 351
Occipital lobes, 57
Olshansky, S., 264, 350organi
Onset of illness: *see* Illness onset
Opiates: *see* Medication, opiates
Organic aggressive syndrome, 195, 198; *see also* Anger
Organization, impaired, 237–239
Orientation
disorientation, 94, 121, 139, 175, 201, 253
reorientation, 140, 201–202
Oscar (Case), 279–280
Overload: *see* Fatigue; Hyperaesthesia
Overprotection, 45, 53–54, 71, 123, 270, 277, 282–284, 301, 315
Overt Aggression Scale, 73, 198, 331, 356

P. T. A. (Case), 253
Pain
chronic, 165, 245, 325, 340, 343, 345
headache, 35, 73, 92, 116, 206, 273
Paranoia, 68–69, 130, 209, 234, 253, 321, 324, 351
Parent: *see* Family, parent
Parenté, R., 133, 292, 298, 299–301, 350
Parietal lobes, 56, 182, 190, 227, 235, 247
Parkinson's disease, 7–8, 18, 22, 159, 182, 190, 217, 268, 317, 351, 354
Partial complex seizures: *see* Epilepsy, temporal lobe
Pathological crying: *see* Reflex crying
Pathological laughter: *see* Reflex laughing
Pathological Laughter and Crying Scale, 185, 330
Patient role, 105, 135, 221, 291–293
Peat, M., 13, 293, 301, 351
Pega (Case), 311–312, 314
Peleo (Case), 118–119, 310
Pepe (Case), 76–77
Perplexity, 55, 57, 58, 85, 94, 168–169, 321, 348
Perseveration, 28, 56, 68, 92, 138, 159, 205, 214, 225–230, 232, 273, 322, 336, 345, 346, 353
Personal reformation, 21, 178–180, 321
Personality,
disorders, 55, 165, 196–197, 295, 310, 351, 356
and executive functions, 213–217, 222
factors of in brain illness, 3, 5–6, 8, 21, 26–29, 198, 321–325, 353
positive change in, with brain illness, 9, 193–195, 351
pre-illness, 34, 36, 47, 63–64, 66–70, 177, 185, 207–208, 285
in temporal lobe epilepsy, 10, 195, 197, 208–211, 340, 344
tests: *see* Assessment, role of personality tests in; Test
Pessar, L. F., 278, 351
Planning, impaired, 56, 159, 175–176, 237–239, 322; *see also* Impairment, organization
PLISSIT (levels of intervention for sexual problems), 272–274
Portland (Case), 230
Post-Stroke Depression Rating Scale, 162, 330
Posttraumatic amnesia see Amnesia, posttraumatic
Posttraumatic stress disorder: *see* PTSD
Pragmatics: *see* Communication pragmatics
Prayer, 143–145
Prevention, 199–201, 319, 355
Prigatano, G. P., ix, 5, 8, 26, 35, 85, 89, 124, 189, 190, 192, 195, 262, 316, 324, 328, 343, 345, 351, 352, 354
Problem
analysis, 91–93
anticipation, 91, 94, 95–96, 148, 152, 203, 236, 268, 287
in assessment: *see* Assessment as a cognitive problem-solving process
behaviors, 91–95, 137, 139–142, 148–151
feelings, 44, 137–152

Problem (*cont.*)
list, and strengths: *see* Strengths and problems list
naming the, 90–91, 119, 211, 239, 310
owning the, 134
solving, 2. 11–12, 61, 64, 99–100, 103, 117, 130, 151–152, 173, 186, 191, 211, 216, 224, 229, 232, 287–288, 304
Procedural learning: *see* Memory, procedural learning
Prognosis, 51, 53–55, 78, 83, 264
Progressive illness onset: *see* Illness onset, progressive
Pseudoempathy, 119–120
Pseudoseizures, 26
Psychiatric medications: *see* Medications
Psychiatry, 89, 314, 345, 346, 347
Psychoanalysis: *see* Psychotherapy, psychoanalytic
Psychopathy. 27, 33, 37, 70, 234, 342, 344
Psychotherapy
approaches to, 33–36
and brain illness, 3–6, 18, 206–208, 249, 262, 341, 348, 350, 351
cognitive, 86, 165
cognitive–behavioral, 41, 118, 340
and dementia, 121, 140, 199–201
-neuropsychotherapy balance, 36–37
psychoanalytic, 35–36, 168, 348
and stroke. 1–2, 52–53, 117, 184–186, 254
validation therapy *see* Neuropsychotherapy; Validation therapy
Pseudobulbar palsy, affect: *see* Reflex crying
PTSD, 155, 174–178, 340, 345, 356
versus TBI, 174–175

R. (Case), 126–127
Raj (Case), 32, 135, 270
Rancho Los Amigos Scale
Ranseen, J., 9, 85, 193, 214, 351
Rao, S., 17 159, 328, 351
Rape, R. N., 264, 351
Raskin, S. A., ix, 40, 70, 176, 344, 351
Reaction, catastrophic: *see* Catastrophic reaction
Record-keeping, 44, 76–77, 92, 104, 146–152
Reflex crying, 1–3, 9, 28, 41, 55, 92, 117, 137, 141, 144, 159, 160, 163–164, 184–187, 330, 340, 348, 322, 352, 356
Reflex laughing, 28, 117, 137, 141, 184–187, 322
Reflex smiling, 184
Reformation, personal: *see* Personal reformation
Reframing, 34, 100, 144, 202, 211, 275; *see also* Behavior, reinterpreting; Self-statements
Rehabilitation
cognitive, ix, 39–48
emotional, 4–6, 37, 138, 146, 211, 315
functional approach, 40
general stimulation, 39–40
natural recovery approach, 44–47
neuropsychological, 293, 339, 341, 343
and neuropsychotherapy 3–5, 8, 39–48
physical, 40
process-specific approach, 41–44
sexual: *see* Sexuality, rehabilitation
vocational: *see* Vocational rehabilitation
Religion, 10, 27, 69, 70, 109, 145, 178, 209, 255, 269, 286
Reorientation: *see* Orientation, reorientation
Repetition, 42, 86, 88–89, 225, 229; *see also* Perseveration
Responsibility
for behavior of person with brain illness, 19–22, 25, 26, 151–152, 199–200
for brain illness, 203–204, 261
continuum of, ix, 17–26, 36, 45, 104–105, 107–108, 149, 309, 313
for intermittent brain dysfunction, 24–26
for success of cognitive compensations, 41, 139, 221
Restoration of function, 42
Restraint, physical, 20, 141–142, 159, 175, 201
Reticular activating system, 247, 256
Ridley, B., 125, 157, 263, 317, 352
Right hemisphere, 52–53, 76, 130, 215, 227, 234, 242, 352
Rigidity, cognitive: *see* Concreteness; Perseveration
Risk, 13, 35, 55, 60–64, 75, 82, 98, 122–129, 199–200, 225, 229, 323–324, 352; *see also* Cost

Roberts, R. J., 210, 292, 325, 331, 343, 352, 353
Robinson, R. G., 121, 161, 185, 187, 330, 352
Roice, J., 312, 352
Role modeling, 99, 173, 205, 219, 293
Role playing, 98, 102, 103, 127, 134–135, 145–146, 173, 188, 204–205, 220, 301, 303
Rolls, E. T., 92, 352
Rosenthal, M., 264, 287, 289, 342, 343, 344, 350, 352
Ross, E. D., 155, 181–182, 184, 264, 316, 344, 347, 352
Rubens, A. B., 253, 352
Ruckdeschel-Hibbard, M., 352
Ruff, R. M., 71, 87, 349, 352

Sachs, P. R., 261, 263, 265, 278, 287–289, 349, 353
SADBD: *see* Structured Assessment of Depression in Brain Damaged Individuals
Salvador (Case), 77–80, 216
Sandson, J., 225, 353
Sbordone, R. J., ix, 18, 175, 285, 346, 353
Schizophrenia, 6, 169, 192, 217, 234, 242, 258, 354
School, 54, 59, 69, 75, 97, 101, 130, 216, 247, 251, 278, 283, 301–302, 304, 340, 355, 356
Seizures, 10, 55, 69, 73, 164, 179, 192, 197, 208–211, 241, 311, 331, 352, 354; *see also* Epilepsy
Self-
  awareness: *see* Awareness
  calming, 143, 204
  control, 7, 20–21, 35, 95, 112, 114, 141–143, 149–152, 193–194, 202–203, 214, 339
  cuing, 41, 143, 149
  esteem, 109, 273
  help, 293, 350
  image, 5–6, 39, 61, 82, 85–86, 265
  instruction, 41
  monitoring, 34, 131–132
  regulation, 28, 91, 137–138, 216–217, 220–221, 224, 228–229, 233, 236–237, 239, 243, 345
  talk, 145–147
Serio, C. D., 265, 353
Session
  agenda, 90, 110, 112
  plan, 108, 110
  summary, 108, 110–111; *see also* Record-keeping
Sexuality
  assessment planning, 273–274, 348
  disinhibition, 48, 126, 215, 273, 275, 305–306, 308
  dysfunction, 272–273, 304, 344
  hypersexuality, 275
  hyposexuality, 275
  interventions for, 287–288
  libido, 69, 159, 190, 275
  problems, 272–277
  rehabilitation, 272, 276–277
  vulnerability, 223, 309
Shame, 135, 172–173, 270, 278; *see also* Embarrassment; Withdrawal
Shapiro, F., 178, 353
Shock
  electrical, 7
  emotional, 53, 324
Sibling: *see* Family, sibling
Sigmund (Case), 89
Silver, J. M., ix, 9, 73, 194–197, 201, 206, 209, 347, 353, 356
Singing: *see* Music
Sister: *see* Family, sibling
Sleep
  disturbance, 159, 161, 163, 206
  insomnia, 166, 174, 175
  need for extra following brain illness, 69, 101, 248, 257
Small, L., 8, 36, 354
Smiling, reflex: *see* Reflex smiling
Social
  appropriateness, 20–21, 46, 89–91, 121, 137, 140–141, 205
  cover-up, 141, 243
  environment, 75, 134, 295, 298, 304, 308
  inappropriateness, 20–21, 66, 95, 138, 207, 214, 221–225, 233–237, 240–243, 306–307, 322
  intelligence, 3
  isolation, 26, 95, 141, 167–168, 188, 243, 265, 270, 302–303
  network, 292, 313, 343

Social (*cont.*)
skills, 39, 45, 135, 182, 216, 273, 283, 292, 302–304, 306, 308 see also Communication pragmatics
stimulation, 39–40, 139
work, 295, 304
Sociopathy: *see* Psychopathy
Socratic dialogue, 97, 100–101
Sohlberg, M. M., ix, 26, 39, 40–43, 107, 218, 248, 250–251, 349, 354
Song: *see* Music
Sonkin, D. J., 142, 354
Sorrow, chronic: *see* Grief
Spanbock, P., viii, 278, 354
Speech, *see also* Communication; Dysarthria; Language; Monotone voice; Word-finding
therapist, 3, 8
therapy, 183
Spiritual, 69–70, 180, 221, 341; *see also* Faith; Religion
Spouse: *see* Family, spouse
Starch, S., 72, 73, 75, 354
Startle, 166–167, 174–177, 258–259, 302, 346, 354
Stimulant: *see* Medication, stimulant
Stimulus-bound, 214, 231, 306–307
Story telling, 97, 100–102, 103
Strengths and problems list, 79, 83, 90, 108–110, 112, 126–127, 131–132, 276
Stress
inoculation, 149, 168, 349
testing, 146
Stroke, 1–2, 9, 33, 52–53, 55, 76, 117, 120, 161, 185–186, 190, 215, 235, 254, 284, 324, 330, 339, 341, 344, 345, 346, 352
Structured Assessment of Depression in Brain Damaged Individuals (SADBD), 161–162, 329–330
Structured Clinical Interview for Complex Partial Seizure-Like Symptoms, 210, 331
Stuss, D. T., 5, 130, 189, 190, 213, 217, 222, 251, 325, 354
Subcortical, 159, 175, 182, 227, 247
Substance abuse, 55, 59, 64, 177, 195–196, 206, 272, 273, 274, 285, 310, 311, 324, 342
Substantia nigra, 217
Sudden illness onset: *see* Illness onset, sudden
Sudden symptom onset, 58, 137–138, 143, 152, 196, 310
Suicide, 53–55, 68–69, 114, 159, 162–163, 179, 324, 330
Sunderland, T., 163, 329, 354
Support
circles of, 78–79, 279, 294–295, 302, 304, 355
groups, 5, 9, 24, 34, 51, 82, 97, 98, 100, 102, 120, 130, 133, 171, 263, 268, 270, 283, 292, 294, 308, 310–311, 318, 339, 350
natural, 288, 292–304
Support group (Case), 184
Supported failure, 131, 133, 158
SWF (Case), 308

TBI, ix, 65, 175, 198, 263, 286, 327, 339–356
mild, 341, 344, 351, 352, 353
Telling others, 26, 134–135
Temporal lobe epilepsy: *see* Epilepsy, temporal lobe
Temporal Lobe Epilepsy Personality Inventory, 210, 235, 331
Temporal lobes, 182, 197
Teri, L., 160, 354
Test, 59, 72–73, 157, 162, 195, 327–331,341, 342, 346; *see also* Assessment
Thalamus, 197, 227, 250–251
The tough case, 11, 12, 354
Things to do list, 41, 218, 221, 252, 300
Thomas (Case), 130–131
Threshold
no intervention/assess/intervention, 60, 61–65, 71, 83, 296
no treatment/test/treatment, 59, 60
Tierno (Case), 283–284
Tillie (Case), 121, 140
Time course of illness, 17–26, 69, 122, 264–271
Time out: *see* Back off
Toluene, 311–312
Touch, 20, 68, 120–121, 140–141, 186, 215, 223, 240, 255, 305–307, 309
Tourette's syndrome, 187–189, 195, 322, 342
Toxicity, brain, 123

Tranquilizer: *see* Medication
Trauma: *see* Amnesia, posttraumatic; Traumatic brain injury; Posttraumatic stress disorder
Traumatic brain injury: *see* TBI
Treiman, D. M., 208, 354
Try again, 138, 141, 142, 144, 149, 168, 202, 229

Udaka, F., 187, 354
United States of America (USA), ix, 11, 13, 105, 263, 302, 319

Validation therapy: *see* Neuropsychotherapy, validation therapy
Victoria Emotion Recognition Test, 183, 330
Video, 45, 74, 80, 87, 97, 98, 103, 107, 128–129, 135, 167, 183, 191, 205, 220, 233, 242, 243, 255, 269, 283, 294, 314
Vigilio (Case), 46–47
Vitaliano, P. P., 24, 263, 285, 287, 354
Vocational
  adaptations, 299
  compensations, 299–300
  job coaches, 133, 297, 299
  placement, 292, 297–299
  rehabilitation, 297
Vygotsky, L. S., 44, 354

Waaland, P. K., viii, 355
Warning signs, 25, 137, 139, 143, 145, 147, 148–149, 200, 211, 224–225, 229, 232
Washington Psychosocial Seizure Inventory, 73, 210, 330, 354
Weber, A. M., 245, 355
Wehman, P., 8, 13, 158, 166, 295, 298, 302, 347, 350, 353, 355
Werner, D., viii, 13, 77, 103, 293, 314, 317, 355
Whatever it takes model, 292, 294, 355
Willer, B. S., ix, 76, 278, 279, 292, 294, 298, 317, 351, 355
Williams, J. M., ix, 26, 73, 87, 287, 346, 355, 356
Wilson, B. A., 17, 41, 43, 72, 88, 239, 251, 343, 344, 351, 355
Withdrawal
  behavior, 80, 123, 168, 169, 171–173, 176, 186, 220, 258, 278, 310
  as intervention, 95, 202, 294
Word-finding: *see* Communication, word-finding
Work: *see* Vocational
World Health Organization, 13, 293, 317, 355

Ylvisaker, M., viii, 26, 295, 301, 355, 356
Yudofsky, S. C., 9, 194–198, 201, 206, 209, 331, 347, 353, 356

Zeigler, E. A., 271, 356
Zone of recovery, 15, 44–46, 111, 149, 152, 164, 171
Zung, W., 73, 356